Proving Homeopathy

Why Homeopathy Works – Sometimes

By Case Adams, Naturopath

Publishers Cataloging in Publication Data

Adams, Case

    Proving Homeopathy: Why Homeopathy Works - Sometimes

    First Edition

       1.   Health. 2. Medicine

    Bibliography and References; Index

    ISBN: 978-1-936251-37-7

Other Books by the Author

ADHD Holistic: Uncovering the Real Causes and Evidence-Based Natural Strategies for Kids and Adults

ARTHRITIS SOLVED NATURALLY: Nature's Answer to Rheumatoid Arthritis, Osteoarthritis, Gout and Other Forms of Arthritis

ASTHMA SOLVED NATURALLY: The Surprising Underlying Causes and Hundreds of Natural Strategies to Beat Asthma

BOOSTING THE IMMUNE SYSTEM: Natural Strategies to Supercharge our Body's Immunity

BREATHING TO HEAL: The Science of Healthy Respiration

THE CONSCIOUS ANATOMY: Healing the Real You

DEPRESSION AND ANXIETY SOLVED NATURALLY: The Science of Mood Disorders with Dozens of Proven Natural Strategies

DIABETES SOLVED NATURALLY: Discovering the Causes, and the Foods, Herbs and Strategies for Type 1 and Type 2 Diabetes

ELECTROMAGNETIC HEALTH: Making Sense of the Research and Practical Solutions for Electromagnetic Fields (EMF) and Radio Frequencies (RF)

THE GLUTEN CURE: Scientifically Proven Natural Solutions to Celiac Disease and Gluten Sensitivities

HAY FEVER AND ALLERGIES: Discovering the Real Culprits and Natural Solutions for Reversing Allergic Rhinitis

HEALING WITH LIGHT: The Science of Natural Light Therapy

HEALING WITH SOUND: The Science of Sound Therapy

HEALTHY SUN: Healing with Sunshine

HEARTBURN SOLVED: The Real Causes and How to Reverse Acid Reflux and GERD Naturally

HOLISTIC REMEDIES FOR ALZHEIMER'S: Natural Strategies to Avoid or Combat Dementia

LEAKY GUT SOLVED: The Real Causes and Real Solutions for Healing Leaky Gut Syndrome

THE BRAIN, MIND AND SUBCONSCIOUS SELF: Unveiling the Ancient Secrets using Science

THE LIVING CLEANSE: Detoxification and Cleansing Using Living Foods and Safe Natural Strategies

THE SCIENCE OF DREAMING: Why We Dream, What Dreams Mean

Table of Contents

Introduction

Homeopathy has had a rough couple of decades. After its acceptance among many conventional medical practitioners in the early part of the twentieth century through the 1970s, and its overwhelming acceptance among parts of the European and British medical communities, scientific research over the past two decades has produced vexing questions about homeopathy.

The primary question that has been raised is whether homeopathy is a proven therapeutic practice or simply a placebo.

A placebo is known generally as an non-active agent that appears to provide a therapeutic effect, when in fact it is not active in the body. One who experiences a therapeutic effect from a placebo will generally be defined as a person subject to the influence of the doctor dispensing the agent, or merely reacting mentally and physically to being given something that may be therapeutic.

Most define this as a mind-body effect, in that the mind's perception of being given a therapeutic agent influences the body's own healing mechanisms. From thousands and thousands of studies, researchers have arrived at a general stance that up to a third of any study population can experience a therapeutic effect from a non-therapeutic substance. In other words, in order to hurdle over a possible placebo effect, a therapeutic agent must typically have effect upon more than about 33% of a study population to convince researchers and their peers that the agent is actively therapeutic within the body.

Many conventional physicians and scientists are convinced, after seeing the research evidence that has been presented over the past two decades, that homeopathy is merely a placebo effect.

On the other hand, hundreds of millions of people – and billions if we include the past – swear by homeopathy. They proclaim that their ills have been treated and cured by the practice.

In addition, there are thousands of practitioners—many of them licensed medical doctors—who have been dispensing homeopathic prescriptions. These practitioners will testify that so many of their patients return to them healed as a result of their homeopathic

1

therapy.

Indeed, Samuel Hahnemann—considered the father of homeopathy—and his successors have conducted and supervised thousands of *provings* that spawned the creation of the homeopathic remedies over the past two centuries. These provings came by dosing healthy people with different doses of various agents, and observing their physical effects and symptoms. These provings were logged in scientific detail into tens of thousands of symptom-agent combinations.

Further clinical experimentation arrived at the notion that when the agent was diluted to the hundredth and thousandth degree it produced the effect of reversing the very symptom/condition that a larger dose of the substance produced.

This "law of similars" is the homeopathic principle whereby when a substance is reduced to an infinitesimal dosage, it produces the effect of stimulating an immune response to the very condition the substance will produce in a larger dose.

In biochemical terms, this infinitesimal dosage used by homeopaths is diluted so many times that it produces a substance that is theoretically devoid of any physical molecules of the original substance. This has been established through laboratory study as we will discuss in the book.

The problem posed by conventional science is that if there are no longer any molecules of the active substance left in the homeopathic medicine, how could there be any real therapeutic metabolic effect when the remedy is taken into the body?

This question—together with the fact that numerous studies over the past two decades have concluded equivocal results with regard to homeopathy—has provided significant doubt in the efficacy of homeopathy among the conventional science and medical communities.

Yet despite this serious charge of placebo effect—and quackery by some—from many conventional doctors and scientists, homeopathy still remains a popular therapy among both patients and their physicians within the alternative community.

Why is this? Why do so many people swear by homeopathy, including clinicians who have collectively treated millions of people? Are we to discount their entire collective successes as a glorified placebo effect? And how about those studies that did show homeopathy is therapeutic for a study population well over 33%?

This book aims to answer this question. Here we will not debate the actual research science that has showed, in some studies, that homeopathy has efficacy while in other cases, that homeopathy does not provide enough therapeutic effect to not be considered a placebo.

Here we will begin by assuming this controversy—that many studies, meta-studies and reviews have concluded that homeopathy may work on in some instances, but is not a proven therapeutic practice.

Rather, in this book we will examine the *potential* for homeopathy to work, and provide a possible explanation as to *why* there are varying results with homeopathic remedies.

We will get to the heart of the matter of efficacy, and explain what would have to take place in order for a homeopathic remedy to have a definite therapeutic effect.

Why is this important? Because in order for homeopaths and their patients to produce a greater likelihood of therapeutic effect, we must understand the *mechanisms* at work in homeopathy. Homeopaths must leave the mysterious language of "vibrations" behind as they discuss and utilize their knowledge.

And in order for conventional scientists to better target the elements of homeopathy that does not provide efficacy, they also must be focused upon the mechanisms that would have to occur in order for homeopathy to be therapeutic. In other words, they also must be armed with the possible mechanisms in order to engage homeopaths in the debate.

Patients of homeopathy must also be versed in the mechanisms to the greatest degree possible if they expect to carry out the prescriptions of their practitioners while being fully informed. This is required not only because patients must know how to handle their remedies. They also need to realize the possible shortcomings of homeopathy from a mechanism perspective.

Another reason why the information in this book is important to understand for anyone considering homeopathy is what I would call therapeutic efficiency: Getting to the heart of whether a particular therapy is worth the cost and the effort in its application to a particular condition.

Added to this efficiency notion is the fact that generally—as the research also substantiates—homeopathy generally comes with few if any adverse side effects, and is typically significantly less expensive than conventional medical treatments.

Using the efficiency formula, this book will scientifically establish a conclusion that will provide a basis for a better focus on those elements of homeopathy that stand a better chance at consistent efficacy, or at least an understanding of what can work and what cannot work.

The reader should note that the author will not conclude with this book whether or not homeopathy is a valid therapy. The information provided here may in itself validate at least the scientific basis for its ability to be valid. Or it may not. The reader must come to his or her own conclusions. This book merely presents the evidence.

Chapter One
Molecular Memory

When we talk homeopathy, we are talking molecular memory. What is molecular memory?

In 1982, a physics research team led by Professor Alain Aspect at the University of Paris determined that subatomic particles exhibited correlating waveforms despite being separated by long distances. This contradicted *Bell's theorem*, which effectively eliminated non-local hidden variables (independent from perception and outside influences) from the quantum mechanics view of the universe. Einstein had issues with non-local influences. Einstein's *principle of locality* proposed that there could be no distant influences: each particle is influenced only by its immediate surroundings.

When two particles split from each other and continue the same waveform, vector and polarity though separated from each other alludes to the fact that either each molecule is continuing to be influenced identically from a distant force, or each particle somehow remembered its waveform activity following bombardment and separation (Aspect *et al.* 1982).

Either way, we have a contradiction between either or perhaps both of the rigid proposals by Bell and Einstein. It would be logical that there were independently local aspects influencing the memory of the particles' former union. It also appears that there is some distant influence maintaining the correlating activities of the estranged pair of particles.

The proposal of a memory of a substance once existing in solution long after the substance is diluted away has been clinically applied over the last 250 years of homeopathic medicine. Homeopaths and researchers have observed clinical success with dilution factors well-beyond one million parts to one: A level at which theoretically no molecule of the substance could remain.

Therapists and practitioners alike can present evidence that homeopathy has documented successful clinical applications with these diluted substances with deeper and more lasting healing responses. With millions of case histories and hundreds of clinical trials illustrating the effectiveness of diluted homeopathic dosing, therapists can selectively offer studies proving efficacy.

At the same time, many other studies, and many review and meta-studies of other studies have concluded quite the opposite. Whether the positive study results are due to what homeopaths describe as 'vibrational memory' or something else is yet to be ascertained. Research on the subject continues to be controversial.

At the epicenter of this controversy lies homeopathic dilution factors. A homeopathic solution labeled as 'c' has undergone a 100th dilution (1/100). An 'x' or 'D' homeopathic medicine has undergone a 10th dilution (1/10). An multiple of the 'x' will be have that 10th dilution multiplied. For example, a 20x dilution will be diluted 1/10 and that solution diluted 1/10, and that dilution diluted 1/10, and so on, for 20 times. An 'LM' homeopathic equates to a dilution factor of 1/50,000 dilutions.

This is quite a small dilution factor. Is there any part of the original substance left in the solution? This lies at the crux of the controversy of homeopathy.

The Case for Molecular Memory

Some rather bold evidence for molecular memory has come from well-respected researchers with no prior acceptance of homeopathy. One of these was a well-known French medical doctor and researcher named Jacques Benveniste, M.D. At one time Dr. Benveniste was the research director at the French National Institute for Health and Medical Research (INSERM). Dr. Benveniste's career was very distinguished, having been credited with the discovery of the platelet-activating factor. Whilst performing research on the immune system—notably the action of basophils—Dr. Benveniste and his research technician Elisabeth Davenas inadvertently observed that basophil activity continued despite extremely low dilution levels: Dilution levels so low it was doubtful any molecules of the biochemical remained in the solution.

Over a four-year period of continual trials, showing repeated confirmation while instituting further controls, Dr. Benveniste and his research team concluded some sort of memory effect was taking place within a former solution following thorough dilution. It was suspected that water might have some faculty to retain and transmit an antibody's biological activity long the biochemical was diluted out of the solution.

Furthermore, as Dr. Benveniste and his team initially diluted a substance, the activity of the substance decreased, as would be expected. At least until the ninth dilution. After the ninth dilution, the activity of the substance began to increase with successive dilutions—as was experienced in the 250 years of clinical homeopathic success.

Dr. Benveniste's research effort was joined by five other research labs in four countries. All of these labs were able to independently replicate Dr. Benveniste's results. After conducting no less than 300 trials, the results were published in 1988 in _Nature_ magazine, authored by thirteen of the researchers. The authors eventually concluded that, _"transmission of the biological information could be related to the molecular organization of water"_ (Davenas _et al._ 1988).

The research became controversial to say the least. This _memory of water_ conclusion had vast implications in the study of medicine and our knowledge of physics. The unintentional byproduct of the research was to inadvertently provide the evidence for the premise of homeopathy—something Dr. Benveniste initially had not agreed with. It challenged others too. _Nature_ magazine's editor assembled a team of outspoken "verifiers" who challenged Benveniste's results and protocol. Initially they observed while the lab confirmed the results.

The "verifiers" then modified the protocols to theoretically remove any bias. With the change in protocol, the team could not duplicate the results. Dr. Benveniste and his associates responded to deaf ears by explaining that the protocol changes themselves eradicated the results. Until his demise in 2004, Dr. Benveniste and other researchers repeatedly confirmed his findings (Bastide _et al._ 1987;

Youbicier-Simo *et al.* 1993; Endler *et al.* 1994; Smith 1994; Pongratz *et al.* 1995; Benveniste *et al.* 1992).

While Dr. Benveniste did not set out to prove homeopathy, he stumbled upon its proof while focused on neurotransmitter research. The issue he enlarged and was eventually discredited for, is one of the most profound issues of science: Is matter solid?

The Promise of Efficacy

Efficacy according to conventional researchers revolves around a premise of whether a chemical molecule had to be present in order to submit a particular biochemical action. This reminds us of the debate regarding the sub-atomic wave theory versus the classical particle theory.

Determining with certainty whether there are any molecules of the original substance left in the water is calculated using probability. Using mathematical probability, the liquid content should be fully displaced with new liquid contents; the likelihood of molecules within that former solution existing in the new contents diminishes substantially, but absence is still only probable.

Viewing the liquid content's molecules and atoms as combinations of interfering waveforms creates a new paradigm. If matter is composed of waveform energy and those waveforms interfere with the solution's other waveforms, there would likely exist a residual memory of original waveforms within the remaining interference patterns. This might be compared with a pond's waves retaining the memory of what was dropped into the pond a few minutes previously.

Over the past two decades and partially in response to the controversial nature of Benveniste's research, the scientific basis for homeopathy has undergone a flurry of research. Most of this research has occurred in Europe, where homeopathy practice is often practiced by conventional physicians. Hundreds of controlled and randomized studies assessing homeopathic treatments have now been accumulated.

Over the past few years there have been four major independent meta-studies that have analyzed this volume of recent research. Three of these reviews concluded that the effects of homeopathy were more significant than the effects of a placebo, while one concluded homeopathy's effects were consistent with the effects of a placebo. However, this later review was also highly criticized for its elimination of studies (Jonas 2003; Chast 2005; Merrell and Shalts 2002).

The implication is simple: Contrary to classical chemistry and physics theory, chemical reactions would not require particles to physically touch within the waveform view. We can observe this because we can create chemical reactions simply by bombarding molecules with radiation. Sub-atomic waveform emissions often exert ionizing influences in much the same manner.

The Electromagnetic Atom

The problem with matter is that it is an illusion. When we look around us, we see objects. What we are actually looking at are electromagnetic waves. Let's start with one of nature's smaller units.

Dalton's atomic theory, put forth by British John Dalton in the early nineteenth century, proposed that the tiniest indivisible piece of matter could be assigned a unit called the *atom*. He concluded that all matter must be made up of these indivisible units. Furthermore, he suggested that the indivisible atoms of different elements must each have a unique atomic weight—and compounds are made up of different combinations of atoms. These combinations, of course, came to be known as *molecules.*

Others had previously envisioned the existence of a smaller unit, the atom. This concept is thought to arise from Sir Isaac Newton and even the Greeks, but it was also written about in ancient Vedic literature thousands of years earlier.

Dalton's theories—with his notions of atomic character—brought mathematical characteristics to these tiny portions of nature.

Radiation instrumentation further developed, due in part to the pioneering work of T.W. Richards—known for his work on the radioactive transformation of lead, which he called "radio-lead." This produced a better understanding of atomic reactivity, and the possibility of the existence of subatomic parts within the atom.

In the late nineteenth century, Joseph John ("JJ") Thomson—winner of the 1906 Nobel Price for Physics—measured cathode rays passed through slits within a vacuum tube. Using magnetic fields, Thomson was able to bend the rays. This indicated to Sir Thomson that elemental matter must have both electronic charge and magnetic field characteristics.

Further cathode ray testing revealed the nature of these rays as subatomic particles. Thomson deduced that the rays must be produced by tiny particles that make up the atom.

Dalton's atomic number soon expanded to subatomic particles, with the notion of electrons, protons and a nucleus. These provided a semblance of balance and a rationale molecular combination.

Several theories of the atom were put forth in the mid- to late-nineteenth century. These ranged from Sir Thomson's *plum pudding model,* to Japanese physicist Hantaro Nagaoka's *Saturnian model.* This of course visualized electrons moving around the nucleus much as the rings of Saturn encircle that planet. This let to the *Rutherford-Bohr model,* which utilized the combined works of Niels Bohr and Ernest Rutherford:

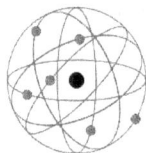

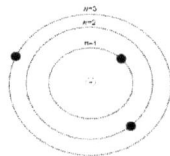

The Rutherford Atom   The Bohr Model

Continued research in the early twentieth century gradually eliminated the Bohr-Rutherford model as an acceptable description of subatomic particle motion. These subatomic 'particles' did not seem to maintain "particle behavior."

J.J. Thomson's cathode ray experiments led to the notion—elaborated on by Paul Dirac, John von Neumann, Max Planck, Louis de Broglie, Max Born, Niels Bohr, Albert Einstein and Erwin Schrödinger—that the reflective effects of the cathode rays indicated that subatomic particles were actually wavelike:

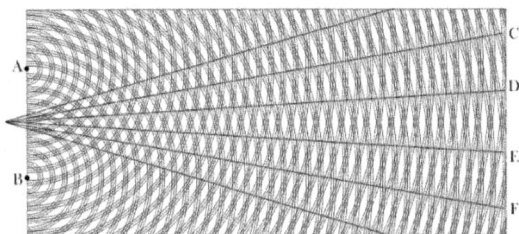

Cathode rays indicate that subatomic particles are wave-like

Subsequent subatomic particle experiments have confirmed that the smallest atomic parts contain electromagnetic properties. As the calculations of wave mechanics led to quantum theories, driven by the research and equations of Rutherford, Plank, Einstein, Born, de Broglie, Bohr, Schrödinger and Neumann, a new reality of the atom gradually came into view: Atoms maintain subatomic electrons in the form of *particle-waves*. The current picture of the atom is an immensely small nucleus surrounded by electromagnetic electron orbital clouds:

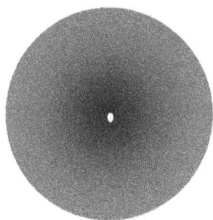

The electromagnetic atom's electron orbital cloud

Electromagnetic Waveforms

Energy moves in waves. Thus the notion of electromagnetic waves has gradually gained scientific confirmation. The realization that light, radio and atomic energy were composed of energy pulsing at regular cycles led to the quantification of electromagnetic radiation using waveform mechanics. The basic waveform parameters are *frequency, wavelength* and *speed*. Furthermore, scientists have arrived at the following relationship between these three characteristics:

WAVELENGTH = SPEED divided by FREQUENCY

This formula has allowed scientists to calculate and categorize the various waveforms that surround us. Today, many of nature's energies—atomic energy, heat, visible light, radiowaves, color, cosmic rays, gamma rays and more—have been quantified in their respective frequencies and wavelengths. As a result, we can present the electromagnetic spectrum within waveform specification:

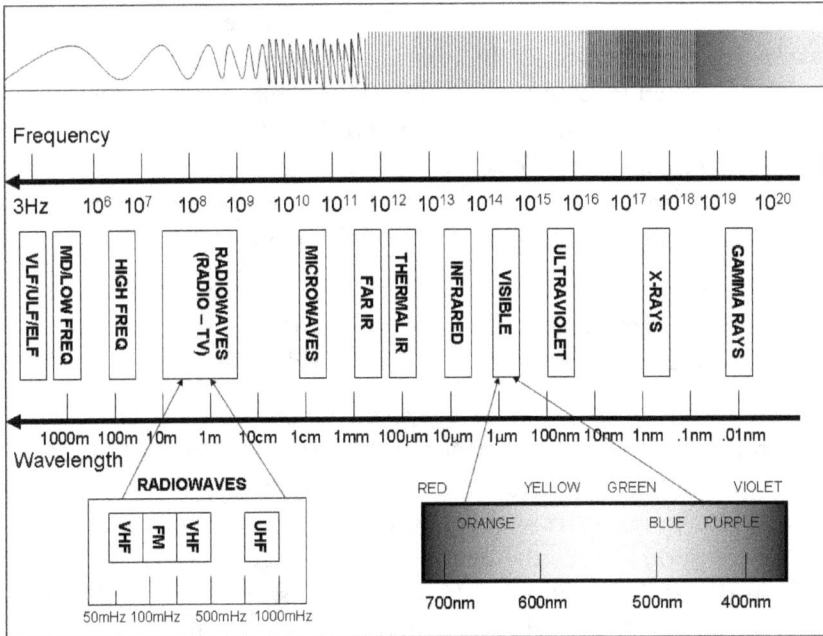

Frequency

3Hz 10^6 10^7 10^8 10^9 10^{10} 10^{11} 10^{12} 10^{13} 10^{14} 10^{15} 10^{16} 10^{17} 10^{18} 10^{19} 10^{20}

VLF/ULF/ELF | MID/LOW FREQ | HIGH FREQ | RADIOWAVES (RADIO – TV) | MICROWAVES | FAR IR | THERMAL IR | INFRARED | VISIBLE | ULTRAVIOLET | X-RAYS | GAMMA RAYS

1000m 100m 10m 1m 10cm 1cm 1mm 100μm 10μm 1μm 100nm 10nm 1nm .1nm .01nm
Wavelength

RADIOWAVES

VHF | FM | VHF | UHF

50mHz 100mHz 500mHz 1000mHz

RED   YELLOW   GREEN   VIOLET
ORANGE   BLUE PURPLE

700nm   600nm   500nm   400nm

THE ELECTOMAGNETIC SPECTRUM

In other words, our universe is pulsing with waves of different types. So what is a wave?

While every electromagnetic frequency is a waveform, not every wave in nature is an electromagnetic wave. Throughout nature, we see repeating rhythmic occurrences. Each day we observe the sun's rise and set, establishing a cycle that is repetitious, adjusting slightly with every cycle. Seasonal changes with the rotation of the earth in respect to its orbit are also waveforms. We see this seasonal rhythmic rise and fall reflected in plant-life—waxing in the spring and waning in the fall. We see birds and other migratory animals move with similar rhythms, traveling periodically with the seasons to amazingly exacting locations.

We also see nature's waveforms pulsing through the oceans, causing waves and weather conditions. We see larger periods of ocean tidal rhythms bringing an exchange of ocean creatures and their food to and from the seashore. We see the rhythmic upwelling of cold waters from the ocean depths rotating and recycling the ocean's various biochemicals and marine life. Meanwhile, these surface waters are spun and rotated by the wind through a recycling temperature gradients. We see a similar rhythmic pulsing of waveforms throughout our atmosphere; recycling temperature, water vapor, and various gas mixtures with periodic precision.

These pulses of nature are waves from a macrocosmic and microcosmic view. The distinct and precise rhythms repeat and cycle, and their variances also repeat in a cyclical fashion.

Nature's waveforms extend to the electromagnetic spectrum. The waveforms pulsing through space in the form of electromagnetic light waves, radio waves, gamma waves, cosmic rays, infrared waves, ultraviolet waves, x-rays and other forms of radiation. These have been produced by the billions of suns of the cosmos for billions of years. Radiation is also produced by the earth, and by our own bodies. We also find geomagnetic field waves and proton storms from cyclic solar storms, and rhythmic magnetic influences around our planet.

The waveform order of nature is evident when considering the accuracy of the atomic clockworks. In today's standard for timekeeping—the atomic cesium clock—radioactive cesium provides a steady stream of radiative waveforms that pass through a magnetic field to routinely oscillate a crystal. The emission from cesium is so rhythmically accurate that we now quite literally set our clocks to these electromagnetic pulses.

When most of us think about waves, we think of the ocean. We think of waves pounding onto the beach. Stirred up by the forces of wind and weather, large waves will march onto the reefs and beaches, standing up with ferocious crests. The beauty and power of a large wave lifting and crashing onto the rocks or beach is often the subject of popular photography and film. What we may not realize is that each single wave is communicating an event that took place thousands of miles away: A particular mix of wind, temperature, atmospheric pressure and moisture combining in just the right way to instigate a weather system.

This weather system converts its potential into waveforms in the surrounding ocean waters. Should we look at a storm's confluence of elements from space, we will see nature's characteristic spiral. Harmonically, we see this same spiral shape within a cross-sectional view of an ocean wave.

A wave is a repeating oscillation of energy: A translation of information through a particular medium. Waves can travel through solids, fluids, gases and space. Waves are not restricted to a particular medium, either. Most waves will move through one medium and continue on through the next medium where those mediums intersect. A sound, for example may vibrate a drum skin first. Where the drum skin meets the air, it oscillates the air molecules to translate the sound information throughout the medium. Where the air connects with the tympanic membrane, the information waveform is translated through the malleus, incus and stapes of the middle ear. After vibrating through to the round window, the oscillation is translated through the cochlea into electromagnetic nerve pulses. This means that the original wave of the drum beat transversed several mediums before being converted to electromagnetic pulses.

A repeated oscillation or waveform through a medium against the backdrop of time is a rhythm. This repetitive and rhythmic pulse translates to a recurring waveform. It also translates to information. Any recurring result is associated with a causal event. In other words, a wave must be initiated by an original event. The waves in a pond originate from a pebble thrown in, for example.

Every movement in nature has a signature rhythm: The earth oscillates in specific types of seismic waves—some causing damage but most hardly noticeable. We each walk with a signature pace as our feet meet the ground. Our vocal cords oscillate to the reflection of our thoughts with a unique pace and timing. Our heart valves oscillate with the needs of circulation. Our lungs oscillate as we breathe in and out—unique to our lung size and cells' needs for oxygen. Even rugged, seemingly solid structures like rocks oscillate—depending upon their position, size, shape, and composition. A cliff by the seashore will oscillate with each pounding wave. A building in a windy city will uniquely oscillate with the movement of the wind through the streets. Each building will oscillate slightly differently, depending upon its architecture and location.

All of these movements—and all movements in nature for that matter—provide recurring oscillations that can be charted in waveform structure. Moreover, the various events within nature come complete with recurring cycles. While many cycles obviously repeat during our range of observation, many cycles have only recently become evident, indicating that many of nature's cycles are still beyond our current observation range.

Natural oscillations balance between a particular pivot point and an axis. The axis is typically a frame of reference between two media or quanta. An axis showing quantification may illustrate time in reference to height, time versus temperature, time versus activity or time versus other quantifying points of reference. Waves will also transist between media. The ocean wave is the transisting of waveforms between the intersection of the atmosphere and the water: the storm system. The water's surface tension gives rise to the ocean wave as it refracts the pressure of the storm system. The storm system's waveform energy will be radiated through the ocean to the rocks and beach.

Nature's waves are relational to the rhythms of planets and galaxies. These rhythms translate to electromagnetic energy and kinetic energy, which translate to the elements of speed, distance, and mass. Momentum, inertia, gravity, and other natural phenomena are thus examples of the cyclical activities that directly relate with nature's wave rhythms. Every rhythm in nature is interconnected with other rhythms. As a house is built with interconnected beams of framing, the universe's waveforms are all interconnected with a design of pacing within the element of time.

The most prevalent waveform found in nature is the sinusoidal wave or sine wave. The sinusoidal wave is the manifestation of circular motion related to time. The sine wave thus repeats through nature's processes defined by time. For example, the rotating positions of the hands of a clock translate to a sinusoidal wave should the angles of the hand positions be charted on one axis with the time on the other axis.

Sinusoidal waveforms are thus the typical waveform structures of light, sound, electromagnetic waves and ocean waves. Late eighteenth and early nineteenth century French physicist Jean Fourier found that just about every motion could be broken down into sinusoidal components. This phenomenon has become known as the Fourier series.

The cycle of a sine wave, moving from midline to peak, then back to midline, then to a trough, and then back to midline completes a full cycle. If we divide the wave into angles, the beginning is consistent with 0 degrees; the first peak is consistent with 90 degrees, the midline with 180 degrees and the trough with 270 degrees. The cycle repeats again, as we make another revolution around the sine wave circle.

Other wave types occurring in nature might not be strictly sine waves, yet they are often sinusoidal in essence. The cosine wave, for example, is sinusoidal because it has the same basic shape, but is simply phase-shifted from the sine. Other waves such as square waves or irregular sound waves can usually be connected to sinusoidal origin when their motion is broken down into composites.

We see so many circular activities within nature. We see the earth recycling molecular components. We see the recycling of water from earth to sea to clouds and back to earth. We see planetary bodies moving in cyclic fashion, repeating their positions in periodic rhythm. We see the seasons moving in cyclic repetition. We see organisms living cycles of repetitive physical activity.

While not every cycle in nature is precisely circular—the orbits of planets or electron energy shells for example—they are nonetheless linked within a grander cycle. Linked cycles often contain various alterations as they adapt to the other cyclic components. This modulation can be described as adaptation—a harmonic process between waveform matter and life.

This all should remind us of the notion of the circle of life, which has been repeatedly observed throughout nature in so many respects that it is generally assumed without fanfare. Circles recur in human and animal activity, social order, customs, and individual circumstances. The tribal circle is common among many ancient cultures—and for good reason. In modern society, we have circular conferences, round-table meetings, and cyclical ceremonies. The potter's wheel, the grinding wheel, and the circular clock are all examples of circular symbols in our attempt to synchronize with nature. Just about every form of communication and transportation is somehow connected to circular motion. For this reason, it is no accident that the wheel provides our primary and most efficient means for transportation. The motion of walking is also circular and sinusoidal, as the legs rise and fall forward, rotating the various joints.

In nature, we observe two basic types of waves: mechanical and electromagnetic. A mechanical wave moves through a particular medium: sound pressure waves as they move through air, for example. Mechanical waves can move over the surface of a medium. Ocean waves and certain earthquake (seismic) waves are examples of mechanical surface waves. Another type of mechanical wave is the torsional wave: This mechanical wave twists through a spiral or helix.

The electromagnetic wave is seemingly different because it theoretically does not move through a medium of any composition. Einstein assumed space is a vacuum and the ultimate electromagnetic wave—light—moved through this vacuum with constant speed. Dr. Einstein's theory supposed that time is collapsed within space: Instead of time and distance being separate, he supposed a singular element called space-time.

Yet in 2001, collaborative research led by Texas A&M University physics professor Dr. Dimitri Nanopoulos, Dr. Nikolaos

Mavromatos of King's College in London, and Dr. John Ellis of the European Center for Particle Physics in Geneva confirmed that additional influences can alter the speed of light. Their calculations showed that the speed of light varies to frequency. Furthermore, in 1999, University of Toronto professor Dr. John Moffat calculated that the speed of light has actually slowed down over time. Space may actually be a bona fide medium after all.

Nature displays two basic waveform structures: transverse and longitudinal. Visible spectrum, radio waves, microwaves, radar, infrared and x-rays are all transverse waveforms. As these waves move, there is a disruption moving at right angles to the vector of the wave. For example, should the wave move along a longitudinal x-axis, its disruption field would move along the perpendicular y-z axis. This might be compared to watching a duck floating in a lake strewn with tiny waves. The duck bobs up and down as the waves pass under the duck's body. In the case of the transverse electromagnetic wave, the disruption field is the magnetic field.

In the longitudinal wave, pressure gradients form regular alternating zones of compression and rarefaction. During the compression phase, the medium is pressed together, and during the rarefaction, the medium is expanded outward. This might be illustrated by the alternating expansion and compression of a spring. Instead of the wave disturbing the medium upward and downward as in the case of a transverse wave, the medium is disturbed in a back and forth fashion, in the direction of the wave. Examples of longitudinal waves are sound waves and most seismic waves. In the case of sound waves, air molecules compress and rarefy in the direction of the sound projection.

These two types of waves may also combine in nature. An ocean wave is a good example of a combination of transverse and longitudinal waveforms. Water may be disturbed up and down as it transmits an ocean wave, and it may convey alternating compressions and rarefaction as it progresses tidal currents.

Waves are typically referred to as radiation when the waveform can translate ("radiate") its energy information from one type of medium to another. In this respect, ocean waves can be considered radiating as they translate their energy onto the sand. In the case of seismic waves, they translate through land to buildings and people. The classic type of radiation comes from electromagnetic waves such as x-rays or ultraviolet rays, which can travel through skin or other molecular mediums after transversing space.

Waves are typically measured by their wave height from trough to crest (amplitude), rate of speed through time (frequency) and the distance from one repeating peak to another (wavelength). Waves are also characterized by their wave shape. Examples of wave shape include sinusoidal waves and square waves, as we've mentioned.

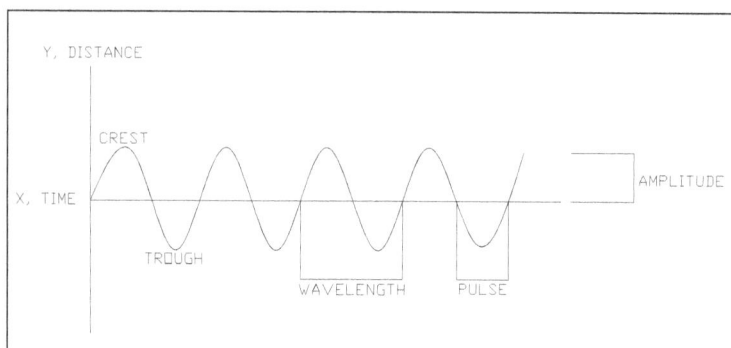

The frequency of a wave is typically measured by how many wave cycles (one complete revolution of the wave—a wavelength) pass a particular point within a period of time. Therefore, waves are often measured in CPS, or cycles per second. The hertz is named after nineteenth century German physicist Dr. Heinrich Hertz—who is said to have discovered radio frequency electromagnetic waves. Note that hertz and CPS are identical: Both identify the number of complete waves passing a given point every second. Other frequency measurements used include machinery's RPM (revolutions per minute), special radiation's RAD/S (radians per second), and the heart's BPM (beats per minute).

When we describe a sinusoidal waveform, we can state either its frequency or wavelength, since the two will be inversely related. Wavelength is typically measured in meters, centimeters, or nanometers to comply with international standards. Each radiation type is classified by its wavelength. A wave's wavelength has an inverse relationship to its frequency. This is because a shorter wavelength wave will travel faster through a particular point than a longer wavelength wave will. Note also that speed is the rate measured from one point to another, while frequency is the rate of one full repetition of a pulse past a particular point. Therefore, a wave's wavelength can be determined by dividing its speed by its frequency, and a wave's frequency can be derived from dividing its speed by its wavelength.

A wave's amplitude is also an important consideration, as this relates to the height of the wave—its magnitude. The amplitude is measured from the wave's baseline to its peak. Among sinusoidal waves, greater frequency will accompany a shorter wavelength but amplitude is independent.

Other considerations among waveforms include phase, medium of travel, and wave shape. These together characterize a particular wave's effect and conductance.

Waves travel with repetition or periodicity. The very definition of a wave describes a repeating motion. This repetition, occurring with a particular pace and particular time reference, forms a rhythm. Can waves be chaotic? To the contrary, it is their consistent rhythm that allows us to interpret light, color, sound, or warmth with duplicatable precision. All of these waveforms connect with the senses because they have consistent and congruent oscillations. In sensing the world around us, we do not perceive each wave individually. Rather, we sense waveform interaction.

When a waveform collides or interferes with another waveform, the interaction yields a more complex waveform. This creates information. As waveforms collide throughout our universe, they comprehensively present a myriad of information via their interference patterns. Our brains and minds translate those interference patterns that resonate with our sensory neurons.

Depending upon the characteristics of the incoming waveforms, wave interference can result in larger, more complex waveforms. These are *constructive interference patterns*. Alternatively, should interactive waveforms contrast each other; their meeting can result in a reduction of magnitude—creating *destructive interference patterns*.

The interactive quality of two waves as they collide often lies within their wave phase similarity. If one wave is cycling in positive territory while the other is cycling in negative territory, they will most likely destructively interfere with each other, resulting in a reduction of amplitude. However, if the two waves move in the same phase—where both cycle with the same points on the curve—then they will most likely constructively interfere with each other, creating a greater amplitude—and a greater magnitude.

As a result, interacting waves are identified as either in-phase or out-of-phase. In-phase waveforms will typically meet with superposition to form constructive interference and greater intensity. Out-of-phase waveforms will often conflict:, reducing their intensity. The canceling or reduction during destructive waveform interference is not necessarily bad, however. Depending upon the type of radiation, destructive interference can also produce healthy effects.

The degree that two or more waves will interfere with each other—either constructively or destructively—relates to their *coherence*. If two waves are coherent, they are either completely in-phase or out-of-phase. They will thus increase in intensity or undergo significant cancellation. Waves that are different but not completely out-of-phase are considered incoherent.

Waveform coherency might be loosely compared to speaking coherently. Coherent speaking refers to sounds that are better understood by the listener. Whether the communication is interpreted by the listener as positive or negative information is not relevant. The clarity of the communication indicates its coherence.

In the same way, coherent waves interact to produce significant results as they interact—either constructively or destructively.

Destructive Interference

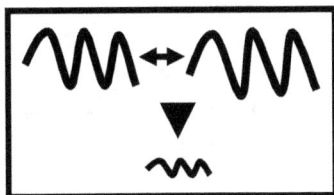

Resonance occurs when individual waves achieve a balanced state—one where phase and periodicity are consistent within that waveform system. Thus, resonating waves typically occur when waves come together in constructive interference.

This results in an increase in their respective amplitudes. This is illustrated when two tuned instruments play the same note or song together. Their notes will resonate together, creating a convergence with greater amplitude, typically resulting in a louder, clearer sound. We also hear this when we create the familiar whistling sound of blowing into an empty bottle: To get the loudest and clearest sound, we must blow with a certain angle and airspeed. Once we find the right positioning, angle and speed, we will have established a resonance between the shape of the bottle and our breath.

Constructive Interference

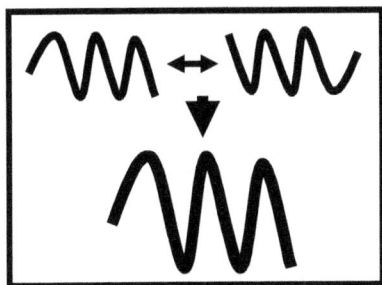

As waves move from one type of media to another, they will often reflect or refract. Reflected waves will bounce off the new medium, while refracted waves will move through the new medium with a different vector and speed. This of course depends upon the density and molecular makeup of the medium. Mediums are thus quantified by their index of refraction, absorbance or conductance levels when it comes to waveform interaction. Some mediums will reflect certain waveforms while refracting others. Thus, the media is as important as the waveforms when it comes to characterizing the positive or negative effects of a type of radiation.

Refraction (A) and Reflection (B)

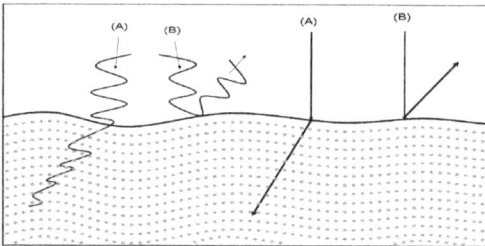

This is illustrated by the passage of UV radiation through the atmosphere. The stratosphere contains higher levels of ozone, which absorb and reflect ultraviolet-B rays in the 270-315 nanometer (NM) range. Ozone's filtering effects absorb or reflect over 98% of the sun's ultraviolet-B rays, as well as some far-infrared radiation.

Surface waves are typically seen at the surface of a particular medium where that medium interfaces with another medium. Surface waves are seen on the surface of mediums—for examples, on the surfaces of oceans and lakes. Surface waves are mechanical in nature and thus tend to respond to surface pressures from the interfacing medium. In the case of surface seismic waves, the collision of the wave with some soils may mute the waveform amplitude while other soils (looser, with more water content) may exaggerate the waveform amplitude.

Surface waves are divided into two basic types—the first being a capillary wave. The capillary wave is a carrier wave that forms during the beginning of the build-up process. Therefore, it is considered a low-amplitude wave—often seen as smaller ripples on the water as the wind freshens. The second type of surface wave is a gravity wave, typically having a larger wavelength and amplitude than the capillary wave has. It is the gravity-type rogue waves that seafarers respect for their shipwrecking abilities, for example.

In deeper water, a combination of transverse and longitudinal wave motions combine to form monochromatic linear plane waves. This forms a type of wave called an inertial wave. Inertial waves are typically moving within rotating fluid mediums. Inertial waves are common in not only the ocean and among lakes, but also within the atmosphere and presumably within the earth's core. The various currents and winds within the atmosphere all travel in inertial waves of varying lengths. Surface waves will interact with these inertial waves to move energy over the surface of their medium. This energy movement allows surfers to ride a wave from the outside to the inside of the tidal region, for example.

A *simple harmonic* is a recurring wave (in nature, usually sinusoidal or cosinusoidal) that repeats in rhythmic frequency. A *combined harmonic* occurs when different waveforms converge and their wavelengths become aligned—their wavelengths are multiples or integers of each other.

In other words, harmonic convergence is achieved when different waveforms with a multiple of the same wavelength-frequency proportions interfere. Other coherent interference among waveforms can also create a harmonic. Though the source waveforms might not be harmonic, a combined harmonic convergence can be created through a combination of natural waveforms and media.

As forward-moving waves interact with returning waves, both

waves will become compressed and dilated. This effect is known as the *Doppler Effect*—named after nineteenth century Austrian physicist Johann Christian Doppler. If the incoming waves have the same waveform, frequency, and amplitude, this will create a standing wave. If they do not, either the incoming or the outgoing wave will divert the waves it meets, and distort those waves in one respect or another. This distortion would be analogous to the oblong or parabolic orbitals of solar systems and electrons, which are distorted by the interference created by surrounding fields or waveforms.

Standing waveforms will typically be created by interacting waves with precisely the same frequency, wavelength, amplitude, and shape.

As suggested by Zhang et al. in 1996, and confirmed by multiple physicists over the last decade, multiple electrons within shared orbitals (or valences) among multiple atoms situated within a close-range matrix are best described as multiple standing waves: These standing waveforms create structure. They also create some of the strongest forces in nature, as they produce the illusion of physical solidity. The convergence of multiple waveforms standing together in a harmonic resonating interference pattern over a period of time is best described as architecture.

In other words, standing waves among molecules interact with and reflect certain types of electromagnetic radiation. These reflected rays resonate with our retinal neurons to produce the illusion of a solid physical world.

Standing waveforms also continually undergo interference displacement. This alters their energy through convergence or interference with other waveforms. This is illustrated by the effect of certain types of radiation upon certain types of materials: The incoming waveforms may produce changes to the molecular structure of the material as they interfere with the standing waveforms existing within its atoms and molecules. As the architecture of the molecules changes, energy may be produced. Heat, for example, is often produced when the sun's radiation begins to interferes with the molecules within our skin cells. We've all experienced this as we've stepped outside into the sunlight.

This interference displacement conveys the energy and information traveling within radiation on to new media. New waveform interference patterns, energy and information are the result. These interference conveyances render the transfer of energy, motion and information within the physical universe.

As researchers have probed deeper into the nature of energy and matter, we have found that everything around us is oscillating at a particular waveform or rhythm. All information is conveyed within waveform interference patterns. It is these interference patterns that our bodies and minds utilize for sensory perception.

This might be compared to the bits and bites of computer code. A bit of computer data is an on state or off state. In itself, neither an off state or off state produces any information. But when a particular pattern of on and off states is put together into a byte, information is created. In the same way, waveforms in themselves do not produce information. It is their interference patterns with others that create the information.

We might consider this in light of the development of telecommunications. Radio wave signaling from the ingenious research of Gugielmo Marconi and Ferdinand Braun during the late nineteenth and early twentieth centuries led to the 1909 Nobel Prize in Physics for the wireless telegraph. This built upon the development of the cable telegraph more than a century earlier through the combined tinkering of Francisco de Salva, Alessandro Volta, Samuel von Soemmering and Johan Schweigger. These efforts began with simple electrostatics—the use of radiating pulses through conductor materials. Electostatics gave us the ability to manipulate currents and voltage to transmit information.

Heinrich Hertz introduced the methodology to measure electromagnetic radiation in the late 1880s. Italian physicist and university professor Augusto Righi investigated and published no less than 200 papers on the transmission of information via electromagnetic propagation. While Marconi developed methods of electronic wave propulsion, it was Righi who meticulously exacted the technology. Through his research, Righi was able to increase the wave stability and the reception clarity of radio transmissions.

Edouard Branly, utilizing some of the work of Italian physicist Temistocle Calzecchi-Onesti, eventually assembled a crude radio wave transmitter. This became referred to as the *Branly coherer*. It utilized current resistance to transmit radiowaves across an electrode conductor through space. Englishman Dr. Oliver Lodge coined the term coherer—postulating that the coherent medium through which the radiowaves transmitted was the aether. Dr. Lodge is thought to have demonstrated wireless transmission prior to Marconi. It is also thought that Nikola Tesla demonstrated the first wireless radio wave communication in 1893—but this claim has proved to be controversial over the years.

Reception was still a missing link. This piece was introduced around 1898 by the German Ferdinand Braun. Braun invented the cat's whisker crystal diode rectifier. This formed the basis for the crystal radio receiver semiconductor. A naturally mined crystal was positioned to receive and conduct radiowaves through contact with a thin bronze wire—the cat's whisker.

Eventually a tuner was installed to fix the radio crystal and whisker upon a particular frequency—one matching the radiowave pulses emitted by the sender. The crystal semiconductor converted these waveforms into electrical pulses, driving a speaker. Marconi, the ultimate businessperson, assembled the various equipment—much of it under patent by the original inventors—and combined them with existing cable telegraph technology to send and receive real-time radiowave communication.

It should be emphasized that the signaling system on both ends must be grounded to the earth: Nature provides not only the facility for semi-conductance, but also the grounding for the electrical pulses to provide the right polarity. Early semiconducting devices were made from crystals of natural minerals such as galena or pyrite. Prior to the cat's whisker crystal radio, other minerals like silicon carbide and vitreous silicon were also used as crude semiconductors. All of these of course preceded the use of synthetic silicon crystals for the semiconduction of modern-day integrated circuits and microchip processors.

In other words, the ability to broadcast communications rides on the bandwidths of nature's radiowaves and the earth's semiconductors. The assembly of these natural components enabled humans to utilize natural radiation as a *carrier* for information communication. With various experiments and mechanisms developed through trial and error, inventors and physicists have been able to piggyback upon nature's technologies.

Electromagnetic technology is also utilized by nature for the transmission of vision, sound, heat, light, chemical reaction and atomic energy. If we examine the timeline of the equations and theories presented by Bohr, Einstein, de Broglie, Planck and others, the mechanical application of electromagnetic radiation thoroughly preceded humankind's understanding of the technologies. Furthermore, we are still trying to fully understand electromagnetic radiation. In other words, we still do not completely understand nature's electromagnetic technologies.

Radiation transmission is an innate rhythmic process natural to all living beings. Radiation communication can be compared to the barking of a dog, or the tapping of Morse code. The sending of a radiowave signal is no different in principle from the act of tapping or barking. The receiving of the signal is the act of sensing or hearing those pulses, followed by a translation of interference patterns into information. This allows the sender and receiver to have intentional communication by filtering out other interference patterns with a handshaking protocol. As long as each party agrees on how the rhythm is to be converted, communication can be pervasive amongst all participants.

A television camera, for example, converts visual radiation into a series of digital pulses. Those pulses are amplified with alternating current and converted into broadcast radiowaves. A television set is the receiver and converter of those radiowaves, translating the waves back into digital pulses. As long as the television receiver is set up with the same conversion pulse coding (or handshaking) used in the camera to broadcast signal conversion, it can convert the pulses into a facsimile of the original visual images.

If we were to analyze voice or even Morse code on a two-dimensional oscilloscope, we will see the same process: A series of pulses translating to information.

Photosynthesis is also a waveform transmission and conversion process. Ultraviolet radiation stimulates photosynthesis to produce the nutrition and energy needed by the plant. Chloroblasts within chlorophyll molecules utilize the sun's radiation to split water into hydrogen and oxygen atoms. The hydrogen atoms combine with carbon dioxide to form carbohydrates (such as CH_2O and $C_6H_{12}O_6$) while releasing oxygen. The carbohydrates make up the plant's sugars, starches and cellulose.

Each living organism has this capability of converting radiation through genetically driven biomolecular reactions. The conversion of the sun's radiation is a fundamental metabolic process common among most organisms.

All organisms are receivers, converter and transmitters of informational waveforms. Dolphins and many whales, for example, can not only code and transmit though sound, but they can utilize informational waveform signals to *echo-locate*—obtaining three-dimensional pictures of surrounding objects or creatures. This sense is typically referred to as sonar, which stands for SOund Navigation And Ranging. Sonar allows these intelligent creatures the ability to analyze an object's shape, movement and location from very long distances. While research has long confirmed that dolphins and whales use sonar, it now appears they may have the ability to sense the feelings and emotions of other creatures during these complex sound wave transmissions.

Other animals can broadcast reports and emotions over many miles. They can announce their proprietary territories along with their state of affairs with complex sounds. When a dog's domain is faced with a threatening situation, for example, he can broadcast that situation to many other dogs in that area. Those dogs can in turn broadcast the information to other regions if necessary. Theoretically, remote dog populations can almost instantly know a single dangerous situation through a relay of sound transmission. This is not unlike the broadcasting feature of radio or cell phone transmitting systems.

This illustrates how broadcasting and reception technologies are simply an extension of natural processes. Just as the ears are equipped with a converting mechanism in the form of the bones of the ear and the cochlear hair that translate sound frequencies into nervous impulses, our cell phones are equipped with antennas, crystals and digital circuits that receive and convert radiowave transmissions into sounds. The same basic operation is taking place, except that cell phone technology requires an external power source. This external power source also happens to be one of the causes of the synthetic radiation put out by these devices. The reception and conversion process is similar nonetheless.

The question, however, is whether these technological uses of natural waveforms interfere in the body's natural processes. Do cell phone towers interfere in the cells' ability to communicate with other cells within the body? Do cell phone radiowaves interfere with the brain's own wave signaling processes?

Different sense organs translate light, sound and tactile waveforms. These waveforms allow us to receive information from a variety of energy sources. These information waveforms provide the basic platform for structure within our universe. The information carried through waveforms of various types connects everything together with resonation and coherence—aligning molecular waveforms into sequential progression. This provides an environment designed for information exchange.

Humans are riding on the back of nature's existing technologies with our electromagnetic appliances. The technologies we are using are not new. The ability to broadcast intended information through waveform radiation is well established by nature. Our technologies deliver information utilizing radiowaves, lasers, x-rays, infrared and atomic energy. These waveform frequencies existed prior to our appliances.

The laser is one such example. LASER means *Light Amplification by Stimulated Emission of Radiation.* Nature's crystals (the ruby was used to initially develop the laser) are used to step up and duplicate light waveforms in a way that concentrates their electromagnetic intensity.

This might be compared to shining the sun's light through a magnifying glass in order to produce fire. Today, lasers are being used for communications and for non-invasive surgery. These purposes present to us the positive effects of their waveforms. Just as the sun's rays intensified through a magnifying glass can light a forest fire that will burn down houses, it can also be used to light a campfire that will cook our food and give us light and heat for the night.

Radiowaves transmitted between cell phones and cell towers or from transmitters to television sets present similar possibilities. They present the ability to communicate information between humans located many miles apart. They also present some the ability to steal money from others (ergo, internet crime).

In other words, electromagnetic technologies can be used intelligently for the good of others—or not.

Our latent realization of the informational wave technology exhibited by nature is illustrated by the nineteenth century research of Oxford University physics professor Henry Moseley. Professor Moseley followed Mendeleev's chemical periodic table formulation with radiation emission measurements.

Using x-ray diffraction, he determined that each element emits a unique frequency of radiation. These frequency relationships, he found, also correlate with their orbital valence relationships. As atomic number count increases among the elements, the wavelengths decrease and the frequencies increase. Moving along the elements of the periodic table, frequency measurements increase in a stepped fashion and taper with elements with completed electromagnetic valence shells.

Diffraction is a type of interference pattern created when one waveform interacts with another waveform or interacts with a medium (a body of waveforms).

When a waveform diffracts, it splits up into sub-waveforms. Assuming there is no energy absorbed or released by the intercepted waveform (or medium), the diffracted set of sub-waveforms exhibit the partial characteristics of the initial interfering waveform. In other words, because energy is conserved, the sum of the energy of the diffracted waveforms must equal to the initial interfering waveform.

This brings us to the extraordinary arrangements displayed by nature resulting from the innumerable interference patterns produced by the electromagnetic waveforms surrounding us.

Spiraling Currents

Just as energy moves in waves, energy interaction produces spirals. As coherent waveforms of nature interact and interfere, spirals develop. For example, when we see the rhythmic spiraling growth of leaves or branches around the trunk of a tree, we are presented with an interference of radiation that result in a spiral of Fibonacci proportions.

This spiral or helix pattern of leaves and branches growing upward and outward is produced by the interference patterns created by nature's conjunctive waveforms. Should we spread out the spiral orientation of a plant into two dimensions—x and y coordinates—we would find that the branching reflects a sinusoidal wave pattern.

Should we look down at the plant from its apex, we would see this spiraling or helical effect, depending upon the size and nature of the plant. Looking at a younger plant—where we could see the top shoots with respect to the bottom trunk—we will likely perceive a spiral. Should we look at a larger tree with a large trunk at the bottom with its branches swirling and widening to the top, we will likely perceive a helix.

These helical and spiraling forms provide the basic structures for function within the physical world. We see these structures present within nature's smallest elements to her largest, most complex organisms. From the double helixed DNA molecule to the spiraling galaxies of the universe, we see the spiral within all types of anatomical shapes. The nautilus shell is most famous, but just about every shell and sea formation also reflects this spiral—illustrated by the swirling of water spouts, hurricanes and weather systems.

Other displays of nature's spiraling waveforms include the biological spirals within claws, teeth, horns, irises, ear pinea, and fingerprints.

Our senses utilize these rotational spirals to channel and conduct information waveforms. Our cochlear anatomy utilizes a spiral to convert air pressure waves to neuron impulses. Our eyes are circular, with spiraling irises to the pupils through to the retina.

As illustrated on page 30, the nature of the electromagnetic wave is also spiraling.

Just as the sinusoid wave is derived from the circle, the classic spiral may be derived from the sphere. Beginning at any one of a sphere's apexes or poles, a spiral is formed if we move around the curvature of the sphere towards opposite poles.

This most basic type of spiral is known as the *spherical spiral*. The spherical spiral is also known as the *arithmetic* or *Archimedean spiral*, named after the third century B.C. Greek mathematician Archimedes of Syracuse. In this spiral, the distance between each layer (and spiral arm) is held equidistant. This creates an angular moment that is consistent throughout.

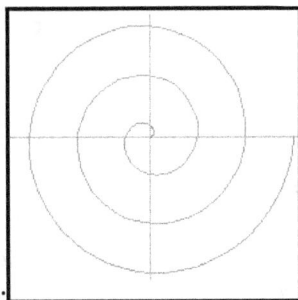

Archimedean spiral-single arm:

There are various other types of spirals appearing in nature. The Fibonacci sequence is either helical or spiral, depending upon the relative perspective. *Fibonacci spirals* are close relatives to the *logarithm spiral*. *Fermat's spiral*—named after sixteenth century Frenchman Pierre de Fermat—is related to the arithmetic spiral. In 1979, Helmut Vogel proposed a variant of Fermat's spiral as a better approximation of nature's Fibonacci spiral. This is the spiral observed within *Phyllotaxis*, which include sunflowers, daisies and certain spiraling universes.

Rene Descartes revealed the *equiangular spiral* around 1868. This spiral reflects geometrical radii outward as polar angles increase. The relationship Descartes discussed (S=AR, which Evangelista Torricelli also developed independently during that era) has also been called the *geometrical spiral*.

Edmond Halley's seventeenth and eighteenth century work revealed the *proportional spiral*. Jacob Bernoulli developed its logarithmic basis, revealing the *logarithmic spiral* shortly thereafter. Bernoulli gave it the namesake of *spira mirabilis*, meaning "wonderful spiral." It is said Bernoulli's fascination of the spiral led to his request it be engraved on his tombstone.

As pointed out by Giuseppe Bertin and C.C. Lin in their 1996 book, *Spiral Structure in the Galaxies*, the spiraling galaxies may well be generated through a combination of density waves that rotate in a slower rhythm than the rest of the galaxy's stars, planets and gases. This *density wave theory*, first proposed in 1964 by C.C. Lin and Frank Shu, explains that the harmonization of the angular paths and the mutual gravitational attraction of the galaxy's components form areas of greater density: This allows the spiral arm formation without a *winding problem.*

Much of nature is arranged in helix or spiral shape. What may not appear to be spiraling is likely requiring us to peer through its cross-section. For example, an ocean wave breaking over a reef may appear to be a half waveform as it is looked at straight on from the beach. However, a cross-sectional view of the same wave reveals its spiral motion:

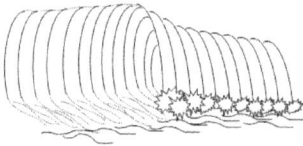

Ocean wave breaking (and spiraling) through to the beach

The combination of the forward movement of the wave to the beach and the sideways movement of water along the crest creates the surfer's classic spiraling *"tube"* or *"barrel."* To ride the tube or barrel requires the surfer to stay just ahead of the final eclipsing of the water with the trough. Should the surfer lapse into the center point of the spiral, the surfer will most likely be separated from the surfboard and experience the dreaded *"wipe out."*

The hurricane provides an additional example of this effect. Waves from two different pressure and temperature fronts interact to form the classic cyclone effect as seen from satellite.

The hurricane's spiral is only visible from above. This means that for thousands of years, humankind had little direct awareness of this spiraled form. Looking at a hurricane front from the land renders a view of the coming wall of rain and wind from the storm. This is why it has been called a 'storm front.' Many have speculated about weather systems as they experienced the 'eye of a hurricane.' They have compared this with other spiraling interactions of waveforms—the tornado. However, it was only when humans began to take to the air that these beautiful spiraling images began to unveil themselves.

This is the same dynamic we see when we flush the toilet or watch water draining a basin. The water's swirling motion reflects the interference pattern of multiple waveform forces. Because the earth is magnetically oriented with north and south poles, the direction of the spiral formed in the basin is clockwise when we flush the toilet in the southern hemisphere. In the northern hemisphere, the same flush rotates counterclockwise. This is caused by the earth's magnetic orientation; effectively "pulling" the water outward one way or another as it is being pulled downward by gravity.

D'Arcy Wentworth Thompson's 1917 classic *On Growth and Form* and Sir T.A. Cook's 1903 *Spirals in Nature and Art* illustrated the many examples of nature's spirals. Mr. Thompson detailed how elements and organisms within nature have a tendency to coil. These include hair, skin cells, tails, elephant trunks, roots and cordiform leaves among others.

Other interesting helix and spiral movements include the spiraled burrowing of rodents and the spiraled swimming of dolphins and whales.

In 1973, Dr. Michael Rossmann reported the finding of a protein structure where multiple coiling strands are linked together with two helical structures. The connection between the strands and the helices were found to be alternating, forming an available structure for nucleotide bonding.

This structure proved to be one of many important helical molecules: Nicotinamide adenine dinucleotide (NAD), a critical coenzyme involved in cellular energy production and genetic transcription within every living cell.

Numerous other biomolecular structures are helical when we are able to observe their *tertiary* structure. Various polysaccharides, polypeptides, hormones, neurotransmitters and fatty acids produced by metabolism have helical-spiral molecular structures.

We can't forget the king of spiral biomolecules, DNA. DNA and its related RNA are protein molecules known for the storage and dissemination of the programming of the body's metabolism. Their helical-spiraling structures have mesmerized the scientific community for nearly six decades.

As we look closer, we find that electron clouds (orbitals or energy states) have helical-spiral dimensions. This spiraling micro-universe of subatomic particle-waves is still beyond the grasp of today's leading physicists.

At the same time, some physicists have been disturbed by the *paradox of the spiral*. This issue was discussed by Dr. Einstein, who concluded this as a radial conductance in his paper on the Faraday disc problem:

"It is known that Maxwell's electrodynamics—as usually understood at the present time—when applied to moving bodies, leads to asymmetries that do not appear to be inherent in the phenomena."

He went on to propose *"asymmetry"* arises when the currents are produced without a *"seat"* of forces. As we have previously discussed, the magnetic field tends to exert a force vector moving perpendicular to that of electrical current. As this happens, angular momentum is inferred from the induction.

When the torque of angular momentum arising from the conducting Faraday disc is considered together with coherently interacting currents and fields, the dynamic of the electromagnetic spiral becomes evident (Serra-Valls 2007).

These waveform forces are precisely mirrored by the classic electromagnetic structure: As the electronic vector pulses forward in one plane, the magnetic vector pulses outward into another plane. Consider a two- and three-dimensional representation:

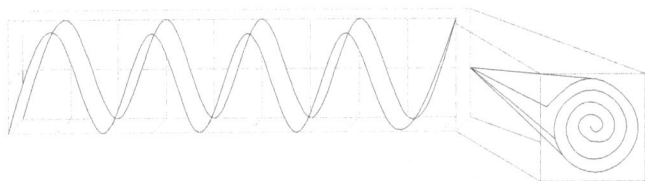

Electromagnetic wave in second and third planes

Electronic radiation is not that different from the motion of water. In both, we see a motion in three dimensions: Playing out the third dimension illustrates the magnetic field moving away perpendicular to the electronic vector of the electromagnetic wave. Because the electronic motion is radiating in an alternating fashion, the magnetic vector moves with a helical, spiraling formation around and outward of the electronic vector. This above representation of this effect shows the electromagnetic waveform from side and cross sections.

Regarding the apparent differences between the spiral and the helix, we point out that when cross-referenced with the axes of time and space, a helix will convert to a spiraled helix. This may require a cross-sectional view to complete the image, however—just as was illustrated earlier with the beach break wave. If we are looking at the wave breaking from the front view, we see a cylinder from the beach.

It is the cross-sectional view of the wave looking down the length of the wave from the side that brings its spiraling motion into view. In the same way, as time and space accumulates helical motion along one axis or another, we observe that one end of the helix will be more relevant than the other end with time. This progression may also be perceived as spiraling arms expanding outward as the helix approaches.

The three dimensional wave presents a helical spiral when the relativity of motion towards the perceiver is considered. We can illustrate the effect of time and space in motion by observing a train approaching us. The front of the train as it approaches us is closer and thus appears larger than the rest of the train.

Though the train size is consistent through all cars, our perception at that point of time is of a large locomotive and small caboose. In the same way, traveling through time within the motion of a spiral would arrive at a helixed perspective: And vice versa for the inverse. Likewise, a person caught in the eye of a hurricane or tornado will not perceive the funneling shape of the storm. The helical or spiral view would only be perceivable from a distance or from above, respectively.

As we peer deeper into the electromagnetic interactivity between electronic current and its reciprocating magnetic field, we unveil through analysis the potential disturbance they create. This implies a designed functionality between conduction and induction. All of nature's waves and spirals oscillate within this sort of cooperative context.

The fields of one electromagnetic rhythm will affect surrounding electromagnetic rhythms. The inter-relationship between natural waveforms within the same environment indicates nature's harmonic organization on a grander level. A chaotic arrangement of replicating depth and organization would simply be an oxymoron.

We can ponder more deeply the nature of matter as we see the elements of multiple dimensions: The waveform and polar mechanics of molecules, combined with the waveform nature of their orbital subatomic content, produces interactive radiation vectors.

This helical-spiral relationship between time and motion also applies to polarity. As polarity bends the electromagnetic spiral motion in one direction or another, the helical orientation turns away or towards the polar application.

Because this is a waveform interaction, this bending creates the facility for information flow along the intersection region. This intersection of pulses and polarity is how combined atoms provide bonding character and structural architecture among their molecular combinations.

As we've discussed, interfering waveforms are information carriers. Spirals, then, are simply a conglomeration of waveform interference patterns under a polar influence. This provides a complexity of information and the facility for resonance.

We might compare a waveform to a letter, a waveform interference pattern to a word, and a spiral to a paragraph or even a book. We could pull a letter out of a book, but its context and meaning would be lost without the rest of the arranged letters and words of the book. While combined waveforms form interference patterns, spirals provide the platform for the flow of information and structure within nature.

In other words, information is conducted through spiraling waveform interference patterns. The medium or space-time may be disturbed by information waveforms, but the information does not move the medium.

The information-waves *pass through the medium.* In *The Evolution of Physics,* Dr. Einstein and Dr. Infeld compared a wave to gossip that travels from one person to another over large distances, yet the people who communicated the gossip did not move. Only the gossip moved. In the same way, we can understand that the spiraling waveform interference patterns of nature serve to conduct complex information through the universe.

Dr. Einstein proposed we accept that the movements of nature are either moving relatively too fast or too slow for us to observe. We can apply this to our understanding of the universe's wavelike, spiraling interference patterns. For this reason, we find out that human research only gives us fleeting glimpses of the complex waveform harmonic existing within the universe.

How does this relate to the electron clouds we discussed previously? The interactions of nature's waveforms to form resonating and sometimes standing waves are harmonic with those of atoms and molecules. Like spirals, electron clouds are created by wave interference and confluence.

The shape and angle of the cloud depends upon the confluence of reciprocating electromagnetic waveforms. How do we know that electron clouds maintain harmonic scale? The valence shells of twos and eights specify this sort of harmonic: Harmonic frequencies of standing waveform orbitals create interference patterns with spiraling frequency.

We also know that certain types of radiation can interfere with these complex spiraling standing electron clouds. This has been repeatedly shown with the bombardment of radiation in particle accelerators. As the resonation of polar interference patterns is disturbed by radiation, the molecule or ion undergoes structural change, and subatomic particles are released (or absorbed) with concurrent energy state changes.

Consider observing standing waves within a small pond of water caused by dropping a couple of small pebbles into the pond. While we see waves appearing to be standing in the same place as they meet each other, their motion is still reflecting the original pebbles that disturbed the water in the first place. In other words, whatever motion is on the water reflects the original cause of the motion.

If we were to drive a car over a cliff into the pond below, the resulting large waves within the pond will also reflect the weight and volume of the car. These waves would reflect onto the basin at the side of the pond to form interfering wave patterns. These patterns eventually become standing waveforms as they resonate with each other and the edge of the pond over time. These standing wave patterns would 'memorize' and reflect the impact of the car upon the water for a period of time.

The 'solids' of nature are all standing, spiraling waveform interference patterns. Each part is made up of a unique combination of specifications which include waveform characteristics such as wavelength, frequency, amplitude, field, and phase—as well as spiral characteristics such as radius, loci and angular velocity. As spiraling waveforms interfere, complex interference patterns form among molecular electron clouds. The radiation they emit or reflect gives them the appearance of solid objects.

This might be compared to looking at the surface of the ocean from far away. From a distance, the ocean looks like a solid, flat object. But when we get closer to the coast, we begin to see that the surface is actually made up of a series of moving, spiraling and standing waves of water.

They 'stand' in this case because while the water waves may be moving through the ocean, the waves themselves are contained within the ocean. When we look at repeating waves onto the shoreline, we are seeing an approximation of standing waves. The waves are vibrating virtually the same water molecules repeatedly.

As we get even closer, we find that these ocean waves are made up of water molecules, which also contain their own electromagnetic waveform interference patterns. These waveforms and interference patterns are harmonically resonating with the spiraling larger waveform interference patterns of the larger ocean waves.

Resonance

The concept of resonance is important to the homeopathic model because this is how electromagnetic radiation is transferred.

Every type of element and every molecular combination emits a unique frequency. These signature frequencies translate to each element, giving off a unique visual experience. This is why gold appears shiny yellowish and silver appears shiny whitish. We have discussed how specific waveform measurements and comparisons have been made possible over recent years with various instruments.

X-ray crystallography and mass spectroscopy are two methods used by chemists to identify different compounds because these instruments read the particular frequencies given off by bombarding those compounds with radiation. After decades of looking at the frequency emissions of various compounds, chemists have cataloged the emission readings of each atom, allowing molecular structures to be identified by their frequencies. This of course indicates that each type of atom and each type of molecule emits a precise and unique *signature* waveform.

Signature waveforms can also be seen across space. For this reason, we have been able to identify a number of different types of elements existing on other planets and stars. Of course, the accuracy of these measurements is limited to the scope of the equipment and our perception. These observations nevertheless illustrate how precise nature can be.

(start here)Over the past few years astronomers at large array radio telescopes have been tracking the existence of persistent intergalactic rhythmic pulses. One of the most puzzling is the *gamma ray burst,* a consistent signature waveform originating from deep space. Gamma rays were discovered at the turn of the twentieth century by the French physicist Paul Villard while working with uranium.

The cyclical yet persistent gamma ray bursts are puzzling to researchers because they stream through the universe from the most remote regions of space, yet maintain a consistent pulse strength throughout that range. Cosmologists have difficulty with these gamma ray bursts because their extreme energy pulses do not seem to be related to a known *physical mass.*

This point is critical to these researchers because the famous postulation of $E=mc^2$—relating energy to mass and the speed of light—is contradicted should there be no physical mass related to these intergalactic oscillations. As a result, cosmologists cannot explain these tremendous rhythmic energies pulsing through the cosmos, opening the door to various speculations about their origin. Regardless of these speculations, the fact remains that gamma ray bursts are macrocosmic pulses out of our range of comprehension.

Humans have figured out how to electronically manipulate rhythmic energies for various purposes. Consider the sonar toothbrush, which sends rhythmic frequencies into the gums to deter certain bacteria. Consider electronic insect and rodent repellents, which plug into the electric circuit of a house, sending pest-irritating waveforms throughout the house. Lasers (**L**ight **A**mplification by **S**timulated **E**mission of **R**adiation) are now seen in just about every household, business, and hospital in one appliance or another. DVD and CD players utilize tiny lasers.

Indeed, there are so many other examples of how we have learned to manipulate rhythmic energies using electronic technologies: Microwaves, x-ray equipment, radios, cordless devices, magnetic resonance imaging equipment, televisions, satellites, and so many other electronic devices utilize and manipulate waveform technology today.

Over recent years, we have determined that many of these electronically manipulated frequencies can be damaging to our physical health. Electromagnetic frequency (EMF) radiation emitted by microwave appliances has been intensely studied for their potential for causing cancers and other disease. For this reason, most wire is shielded by twisting and heavy gauge shields to protect our skin from damage.

Hospital staff wear lead aprons to avoid negative health affects from excessive x-ray exposure. Shielding devices have been installed in cell phones to try to filter their radiation from the ear. All of these attempts have certainly created more safety amongst EMFs. Whether we are out of danger is questionable, as we will investigate later. In general, this research indicates that some waveforms are beneficial to the body while other waveforms may be harmful.

For example, the radiation from sunlight is a beneficial waveform to most living organisms, while the radiation from uranium isotopes or x-rays can be very harmful. Still other waveforms appear to be neither harmful nor healthy as far as we can tell.

Let us consider these issues relative to the rhythmic theory. Why are some waveforms healthy while some are harmful? This question brings us back to the issue of *resonance*. If a particular waveform vibrates in such a way that synchronizes with the natural vibrations occurring within our bodies and around us in nature, this vibration would create a larger, stronger interference pattern. Assuming these stronger resulting waveforms are harmonious to the other vibrations pulsing through and around our physical bodies, these waveforms should lead to greater vitality.

Should the waveform be contradictory to the natural wavelengths occurring in our environment, those vibrations would be considered disruptive. We can easily see this phenomenon when we look at ripples or waves on the surface of water: If a pebble is dropped into a still pond, precisely concentric waves will expand outward from the point of contact on the water surface. If a larger rock were then dropped into the spreading pebble waves, larger waves from the rock drop will collide and overwhelm the waves from the small pebble. This will cause a disfiguring of the concentric design, leaving a host of angled wave collisions.

This illustrates how waves can collide and disrupt other waves, creating unique successive waveforms. While some waves will not interfere because they lack coherency, other waves may interact, leading to a cascade of either constructive or destructive interference patterns. As these waves continue to collide, they may form standing waves or simply create more collisions. Either way, they transmit information through their interference mapping.

Chapter Two
Electromagnetics and Homeopathy

A New Reality

The essence of homeopathy is electromagnetic radiation. Radiation? Like microwave radiation or the sun's radiation? No. We're talking radiation between the smallest of units—the atoms and subatomic elements. Atomic and subatomic radiation maintains the information of the universe. Radiation at this level is the programming of the universe.

In 1175, English monk The realization of the relationship between electricity and magnetism donned on Michael Faraday in 1831 when he coiled wire around an iron ring and demonstrated induction by passing a magnet through the ring. Faraday followed these demonstrations by calculating the relationships and proclaiming four formulas as the basis for what is now known as the *Field theory*. Faraday's proposed that a combination of current and magnetism formed a strange yet universal notion soon dubbed *electromagnetism*.

As many discoveries are, Faraday's theories were not accepted for many years. This didn't stop Faraday from further research into this strange substance. He soon developed the *homopolar generator*—still in use even today as the primary method of advancing direct current through a circuit. This is the most basic form of electrical generation—referred to as induction. Should it be directed through a circulating magnetic disk, the induction begins to alternate with the rotation. This phenomenon is was coined *Faraday's disc*.

Within a few years of Faraday's work, Heinrich Ruhmkorff developed a higher-voltage pulse from DC current. The *Ruhmkorff coil* consisted of copper wires coiled around an iron core—very similar to Faraday's disk. As a DC current was passed through one of his coils, current potential increased. When the pulse was shorted or interrupted, the immediate magnetic field decrease drove the voltage to jump into high gear onto the second coil. This could be arced out to an outlet line, producing a large spike in the voltage with a pulsed, alternating flow of current.

The distribution of this strange alternating current called electricity took a big leap when physicist and fire alarm designer William Stanley conjured a crude AC electrical installation at a New York Fifth Avenue store. Prior to that, direct current distribution technology had been dominated by the marketing and scientific genius of Thomas Edison.

The mid-1800s research of Scottish physicist James Maxwell cemented the notion that light moved through space in the form of waves. Maxwell utilized the notions of Faraday and Hans Christian Oersted to mathematically establish the relationship between electric and magnetic fields. Maxwell's equations also utilized the velocity of light as a constant, to establish what is now known as the *electromagnetic theory*. Maxwell, also given credit for producing the color photograph, should probably have the distinction as the father of electromagnetism. Maxwell published his research in a 1864 book entitled *A Dynamical Theory of the Electromagnetic Field*.

Albert Einstein, Max Plank, Niels Bohr and others followed Maxwell's mathematical approach as they further investigated the electromagnetic nature of atomic radiation, gravity, space and light. Maxwell was a mathematician by training, so his use of formulation assumed that a proof existed when each side of the equal sign was in fact, equal. This method of using *equations* to determine the properties of radiation became the standard: An equality between two or more conditions within nature. This of course assumes that nature is geometrically and harmonically balanced—a proposition famously presented by Pythagoras two thousand years earlier.

EMF refers to the fields that are created by electromagnetic radiation (EMR). The plural is used here because EMR actually produces two fields concurrently. One is an electric field (or vector), caused by the motion of electrons. The second field is a magnetic field, which typically moves perpendicular to electron radiation. While electric fields can "leak" from the flow of electric currents, most wires are insulated and grounded. This can significantly reduce electron fields. Magnetic fields are typically another story.

Electromagnetic fields are caused by the *waveforms* of the electronic and magnetic vectors of radiation. So what are waveforms? Here we will illustrate that not only are we surrounded by waveforms, but matter is quite literally made up of waveforms.

A Magnetic Planet

In 1175, English monk Alexander Neckam experimented with and eventually described how a magnet could be used to make a compass. In 1269, Petrus Peregrinus de Marincourt described the pivot compass. William Gilbert's sixteenth century *De Magnete* described many other uses for the magnet. He also proposed that the pointing of the magnetized needle of a compass in the downwardly north direction meant that the earth must have a *"magnetic soul."*

Polarity is the key ingredient of magnetism, and shifting polarity is a driver of alternating current. In any organism, the polarity of the molecules and atoms making up living cells are arranged in such a way that the poles of each molecule balance each other. This is driven by the reality that negative and positive poles tend to attract each other. Solid structures have latticed patterns founded upon this polarity balance. A polar balance creates stability between intercellular organelles, inner and outer cell membranes, organ tissues, and other cooperative components of the body.

Most biomolecules are either *paramagnetic* (attracted to a magnet) or *diamagnetic* (repelled by a magnet), depending upon which way their polarity balance is trending. In a lodestone or ferro-magnet, however, there is a little less balance in the structure. Groupings of magnetic atoms align together with their poles pointing in one direction or another.

These aligned groupings tend to overwhelm unaligned atoms of the substance, rendering one end a polar negative and the other a polar positive. The ability of a magnet to attract or repel other materials works via this polarity difference on one end or another. As a result, the polarity difference on one side will produce a field that attracts the opposite polarity among other materials. This polar attraction of a magnet is strong enough to drive the rotors of an electric motor.

The strength of the field created by this polarity difference is typically measured in gauss or Teslas. A Tesla is 10,000 gauss.

When an electronic pulse moves through a magnetic field, the electron flow will be drawn either away from or towards the magnet, depending upon the polarity. The forward motion of the electronic current creates an arc. This arc is a representation or byproduct of angular momentum. As electronic currents and magnetic fields interact together in nature, this angular momentum effect creates the spiraling of orbital clouds and matter in general.

The dynamics of magnetic induction between the sun and the earth also creates a pathway for the arc of gravitational orbits.

Consider the trajectory of an arrow shot upwards. It would continue in a straight line until it was acted upon by gravity. Since an arrow's path typically curves upward, arcs, and then curves downward, we can see that the force of gravity was acting in a direction opposing the (upward) direction of the arrow. This interfering combination of vectors produces the perfect arc of the arrow as it heads back to earth. In the same way, the arcing of geomagnetism within the solar system adjusts the vectors of the electromagnetic waves pulsing from the sun.

The earth is a giant magnet, and so are all living organisms. Geologists propose that the earth is magnetic due to the motion of magnetic metals within the surface—a sort of liquefied magnetic core. The concept of a core in motion stems from the fact that the earth's magnetic fields are not static, but are changing. Findings from mountain and desert core samples show that the earth's magnetic north and south poles have varied from the current poles over the past few million years.

The magnetic North Pole is now near Bathurst Island—equidistant from the north geographic pole and the Canada's Arctic Circle. The magnetic South Pole is located close to Hobart, Tasmania. In the late sixteenth century, William Gilbert measured the north magnetic declination at 10 degrees east. By the early nineteenth century, it was 25 degrees west. Now the north magnetic pole lies about 6 degrees west. The magnetic north pole is by no means static.

The earth's physiology is intimately connected with the geomagnetic flows from the sun. This becomes especially apparent when considering the moon's relative effects upon the planet, and the *aurora borealis*—or northern lights. The later is caused by the interaction between atmospheric ions and the electromagnetic radiation from solar activity with the earth's magnetic fields. A glorious light show from nature's EMF arsenal.

Scientists have long thought the earth's magnetic fields rotated above the earth's surface like a band of atmosphere. However, anisotropic scaling has modeled and measured magnetic fields flowing both vertically and horizontally, cross-sectioning the earth's crust. It has also been proposed that these changing magnetic fields predispose movement of magma and/or tectonic plates (Moshe 1996).

The amount of the earth's magnetic field ranges from 45,000 to 60,000 nT (nanoTeslas) over the U.S. This huge variance is assumed to be created by the existence of "buried magnetic bodies" under the earth's surface. This is consistent with surface magnetic field variances found in areas where underground tanks or other fixtures are buried. Steel underground tanks, for example, will result in magnetic field variances of thousands of nanoTeslas.

Core samples with magnetometer readings have confirmed that the earth's magnetic flow has maintained the same approximate direction over the past 700,000 years. Before that, the magnetic field direction of the earth changed a number of times. More than once, the poles have completely reversed. Several times in the planet's history, the earth's major magnetic field has traveled from east to west. Measurements are now illustrating that there is an overall weakening of the magnetic field—some 16% since 1670. This indicates that there is a reversal or another abrupt change in progress. Some estimate a complete phase change—or reversal—

could come as soon as 2000 years from now.

The moving core theory is not the only theory that attempts to explain the earth's changing polarity and magnetic fields. Some have proposed magnetic direction changes are caused by the motion of magnetic field loops circulating from east to west within the earth's interior. This rhythmic field looping has been compared to the rotating magnetism apparent between each side of a bar magnet as it changes polarity. Still others have proposed that an impact from a large meteor might be strong enough to change the earth's magnetic field. The emerging possibility is that the rhythmic geomagnetic fields created by solar storms produce the earth's magnetic changes. Certainly, the sun's solar storms are a contributing factor.

Research on animal migration has confirmed that migratory movement is directly related to the earth's magnetic fields. Cornell University research in 1974 disclosed migration's link to geomagnetism. Researchers tied magnets on bird's heads and let them fly. The birds became disoriented and could not navigate.

Further testing with other migrating species such as lobsters and turtles have since confirmed that all migrating organisms find their direction using tiny magnetic elements within certain cells. Magnetite metals within their cells orient with the earth's polarity to guide their migratory path—much the same way a compass might be used by a ship's navigator to steer a course over the sea.

Magnetic cells have been found in the smallest of species. Bacteria have been found to contain tiny magnetic metals, for example. In fact, many bacteria could very well be compared to a living bar magnets. Tiny pieces of magnetite material will line up within the center of the bacterium—approximating a rudimentary spine. This observation has led some researchers to speculate that the human spine is also magnetic. Indeed, researchers have recently discovered magnetic molecules such as iron oxide within certain human brain and spinal nerve cells. Thus, we might conclude that our bodies also contain little magnetic compasses.

Electromagnetic Circuitry

A circuit consists of a closed loop of current running from one terminal point to another through appropriate grade wiring, often together with various switches, fuses, resistors and grounding mechanisms. The utility power grid is a network of electrical circuits connecting houses to power generating facilities. This is also a circuit—albeit a larger one. Once power is delivered from the grid to a house, it is led into a number of smaller circuits—each distributing power into the different regions of the house.

Each circuit is opened and closed with a circuit breaker wired into a main panel: The current for each circuit travels from the distribution panel through that area of the house and then back to the panel. Outlets and switches allow the electrical circuit to distribute current to electrical appliances. Assuming the appliance has the right capacity, resistance and conductance; it will utilize this incoming current to power its operations.

All electricity has a power source. Modern electricity is produced from nature's elements. This includes hydroelectric (water), solar (sun), or the combustion of carbon (coal or gas).

Many power generating plants will produce and send alternating current through their grid circuits. Transformers will step down the voltage as it enters houses and buildings. Alternating current has become the standard because alternating current can be fairly efficiently transmitted over long distances in higher voltages and stepped down through transformers. In more recent years, high voltage direct current has become the preferred method of long distance power transmission, because direct current produces less resistance within wire conductors. This allows power to be transmitted over longer distances with less power loss and smaller wires.

Because every conductor provides some resistance to a current, power loss is a critical issue. Alternating current produces a *skin effect,* which pushes its conduction outward. This utilizes less of the conducting material, producing more resistance. Nonetheless, alternating current is the norm for appliances and household currents. An alternating current's waveforms pulse in one direction before reversing direction. Direct currents pulse in one direction only.

As power moves through the electrical grid, it is stepped down in voltage using transformers, and eventually enters the house with a single-phase three wire circuit. This means a positive wire and a negative wire with a ground or neutral wire. Triple-phase transmission is typically used at generating plants, enabling greater voltages with more stability, as three conductors are placed around each other at 120-degree angles to cancel their magnetic fields.

Electricity is complicated by its magnetic fields. The magnetic field pulses in a direction perpendicular to the motion of the electrical pulse. This affects the local environment of a circuit. For this reason, electrical wires are double-stranded, twisted and shielded. The double stranding and twisting cancels a good amount of the magnetic fields as they destructively interfere with each other. Shielding further prevents leakage and loss of electrical current. These strategies are designed to increase safety and lower magnetic field production within the household environment.

If a circuit were to surge inconsistently, appliances on the circuit may be damaged. Spikes in electrical current can occur during a lightning storm or power interruption. Circuit breakers and surge protectors are often installed into a house circuit to reduce surging and prevent an overloading of current within the circuit.

Most appliances contain their own miniature circuits. Electricity will be filtered through these appliance circuits using a series of resistors, transistors and capacitors. Most of today's appliances use integrated circuits to bring a greater number of resisters and transistors together into a single compact chip. These are designed to modify the waveform qualities of the current, and translate them into the waveform requirements of the appliance. The integrated circuit is thus designed to modulate and translate waveforms from one type to another. Digital appliances convert alternating current into a series of pulsed digital waveforms using integrated circuitry. These digital waveforms contain unique patterns, which create the programming instructions (often called machine code) to operate the appliance. Meanwhile, power will also be channeled directly into the mechanical portions of the appliance to give it the power to execute its hardware operations.

An appliance may also bring other waveforms. A radio or television will use an antenna and a receiver to channel in broadcasted radiowaves moving through the air. For this reason, most radios and televisions have tuners that focus their receivers onto particular waveform frequencies. Once received, these waveforms will have to be modulated and converted as they are brought into the appliance. Once the waveforms are crystallized, integrated circuits will convert them into digital pulses. These digital pulses are converted into the informational pulses that drive the speakers and/or screen—giving sight and sound to our televisions and radios.

Modern electrical circuits conduct current through copper, gold, silver, aluminum or other metals. Various alloys have been created in recent years. Copper is one of the most used conductors in home circuits because of its stability and low heat production. This makes copper less likely to cause a fire. Aluminum was popular for home wiring in decades past. Electrical fires have been found to be more prevalent in aluminum-wired households. For good reason, insurance companies now prefer copper wiring.

Other materials are considered partial conductors of electrical potential. In other words, they allow for only a muted or partial transmission of electromagnetism: These are called *semiconductors*. Most semiconductors have a crystalline structure such as silicon or germanium—whose crystal structure compares to a diamond. Other compounded elements like indium phosphide and gallium arsenide are also used to provide specific semiconductance. Silicon is probably the most popular semiconductor used today, primarily because of its relatively low cost.

The Electromagnetic Homeopathic Response

How does this relate to homeopathy? We must combine this knowledge about electromagnetics with the wave qualities of the electronic orbitals of molecules.

From a wave perspective, there are multiple intersections of resonance when biochemical dilutions are made and succussed. In order to have an effect after it is diluted, the original molecules of the homeopathic remedy must resonate or interfere in one way or another with the water's molecules during its mixing and dilution process.

This electromagnetic resonation or interference may occur with the water itself, the water container or the minerals or other dilutes of the water.

Most likely, it will be the latter, as water is one of the most stable molecules in nature. Even still, water molecules will certainly electromagnetically react with other substances, depending upon the electromagnetic bonding orbitals of the substance. But given water's relative stability, this reactivity can also occur among the other elements within and surrounding the water.

We must establish at this point the reality that water is never 100% H_2O. Depending on its source, it will contain various dilutes of minerals, metals and salts. Any of these—or all of these—may have electromagnetic bonds that interfere or resonate with the bonds of the remedy, producing minute free radical forms of themselves that can later produce responses within the body.

This resonance or interference highly depends upon the particular electromagnetic nature of the orbitals around the molecules and atoms making up the substance. Thus their electrical and magnetic nature, symptomized by their respective atomic magnetic and electrical specifications.

The proof is found in the observation that these same substances will resonate or interfere with the molecules within the human body. The body is composed of well over 90% water molecules, and the rest of the body is composed of many of the same elements normally diluted in water—such as magnesium, calcium and so on. This means there are similar electromagnetic bonding patterns between water's composition and the human body. And since an resonance or interference electromagnetic process will occur in the form of a physical reaction to the substance in its non-diluted form—a diluted form of the substance after being dissolved in water will still maintain the electromagnetic results of this resonance or interference with whatever part of the solution remains.

Let's use an example. The homeopathic Rhus tox—derived from *Toxicodendron radicans* also known as poison oak—causes rash and itching when the skin comes into contact with oils from the plant. But when these oils are diluted homeopathically, Rhus tox has been clinical prescribed for the relief of itchy skin rashes along the lines of eczema. How does this work?

The molecules within the poison oak oils electromagnetically interfere with the molecules within and on top of the skin, producing oxidative radicals. These oxidative radicals in turn damage the skin cells, producing an inflammatory reaction by the immune system. This inflammatory reaction stimulates leukotrienes, substance P and prostaglandins that produce pain and itching sensations around the damaged skin cells. This inflammation is produced to clean up the site, repair or slough off damaged cells, and neutralize the radicals.

Depending upon the specific nature of the water—its container and minute dilutes—the same electromagnetic forces that produced poison oak's oxidative response with the molecules of the skin will also render an electromagnetic change with one or multiple elements within the water. This may produce radical forms of those elements, or at least electromagnetically-affected forms of those molecules.

As the mixture becomes further and further diluted, these electromagnetic effects will remain with one or more of the water's solutes, the water molecules themselves or the water container, even if the macro portion of the homeopathic substance is reduced.

For example, should one or more of the oxidative elements within Rhus tox produce an oxidative reaction with some of the calcium ions or molecules composed of calcium, those oxidative effects would carry on as the solute is diluted.

We could compare this to heating a rock in a fire and then putting the rock into a pot of water and/or food—an ancient cooking method in many cultures. When the rock is removed, the heat remains. Because the electromagnetic orbitals of the molecules and atoms of the rock have been affected by the fire—raised to higher energy states—that same raised electromagnetic energy state will in turn raise the energy states among the molecules of the water and food in the pot, causing the water and food in the pot to heat up.

While this can also be explained using thermal radiation—in that the heat transfers—what is actually transferring is the raised energy state among the orbitals of the rock's elements. And because these energy states are in essence waveforms, their transference to other molecules is produced by wave resonance or interference.

Oxidative reactions are similar to heat because they are also taking place due to relative energy states among the orbitals of the atomic elements. Oxidative reactions can also accompany thermal response, as the change in the electromagnetic bonds will spill off radiation in the form of heat. This is also a waveform proposition.

Other types of chemical reactions—regardless of how intense—that may occur between the constituents of a non-diluted substance and those dissolved elements in the water, the water molecules themselves or the water container will also be an electromagnetic process that changes the relative energy states of those atomic elements. This change in atomic energy states—like the transfer of heat from substance to substance—will transfer through even a repeated dilution process.

This transfer of electromagnetic energy, taking place through resonation or interference, will also transfer through to the body. How does the body receive such resonance or interference? The body, as we'll discuss, is an electromagnetic machine, full of a myriad of electromagnetic processes that interact. This creates a form of circuitry within the body, which transfers and translates those electromagnetic responses through the body.

Chapter Three

Physiological Circuitry

The Living Circuits

In order for any substance—homeopathic or not—to have an effect upon the physical body or mind, there must be a conduit for that interaction. What is this interaction? It is the transfer of electromagnetic information from a substance into the body. Once it enters the body, the information must be conveyed through the body. Let's discuss the body's information circuitry.

The human body also contains living circuits that transmit using molecular and wave technology. The body circulates and modulates electromagnetic waveforms in much the same way a grid, house, computer, radio or television does. The circuitry of the body is infinitely more complex than any of these, however. The human body utilizes a huge array of conducting and semiconducting mechanisms to distribute and translate waveform information throughout its circuitry.

The crystals used by early radio receivers and the various semiconductor materials used in today's digital devices utilize a similar process that particular biochemicals provide in the body. The senses and their specialized neurons receive transmitted waveforms much the same way a radio or television antenna and receiver does. Once received, these waveforms are converted and translated from their generated source transmissions into electromagnetic pulses suitable for nerve transmission within the body's circuits. These converted waveforms are then transmitted through a vast array of cells and biochemicals, to eventually be viewed by a conscious seer—the self. Once the self within reviews the transmitted and converted information, the self responds with emotion.

The emotional response by the self also utilizes specialized cells to accommodate and translate the information transmitted. These responses utilize the facilities of nerves, hormones, proteins, neurotransmitters, enzymes and DNA as crystals and semiconductors, to convert and transmit intention into informational waveforms and physical responses.

The connection between electricity and the body was established in 1937. Harold Saxton Burr, Ph.D. and Professor of Anatomy at Yale University's School of Medicine, began his research on what he described as living organisms' *biomagnetic field.* Later he named these fields *L-fields,* or *fields of life.* Dr. Burr believed the electromagnetic property of living tissue provided its "organizing principle." This, he thought, prevented the cell from descending into chaos. Dr. Burr also established that physical disease in a living organism is preceded by particular electromagnetic changes.

To establish living organisms' electromagnetic properties, Burr developed an instrument and measurement system sensitive to very weak electromagnetic waveforms. From observations using his specialized equipment, he concluded that living organisms conducted and resisted electricity in the 10^{-6} volts range—small enough to be called *microvolts.*

In one trial, using specially designed microvolt meters with transistors, Dr. Burr suspended salamander eggs within a saline solution. To screen out the potential galvanic action of the solution, Dr. Burr inserted minimizing silver nitrate electrodes between the microvolt meter probe and the saline. He also set up a spinning disc with a measurable sinusoidal voltage waveform, which allowed him to establish a net increase in voltage when the egg was added. This design allowed Dr. Burr to accurately measure any subtle changes in electronic potentials. To provide some controls, Dr. Burr also tested and compared electric potentials of salamander unfertilized eggs. The results were compared with the readings of fertilized eggs and salamanders immediately after hatching. Using a control group of about 100 eggs, Dr. Burr's testing provided clear evidence that the salamander eggs possessed electromagnetic circuitry. Furthermore, he established that the eggs exhibited increasing levels of electromagnetic energy as the eggs matured.

Dr. Burr also discovered that a particular point on the equator of the eggs had a higher voltage than anywhere else on the egg. Points 180 degrees from that point on its equator had a significantly lower voltage. As the eggs matured and hatched, it became evident the higher voltage points corresponded with the salamander's head and the lowest voltage points corresponded with the salamander's tail. Dr. Burr duplicated these results with frogs' eggs and chick embryos. It became evident that a voltage circuit occurred along the alignment of the body's nervous system, with the greatest voltage differential occurring between the top and the bottom of the spine.

Dr. Burr's studies with the living bioelectrical field expanded into diverse areas in the following decades. He published or contributed to nearly one hundred scientific papers on the subject. One of the more fascinating studies Dr. Burr conducted was on the relationship between disease and the bioelectric field. Here he discovered that within about two weeks of contracting cancer, mice would experience an abnormal spiking of their bioelectric field. Confirmed with over 10,000 measurements, it became obvious that most organisms emit a bioelectric surge in advance of contracting disease (Burr 1938).

Another notable result from Dr. Burr's research on various animals and humans was the observation of abnormal bioelectric voltage changes during episodes of metabolic stress. For example, notable voltage changes were observed during wound healing, ovulation, drug use, and a variety of illnesses (Burr 1936; Burr 1937; Burr 1972).

The nervous system is not the only bio-electromagnetic system of the body. The entire body contains multiple circuits and conducting mechanisms. This has gradually become apparent to mainstream science with the discoveries of a multitude of various types of *ion channels*. These are tiny *gateways* lying within cell membranes, consisting primarily of proteins. These protein ion channels reside within the phospholipids of cell membranes. They provide the primary passageways through which the cell's electromagnetic balance is established. The ion channel gateways are stimulated through voltage potential changes, which can take place through the conductance of minerals such as sodium, calcium, magnesium, potassium and others.

In other words, voltage potentials are negotiated through these ion channel gateways. As an ion channel gateway is stimulated with a particular ion polarity, it will open or close. As it opens, it conducts specific information into the cell. The process compares favorably to the opening of an electrical circuit to power an appliance. Once we switch on the power to an appliance, we open its circuits. Then we can tune it to the proper frequencies in order to channel in the information we desire. In the same way, ion channels within the body can be opened or closed. Once open, informational signals (or nutrition) can be channeled in. Typically, mineral ion polarities open or close these gateways. These polarities are networked through the body to open many ion channel circuits at once.

The metabolic importance of these ion channels located throughout the body cannot be overstated. Should these channels fail to respond or react appropriately to a particular voltage parameter, or should they close or open at the wrong times, they can signal the wrong action, or perhaps even signal cells to shut down. This would undoubtedly result in a diseased condition.

Ion channels function very similarly to circuit breakers, resistors and capacitors. They are the gateways for the informational electromagnetic currents running through our body. These electromagnetic currents utilize minerals as conductors. Just as copper conducts electricity through our house wiring systems, the various mineral ions like calcium, sodium, potassium and others conduct information and energy through our bodies. They provide the means through which electromagnetic information is passed from one part of the body to the other.

Ions, however, provide only a subsystem of many levels of bio-conductance. Along with ions, *neurotransmitters* provide the conductors for the legions of neurons tied together with synapses and ion channels. These linked neurons create the pipelines that make up our nervous system. The nervous system utilizes synapses and ion channels to conduct information from one neuron to the next.

Other complex molecules such as *enzymes* and *coenzymes* also facilitate the exchange of electromagnetic information throughout the body. Like integrated circuits, these specialized biomolecules conduct and transmit information by stimulating and catalyzing biochemical reactions within the body. Hence they act as the body's resistors and transistors for electromagnetic information.

The body also conducts complex information through the broadcasting mechanisms of *hormones*. Hormones fall within a grouping of specialized proteins called *ligands*. Ligands have molecular structures that transfer unique waveform combinations. These unique waveform combinations provide specific information. Information is transmitted from ligands to specialized gateway biomolecules called *receptors*. Within the body are innumerable types of receptors and ligands, each equipped to send and receive different sorts of information. Receptors are very similar to ion channels. Like ion channels, they are responsive to electromagnetic conductors. By stimulating receptors, ligand 'conductors' can switch on metabolic activities within cells, discontinue metabolic activities, or significantly alter metabolic activities.

For example, on the surface of most cells are insulin receptors. These will respond to the information communicated via the ligand hormone, insulin. As part of a vast array of mechanisms including glucose reception and surtuin instigation, insulin receptors are stimulated and 'switched on' by insulin.

When insulin receptors are switched on, the cell becomes receptive to glucose. This will allow the cell to readily absorb glucose molecules for energy utilization. Should the insulin receptors become altered over time as a result of a poor diet, the receptors can become less sensitive to insulin. They won't be switched on as easily, in other words.

This insensitivity can contribute to the condition of adult-onset diabetes—which is increasingly being seen among modern children.

As a strategy to prevent the surging of insulin into the bloodstream, high fiber foods can be eaten with every meal. These high fibers slow the absorption of glucose into the bloodstream—giving the blood somewhat of a timed release of glucose and insulin (as nature intended). This timed release of insulin and glucose can gradually increase the sensitivity of insulin receptors, thereby smoothing out the cells' utilization of glucose.

Innumerable ligand-receptor transmission circuits conduct information throughout the body. These range from thyroid hormones, growth hormones, cortisol, melatonin, dopamine, serotonin, epinephrine, and so many others. Some ligands communicate specific instructions to cells from endocrine command centers, while others facilitate cell-to-cell communication. Neurotransmitters are examples of the latter. Through neurotransmitters, particular waveforms are transmitted from nerve cell to nerve cell. Neurotransmitters and hormones are functionally the same in that they broadcast information signals. However, hormones tend to broadcast a tighter range of instructions. Neurotransmitters appear to provide a broader range of waveform conductance.

Hormones and neurotransmitters are extremely complex biochemical molecules. Most are proteins, consisting of hundreds of amino acids joined with other elements. We might compare them to miniature radio stations because they will broadcast received information, while filtering and even sometimes distorting the information to fit their particular design and situation.

The Semiconductors

Within each hormone or neurotransmitter lie semiconductors and integrated circuits. They also have their own broadcasting beacons—the ligand portion of the molecule. These ligand portions conduct electromagnetic information. Prior to conductance, information is modulated, filtered or regulated as it is processed through the molecule.

This translation function gives these molecules tremendous power within the body. Incidentally, most of these larger biomolecules are crystalline with helical or spiral molecular shapes. This would compare favorably with some of our integrated circuits with semiconductor crystals such as silicon and germanium.

The complexity of these *integrated bio-semiconductors* reflects the programming involved within the various circuits of the body. Digital appliances use a system of 1s and 0s compiled together into bytes, which translate information. The on and off gateway states of ion channels, hormones and neurotransmitters create groups of on-off states. These provide complex instructions in the same way a gathering of computer bytes in machine code can instruct hardware operations.

Consider again the pulsing—the rise and fall—of a waveform. An on state would be equivalent to the peak of the wave, and the off state would be considered its trough. As different waveforms *interfere* with each other, however, they can form a more complex pattern of on and off states, depending upon how waveforms collided. This combination of waveforms (the interference pattern) provides a larger array of information—comparable to the byte.

As computers have progressed, their byte length systems have increased. Only a couple of decades ago, computer processing programs worked on an 8-bit byte. This meant that a combination of eight 1s or 0s could fit within a particular byte. The 8-bit byte has now been replaced by 64-bit and 128-bit bytes. The increased byte size increases the productivity of the computer by requiring fewer bytes to process complex information.

The intersection of multiple waveforms within the body creates an tremendously larger 'byte size'. This allows for an almost limitless opportunity for information complexity. Suffice to say that our bodies are not limited to 8- or even 132-bit processing. The body has multifarious gateway switches at different levels, with a multiplex of variances at any level. Thus, comparing the 1s and 0s on-off states of digital computer processing with the body's metabolic processing circuitry might be like comparing a game of checkers to a combat war covering multiple continents and millions of soldiers.

Physiological Illumination

The electrical nature of the body was illuminated by the controversial work of Russian researcher Semyon Kirlian. In 1917, Kirlian attended a presentation by Nikola Tesla, who at the time was experimenting with a new phenomenon called *corona discharge*. Working as an electrical equipment technician later, Kirlian noticed a light flash between an electrotherapy apparatus and a patient's skin.

This gave Kirlian another type of flash. For the next few years, he and his wife Valentina worked to develop an oscillating generator. This allowed an observer to look through an optical filter at the electrical activity arising from the skin's surface. This is dramatically similar to the sun's coronal effect as seen during an eclipse through telescopic equipment.

The ability to photograph the body's *corona effect* was developed by the Kirlians shortly thereafter. They began to notice several interesting correlations as they compared coronal images between different people in different circumstances: The color and activity of the corona seemed different between healthy people and diseased people. They also noticed relationship between the corona and the Chinese *meridian* points.

Observations of *auras* have also been recorded in ancient texts, some thousands of years old. Halos and illuminations have been described in various circumstances throughout Biblical texts. The ancient Vedic literature of the Indus Valley described the *pranic aura field* surrounding the body and the observations of certain personalities with significant bodily effulgence thousands of years ago. In addition, the outward effects of *chi* as an effulgence surrounding the body was also described in ancient Taoist texts. Pythagoras recorded the notion of an outer human energy field around 500 B.C., and Paracelsus described it in the sixteenth century as the *"vital force"* that *"radiates round him like a luminous sphere...."*

More recently, Romanian physician Dr. Ion Dumitrescu had a startling discovery in the late 1970s. His discovery illustrated that the living electromagnetic aura also has a holographic nature. Dr. Dumitrescu utilized an electrographic process with a scanning mechanism to photograph leaf images before and after portions of the leaves were removed. Interestingly, the leaf's corona, despite the removal of a section of leaf, would remain in the shape of the entire leaf as if the section were never removed. The phenomenon was even more dramatic when a hole in the center of the leaf was cut out. Through this hole, the electrographic photo revealed a tiny leaf shape, identical to the outer leaf, which also had a hole in it (Gerber 1988).

Electrotherapy

Western medical science avoided the role of electromagnetics in living organisms for many years. This was despite the research of Burr and others. For example, in the mid-twentieth century, Dr. Robert Becker proved that salamander limb regeneration accompanied millivolt potentials (Becker 1985). This and other research has showed the proliferation of electromagnetism throughout the body.

Continuing studies of *electrotherapy* have confirmed the body's electromagnetic qualities. Electrical stimulation for pain relief is now well established, and today hospitals and pain centers regularly implant *electrostimulators* into the spinal cord region to relieve pain.

Current theories regarding the process of pain relief now center around the *gate control theory* first proposed in 1964 by Melzack and Wall. This theory states the closing and opening of pain-relay gates located in the spine determines the level of electronic transduction of pain signal communication to the brain.

Apparent confirmation of this theory has been the successful treatment of lower back neuropathic pain and pain elsewhere. In addition, electrostimulation has proven successful in bone healing. Veterinary surgeons report success rates in the 75% to 80% range for healing fractures and nonunions with electrostimulation (Clark

1987). Healing rates of almost 65% with an 85% effectiveness rate in human patients have also been observed (Heckman *et al.* 1981).

A number of other studies confirm these. Neurostimulation has been proven successful in a variety of human applications. Pathologies have included urinary and bladder issues (Tanagho 1990, Dalmose 2003, Banyo 2003, Kennedy *et al.* 1995); tachycardia arrhythmias (Volkmann 1991); spinal cord injuries (Beckerman *et al.* 1993, Meinecke 1991); low back pain (Shutov 2007); gastric issues (Deitel 2004); pain (Devulder *et al.* 2002, Siegfried 1988); smoking cessation (White *et al.* 2002); and many other conditions.

The research of Dr. Ronald Melzack and Dr. Patrick Wall eventually led to the famous McGill Pain Questionnaire and other gate control applications. These in turn led to the discoveries of some of the body's feel-good biochemical conductors such as endorphins and enkephalins.

The gate control theories also led to hypotheses regarding the *phantom limb* phenomenon. This curious event—in which an amputee continues to feel pain in an area of an amputated limb—is congruent with Dr. Dumitrescu's *phantom leaf theory* mentioned above.

Observation tells us that the body derives energy from food, sunlight, water, and air. However, there is significant evidence to conclude that these are actually different forms of radiative inputs translated from an upstream generating source. A hydroelectric plant—generating electricity for millions of homes—is not actually producing power. The power is being converted from one energy source to another. This is also stated in the conservation of energy law of thermodynamics.

The body's energy sources—food, sunlight, water and air—are more appropriately identified as conductors. Their waveform potentials carry nutrients into the body. Nutrients include amino acids, minerals, vitamins and oxygen. As discussed in the first chapter, these molecules are made up of atoms, which are made up of electromagnetic electron clouds. These electromagnetic waveforms provide the information our body requires to conduct its operations. This is illustrated by the damage a free radical (the anti-nutrient) can do within the body. Free radicals damage arteries and other tissues, producing disease. A free radical is essentially a molecule with an 'free electron'—an unstable electron cloud that damages other molecules as it seeks stability.

Magnetic Physiology

The body is full of polarity differentials. This makes the body a magnet. Most of our cells, organs and tissue systems are also independently magnetic. As electromagnetic biochemical reactions cascade through the body, magnetic fields are generated. These magnetic fields are dispatched through our local environment with polar results. Some fields are by-products of electronic processes, while others maintain polarities that affect metabolism directly.

The anatomical effects of magnetism are not readily addressed by modern medical science. This is odd, noting the extensive use of diagnosis using magnetic resonance technologies. MRIs (magnetic resonance) utilize the body's inherent polarity to visualize its anatomy. Just as electrical currents moving through appliances generate magnetic fields, the currents running through the body's ionic mechanisms utilize magnetic fields.

Magnets were named after the lodestone—a rock found by the Greeks in the province of Magnesia. This was a curious stone, and it was found by early Greek physicians to have healing properties. The Greek philosopher-physician Aristophanes explored this mysterious rock for many years. Hippocrates utilized the magnet for many treatments. Chinese and Vedic physicians had used magnets for healing centuries earlier. Ancient texts show that everything from heart disease to gout was treated with magnets in Chinese, Greek, medieval European, and Ayurvedic therapies.

After suffering from avoidance, the concept of magnetism within the human physiology arose again when the late-nineteenth century Julius Bernstein proposed that nerve impulses transferred through polarization. This *membrane polarization* model became the basis for the conclusive research of Otto Loewi in the early 1920s, which led to a 1936 Nobel Prize for synaptic transmission. Loewi's experiment—which apparently occurred to him during a dream—was to extract two frog hearts and retain each in a separate bath of saline. Some of the solution surrounding the faster heartbeat was extracted and put into the bath of the slower heart. This made the slower heart beat faster. The experiment effectively provided the evidence for biochemical synaptic transmission.

The polarity exchange between ions and biochemicals is unmistakably magnetic. Magnetism is, after all, a polarity issue of ions or atoms aligning in one direction or another. The irrefutable link between magnetism and biological response has been confirmed by study and clinical application during the last half of the twentieth century, as the existence of ion channels has been clarified.

Furthermore, the link between intention and magnetism has become evident. This was illustrated by Dr. Grad's research at Canada's McGill University in the late 1950s and early 1960s, when growth rates of barley sprouts were stimulated by the focused intentions of particularly gifted individuals. Further studies indicated these growth rate effects were similar to the influence magnetism has upon plant growth.

The central subject of these investigations was a Hungarian refugee named Oskar Estebany, who appeared to be able to exert intentional effects with his hands. A number of tests confirmed that magnetism was involved in Mr. Estebany's abilities. In one, Dr. Justa Smith at the Rosary Hill College (1973) compared Mr. Estebany's ability to increase enzyme reaction rates to those of magnetic field emissions. After Mr. Estebany affected an increase in reactivity among enzyme reaction rates, Dr. Smith applied magnetic fields and compared the rates. It turned out that the increased growth caused by Mr. Estebany precisely matched the growth caused by a 13,000 gauss magnetic field. The results indicated that somehow, intention can produce magnetic fields within the body.

Dr. Smith had spent a number of years studying these effects prior to and after her tests with Mr. Estebany. She authored a book on the topic—*Effect of Magnetic Fields on Enzyme Reactivity* (1969). While this research was considered radical at that time, other scientists soon confirmed her findings. In the 1990s, a flurry of research was published around the world showing magnetic fields in the 2,500-10,000 gauss range affecting reaction rates of various enzymatic reactions. By 1996, more than fifty different enzyme reactions were found to be influenced by magnetic fields. In two linked studies by University of Utah's Charles Grissom, (1993, 1996), single-beam UV-to-visible spectrum and rapid-scanning spectrophotometers with electromagnets built in were applied to two different cobalamine (B12) enzymes.

One enzyme (ethanolamine ammonia lyase) had significantly different reaction rates in response to magnetic fields, while the other enzyme (methylmalonyl CoA mutase) had no apparent response. It could thus be concluded that some biochemical processes are sensitive to magnetic field influence and others are not. This effect is still mysterious, but it has become increasingly evident that within the body exists a driver of magnetic fields.

There have been a number of controlled studies showing that major body centers respond to magnetic stimulation. Amassian *et al.* (1989) stimulated the motor cortex with a focal magnetic coil, which rendered movement to paralyzed appendages. Maccabee *et al.* (1991) stimulated almost the entire nervous system with a magnetic coil. This particular stimulation instigated responses from the distal peripheral nerve, the nerve root, the cranial nerve, the motor cortex, the premotor cortex, the frontal motor areas related to speech, and other nerve centers.

Dr. Howard Friedman and Dr. Robert Becker studied human behavior and magnetic fields in the early 1960s. They found *extremely low frequencies* (ELF) such as .1 or .2 Hz affected volunteer reaction times (Becker 1985). This paralleled work by Dr. Norbert Weiner and Dr. James Hamer with low-intensity fields—described as "driving" waveforms existing within the body.

Dr. Jose Delgado's research illustrated that ELF magnetic fields influence sleep and manic behavior.

Furthermore, a substantial amount of evidence demonstrates that magnetic fields generated from power lines and transformers can modulate physiology. This has been especially noticeable in power line and transformer effects upon plants. Research linking cancer and power lines has been controversial. Still, enough evidence enables a conclusion that magnetic fields can alter certain physiological processes, as we'll discuss in more detail later.

The magnetic nature of the body is revealed through *nuclear magnetic resonance* (NMR). Its application of *magnetic resonance imaging* (MRI) is now one of the more useful diagnostic machines used in medicine when a true cross-sectional analysis of the body is required.

The NMR scan is performed on the human body by surrounding the body with strong magnetic fields. The body is guided underneath magnetic fields ranging from about 5,000 to 20,000 gauss (the earth's magnetic field is about .5 gauss by comparison). These fields polarize the hydrogen ($H+$) proton ions in water (as the body is mostly water). As these ions' north poles align, they emit a particular frequency. Radio beams positioned around the body (tuned to this frequency) are shot through the body. As the polarity-altered hydrogen protons become excited by radio signals, a computer calculates the water content differences to form the image. Were it not for the magnetic nature of the body's molecules, the three-dimensional images produced by the MRI would not be possible.

Our entire metabolism is magnetic. Every cell and every tissue system utilizes and produces polarity during instructional transmissions. This is illustrated in the behavior of ion channels, neurotransmitters, hormones, enzymes and ligand-receptors as we've illustrated. While magnetic metabolism is symptomized in migratory travel, it is further demonstrated in our metabolic responses to the sun's geomagnetic fields produced during solar storm activity.

Magnetic Behavior

The awareness of a correlation between human behavior and solar cycles is due largely to the research of Russian scientist Alexander Chizhevsky. Chizevsky is also known for his groundbreaking research discovering the properties of ionized air during the earlier part of the twentieth century.

In the early 1920s, Chizhevsky analyzed the timing of wars, battles, riots, and revolutions among the histories of 72 countries from 500 BCE to 1922. He discovered that 80% of these critical events took place close to a sunspot activity peak. In an attempt to explain the data, Chizhevsky proposed that strong magnetic fields might be emanating from these intense solar storms. He suggested that magnetic influences from magnetic solar storms could trigger mass behavior changes among large populations simultaneously. These magnetic stimulatory effects, he thought, could affect mental propensities, predisposing aggressive or violent behavior.

Chizhevsky's studies demonstrated similar patterns between solar sunspot cycles and mortality rates caused by epidemics and spikes in births. This research was considered novel and controversial during Chizhevsky's lifetime. However, continued research over the decades since Chizhevsky has confirmed a number of significant effects caused by what is now referred to as *geomagnetism* upon behavior and disease.

The relevance and conclusions from Chizhevsky's research have received confirmation in new research by Musaev *et al.* (2007), which studied solar activity and demographic data specific to infectious disease mortality between 1930 and 2000. Disease and mortality statistics related to cardiovascular, neurological, oncological, bronchi-pulmonary, and infectious pandemics proved to be instructive. The data indicated a clear relationship between these pandemics and solar storm cycles.

Recent research has uncovered many other disease associations resulting from the geomagnetic influence of auroras, sunspots and solar storms. The Cardiology department of Israel's Rabin Medical Center (Stoupel *et al.* 2007) studied the occurrence of acute myocardial infarction together with the timing and measurement of solar activity. This study differentiated the effects of higher cosmic ray activity from periods of higher geomagnetic activity (sunspots and solar flares). It was found that myocardial infarction rates inversely correlate with monthly solar activity, and positively correlate with increased cosmic ray activity. Low geomagnetic activity days and higher cosmic ray days are linked with significantly greater rates of fatalities due to myocardial infarction.

Marasanov and Matveev also reported in 2007 that among lung cancer patients having surgery, complications occur more significantly during geomagnetic solar storm periods than during geomagnetic "quiet" days.

In 2006, Stoupel et al. calculated immune system strength by measuring levels of IgG, IgM, IgA, lupus anti-coagulant, clotting time, and autoantibody blood levels among a group of subjects over time. Their levels were correlated with solar activity patterns as measured by the U.S. National Geophysical Data Center. This research found that these immune system levels move with solar geomagnetic activity—reducing with more activity and increasing with less solar activity.

Stoupel's research was confirmed by studies done at Canada's Laurentian University (Kinoshameg and Persinger 2004). Here, rats exposed to induced geomagnetic activity suffered immunosuppression, resulting in higher rates of infection.

In 2006, Yeung analyzed pandemic influenza outbreaks from 1700 A.D. to 2000 A.D. Significant correlations were found between flu outbreaks and sunspot cycles.

Vaquero and Gallego (2007) confirmed the connection between immunosuppression, infectious outbreaks, and sunspot cycles in research studying pandemic influenza A.

A 2006 study from Kyoto University (Japan) researchers (Otsu et al.) reported that a strong correlation existed between sunspot activity, unemployment rates and suicides between 1971 and 2001. Both unemployment and suicides were inversely proportional to sunspot rhythmic periods.

Another study from 2006 (Davis and Lowell) using the birth dates of 237,000 humans, found a positive correlation between the births of children with genetic mental diseases like schizophrenia and bipolar disorder with solar activity. They also found similar correlations between solar activity cycles and 'genetic' diseases like multiple sclerosis and rheumatoid arthritis. These diseases were also closely correlated with being born in a particular season.

In another study done in Israel (Stoupel *et al.* 2006), 339,252 newborn births over a period of seven years were compared to monthly cosmic ray and solar activity. Significantly more babies were born of both genders during periods of greater cosmic ray activity. In other words, fewer newborns were born during high solar activity periods as compared with periods of reduced solar activity.

The Rabin Medical Center (Stoupel *et al.* 2005) also studied Down syndrome cases among 1,108,449 births together with solar activity. With 1,310 total cases of Down syndrome in the data, a significant inverse relationship between solar activity occurred. In other words, Down syndrome—long considered a genetic defect—occurs more often during periods of reduced solar activity, and less often during periods of increased solar activity.

Researchers at the Universidad de Chile's Clinica Psiquiatrica Universitaria (Ivanovic-Zuvic *et al.*) presented a study in 2005 that compared increased hospitalizations of depressive patients and manic patients to solar activity periods. In this study, depressive hospitalizations correlated with periods of lower solar activity, while manic hospitalizations positively correlated with higher solar activity periods.

A study at the Augusta Mental Health Institute in Maine (Davis and Lowell 2004) established that excessive ultraviolet radiation from the sun combined with solar flare cycles correlated positively with mental illnesses resulting from DNA damage.

It also appears from other research by Davis and Lowell (2004) that human lifespan correlates with solar activity. This research illustrated that chaotic solar activity (as opposed to typical pattern cycles) coincide with increases in mutagenic DNA effects. Further exploration into lifespan and birthdates around solar cycles found disrupted solar cycles correlating positively with shorter lifespan.

In an Australian study (Berk *et al.* 2006) of suicides between 1968 and 2002, both seasonal and geomagnetic solar storm activity were investigated using 51,845 male and 16,327 female suicides. Suicides among females significantly increased in the autumn, concurrent with increased geomagnetic storm activity. Suicides were lowest during autumn for males and lowest during the summer for females. The average number of suicides for both males and females were the greatest during the spring.

This connection of seasonal and geomagnetic activity with suicide was also confirmed in research on 27,469 Finnish suicide cases between 1979 and 1999 by Partonen *et al.* (2004).

Cellular Communication

Anyone who has taken a polygraph will report that the examination is complex and requires some technical training in physiology and psychology. A polygraph examiner is thus typically expert in physical-emotion expression. The equipment utilizes primarily *galvanic skin response* (GSR) and electrocardiography equipment to monitor the physical reflections of specific emotions. What polygraph examination techniques have taught scientists over the years is that the skin, heart and many other parts of the body will reveal heightened emotions with particular physical responses. One of the most noticeable physical responses results from the emotion of fear.

Lie detection has thus become recognized as a verifiable science after over thousands of polygraph examinations and hundreds of studies. Even with the occasional variance in specific results, there is undeniable evidence that the body reflects heightened emotional response. Polygraph research has revealed that some people have the ability to cheat the polygraph, assuming they understand how to control certain emotional and physical responses. Here again, this underscores the connection between intention and physical response. Whether cheating the polygraph or not, intention is being expressed through the various responses of the body.

In 1966, Cleve Backster, a former CIA employee and licensed polygraph examiner, began experimenting with polygraph equipment connected to plants. His first plant was a dracaena cane plant. After connecting the polygraph's electrodes, he immediately began to notice that its galvanic skin response readings were not so different from human examination charts. What surprised Dr. Backster was that the plant's exam also registered emotional responses that reflected fear. Furthermore, these responses were highest during moments where an intention to harm the plant came to mind. A simple thought by a nearby human of harming the plant produced a precise fear response in the plant's skin response.

The prospect of a plant responding to a threatening intention was certainly incredible to Dr. Backster—then an owner of a polygraph school and research laboratory. Following this incident, Dr. Backster spent the next thirty years carefully conducting controlled experiments to study conscious mechanisms within plants, eggs, and then human cells. Dr. Backster published two scientific papers on the subject, along with a number of popular magazine articles and a book documenting his years of study (Backster 2003).

Dr. Backster carefully conducted hundreds of experiments on emotional intention, devising automated research equipment to remove extraneous influences. Many of these studies were reviewed by well-known scientists, and some even took part in the research. His results were clear, and many were replicated by other scientists—although this also proved to be difficult to the spontaneity required by consciousness research. Dr. Backster discovered that plants were not the only living organism to sense intention. Through exhaustive tests using various subjects and perspectives, he found that human leukocytes separated from their host and kept *in vitro* somehow had the ability to sense and respond to emotions of fear and excitement that occurred within their former host *remotely*. Furthermore and amazingly, he found this effect can occur at a distance of up to fifty miles.

The human polygraph examination focuses upon our fear of detection. The fear of harm through discovery is the typical emotion being tested. This is also controlled in Dr. Backster's research on plants, eggs and human cells. Because the fear of detection is closely related to the fear of harm, the physiological results of the two emotions are practically identical.

One of the dramatic findings of Dr. Backster's research with plants was that once a person consistently begins caring for a plant, that plant becomes emotionally connected to that person. Dr. Backster discovered that even when the person has traveled miles away from this plant, emotionally charged circumstances occurring in the life of the person would affect the plant. In other words, the plant becomes emotionally tied to the person taking care of it. This sort of emotion is typically referred to as *empathy*.

In vitro cells separated from a human responded very similarly in Dr. Backster's research, but only with their host. Living cells being incubated and electroded with the equipment responded to the heightened emotional activity of their former host, even when the host was located rooms or even miles away from the cells. This indicated the separated cells somehow had the ability to receive remote communication transmissions from the host. How is it that cells have this ability? Furthermore, Dr. Backster's research demonstrated that the cells were able to prioritize their responses specifically for their host, even amongst emotional controls set up to distract the response.

Dr. Backster's research controls were thoroughly vetted by a number of scientists. Still, it is regarded as controversial, and has been difficult to duplicate in some cases. Nonetheless, communications between a remote ex-host is not altogether different from the cell's known ability to instantly receive instructions from the brain and other remote locations in the body—located many feet away, amongst trillions of other cells. Medical researchers recognize that the body's nervous systems and various biochemicals such as neurotransmitters and hormones conduct waveforms from one location of the body to another. This begs the question: How do billions of cells instantly become orchestrated into a particular activity? Nerves are certainly high-speed, but all cells are not innervated. So how do all the cells instantly respond?

Every cell making up a living organism is a waveform receiver. Each cell has the ability to receive instructional waveforms just as any radio can receive a local broadcast. In addition, groups of cells can align and organize to receive and respond to specific types of waveforms. Just as a radio broadcast will reach millions of radios at once, the body's waveform broadcasts reach a multitude of cells simultaneously.

Our entire metabolism is set up to send and receive multi-spectrum waveforms. Groups of cells called the senses have organized around receiving specific types of waveforms. We can perceive waves in the visible spectrum with the eyes, infrared radiation with the skin, air pressure waves with the ears, and subtle electromagnetic waveforms with the tongue and nose. These are only a few of the multitude of waveforms that are received and translated throughout the body. This is compounded by the fact that the cells also conduct various waveforms via ion channels and receptors.

The body's cells pick up waveforms beyond our current technologies. This is the only explanation for cells being able to receive precise information from remote locations. Dr. Backster's research illustrated that these communications are received through insulated and even metal walls.

Waveform communications outside our range of recognition is not a new paradigm to science. The past few hundred years of research have continuously revealed previously unperceivable waveforms.

The body's cells have the ability to perceive a variety of waveforms considered outside the visible wavelengths. There is evidence to the contrary. Wavelengths shorter than violet such as ultraviolet, x-rays, and gamma rays have been observed visually under extraordinary circumstances such as a darkened room penetrated with radiation leakage. Both x-rays and gamma rays have been observed on occasion with the naked eye, as a yellow-green glow. Meanwhile, some have identified nuclear leakage in flashes of blue. As the rods of the eyes sensitize for night vision they also become sensitive to other waveforms. Longer and less damaging radiowaves have also been received by humans in extraordinary circumstances. Hearing radio stations through dental fillings, bridgework, and even bobby pins has been a rare but well-documented occurrence.

The body's cells translate radiowaves into electrical brain impulses just as a radio crystal translates radiowaves into electronic pulses. The senses illustrate this well. Once received through the antenna mechanisms of the eyes, ears, nose, tongue and so on—waveforms are converted through the crystalline structures of nerve cells.

Individual cells have these same antenna systems. Radiowaves influencing single cells and single-cell living organisms is well documented. In 1958, for example, *The New England Institute for Medical Research* published articles documenting that radiowaves could influence red blood cell movement and bacteria motion. Murchie (1978) observed amebas, euglenas, and paramecia aligning their movement with radiating field lines of five to forty megacycle radiowaves. Many other studies have documented similar effects.

The reception and translation of ultraviolet radiation by skin cells is obvious and well understood. The sun's ultraviolet B waveforms stimulate the production of vitamin D_3 when wavelengths of 270-290 nanometers enter the epidermal layer. The *conrotatory electrocyclic reaction* cycles 7-dehydrocholesterol to pre-vitamin D, and eventually to 1,25 dihydroxyvitamin D, or 25-OHD. During this cycle, melanin production is stimulated to provide a filtering and buffering mechanism for additional rays from the sun. Vitamin D is an essential nutrient to the human body. It is important for immunity, cardiovascular health, nerve health and bones and teeth health. Our primary source is through the sun, although a limited number of foods contain small amounts as well.

For many decades, researchers have been studying the effects of light upon other human cells. We all know about photosynthesis—

where plant cells utilize light, water and carbon dioxide to produce starches, sugars and oxygen. The molecular structure of chlorophyll acts as a semiconducting crystal, absorbing some ultraviolet waveforms from the sun while reflecting others. With these absorbed waveforms, the unique biochemical reaction of photosynthesis is stimulated among special chloroplasts— specialized proteins embedded inside chlorophyll.

This process illustrates the intimate connection between waveform conversion and living organisms. The complex transformation of light waveforms to plant nutrition is a conversion related to the intention to survive—a conscious act. This intention creates the impetus for energy transformation. We see a similar transformation process occurring through the human cellular production of energy from oxygen and glucose. Cellular energy production occurs through a waveform transition process called *electron transport* (reminiscent of the characterization of electricity as electron movement). ATP and NADPH are created and water is split, releasing oxygen. Part of this process uses an interesting exchange of phosphorus ions called *phosphorylation*. This process is one of transferring waveform energy through a transport chain to create an NADP+ molecule, after which an additional transformation takes place through a process of *redox* to create an energized NADPH. Some have theorized that the continuing process of ATP conversion and glucose takes place without UV. Further research has revealed that light is at least indirectly involved, as it stimulates the production of some of the enzymes used as catalysts.

In the 1920s, a Russian scientist Alexander Gurwitsch picked up a weak photoemission from living tissue. The emissions appeared stronger during mitosis, so he termed these UV-range wavelength rhythms *mitogenetic rays*. The presence of living radiation emitted from dividing cells was confirmed shortly thereafter by some German researchers. Even still, their conclusions were overshadowed by doubts from skeptics. Nonetheless, ongoing biochemical experiments have continued to confirm that cellular division produces radiation emissions.

The topic did not gain much additional research attention until after World War II. Research teams from Italy, Germany and Britain independently worked on the living photon research. Each confirmed waveform observations from living cells, which they named variously. Two names have stuck: *low-level luminescence* and *ultraweak chemiluminescence*. We'll discuss this research on biophotons in more detail later.

As we survey the empirical evidence, we arrive at the reality that throughout the body—through every cell, tissue system, circulatory system, organ system and nerve center—flow a variety of different waveforms. As we will discover in detail, every type of body waveform has a specific function, and affects metabolism in a distinctive way. Furthermore, the variety of different waveforms are all interacting within the body. These interactions result in the facilities we have come to understand as physiology. For this reason, we will utilize a new descriptor for the body's variety of internal waveforms that stem from consciousness: *Biowaves*.

Datacom Pathways

Cells are like smart radio-driven generators with multi-layered reception and transmission communication systems. As physiologists have delved deeper into the activities of the estimated trillion cells in the human body, they have continued to see increasingly deeper levels of biocommunication activity amongst the electrolyte ions within and around the cell.

The ion channel is an informational device because it establishes an on-off state in the form of an open or closed gateway. Actually, the gateway of most ion channels is a bit more complex. Research has indicated that one of three possible states is produced within the typical ion channel gateway: deactivation, activation or inactivation. Both the deactivated state and the inactivated state are closed, while the activated state is open. The difference between the two closed states is that a deactivated gate is blocked by an opposing open gate, while the inactive gate is simply closed in process after activation. In other words, the latter produces a rhythmic opening and closing adherent to voltage potential changes.

As we've discussed, these ion channels interact intimately with mineral ions such as sodium, potassium and other electron-transporting mechanisms like ATPase. The electro-chemical aspects of mineral ions led to early discoveries of electricity and its magnetic field qualities. This is because ions are electromagnetic conductors. Ions are activated with pulsed electromagnetic fields. This provides a means to carry and exchange waveform information. As the ionic waveforms interact with biowaves from other sources, an interference pattern results. This creates a mapping system that conveys information.

Ion channels have been observed transferring chemical charges and communicating processes such as glucose utilization and immune response between cell membranes and intercellular tissues. These electro-chemical pathways have been correlated with biophoton emissions, illustrating the reality that information-signaling systems exist on more than a chemical basis.

One of the most prominent potential conductors in the body is the sodium ion. Sodium ions negotiate electromagnetic waveforms efficiently. *Sodium channels* thus lie within cell membranes of the most active cells in the body, including muscle and nerve cells. These protein complexes are activated by the voltage potentials provided by sodium ions as they cycle through their biochemical processes. In response to ionic state changes, many sodium channels will generate a change in electric potential inside the cell by conducting sodium ions through the cell membrane. By changing the cell's electrical potential, the cell's inner polarity and reactive potential with various nutrients and biochemicals will change. This will stimulate particular types of biological processes within the cell. Among sodium channels are various sub-types—specialized for a particular cellular activity, organ or tissue system.

Potassium channels exist in almost every cell in the body. They are involved in regulating the secretion and reception of various types of hormones. Potassium channels lie primarily within the cell membrane. Much like the sodium channels, they provide voltage gates through which potassium ion charges can travel. Potassium channels are activated by various means with specific response ranges. A newly discovered type of potassium channel system is the double-pore system, contrasting with the primarily single pore system of other known ionic channels. This double-pore potassium channel is thought to be a complex regulator in vascular cells—it stimulates tone and flexibility to the artery walls.

Calcium channels provide another type of voltage circuit. Calcium ion channels are found among various specialized cells in brain, organ, and nerve tissues. The calcium gateways have been linked with an informational depolarization process. This turns on and off the release of various neurotransmitters and hormones. Like the sodium and potassium channels, calcium channels have various sub-types. These will produce specific results within specialized cells.

Chloride channels appear to be related to regulating the cell's nutritional contents. No less than thirteen different types of chloride channels have been discovered. Each type regulates different nutrients and informational functions within different types of cells.

These are merely the tip of the iceberg. There are likely billions of ion channels located throughout the body. Information flows through each and every one constantly. Other types of channels have been isolated by research over recent years. *Cation channels* are activated through a combination of ions. They predominate within sperm cells. Cation-selective double pore channels provide both inward and outward voltage potential changes. *Rhodopsin channels* are activated open through the reception of light. Another type of voltage channel is the *cyclic nucleotide channel*. These are thought to regulate the entry of ions and nucleotides that drive energy use and cellular clock activity. The heart's pacemaker neurons function extensively with cyclic nucleotide channels, for example. *Transient receptor potential channels*—also called TRPs—have so far been observed among fruit flies, but many scientists suspect that these also exist within humans. TRP channels respond to photoelectric waveforms. There are a number of different types of TRPs with various functions. To the billions of channels of the types mentioned above, we can add the cAMP and IP3 channels, along with many others.

There are about 80 known macro and trace minerals in the body. As nutritional research into macro minerals has progressed, we have gradually come to understand that every mineral plays an important role. Should the human body be lacking in any of these elements, imbalances in metabolism begin to occur. Some of the more prevalent macro minerals include, among others, calcium, potassium, magnesium, sodium and phosphorus. These are called macro because they exist in larger quantities in the body. These minerals contribute to the ionic informational activities of the vast legions of catalysts, proteins, enzymes, cell walls, artery walls, and so many other structural elements of the body's anatomy. And of course, they also facilitate communications between cells through ion channels.

All the trace and macro minerals are subject to ionization within the polarity of the body's metabolism. Ionization produces conductivity, as ions can connect and pass on electron waves. This also explains why negative ions in the atmosphere appear to increase well-being. Positive atmospheric ions—in advance of storm fronts or accompanying Foehn winds—will often bring about an array of health problems such as inflammation, headaches and allergies.

Ions are also produced by the body's trace minerals, including fluorine, cadmium, copper, chlorine and even uranium. In larger quantities, these elements can be toxic. They become ionized during metabolic reactions. They are each involved directly or indirectly in innumerable enzyme functions, protein sequencing, immune cell composition and many other functions. Without a consistent supply of trace elements, our body's ion operations quickly become handicapped.

Each mineral ion provides a specific polarity and covalence for subatomic bonding. Each also provides a unique facility for waveform conductance. Conducting ions provide a bridge for information transmission throughout the body. Mineral-conducting biowaves converge through a variety of ion bridges and channels into interference patterns. From these interference patterns, instructional signals emerge.

Just as 110 household current is conducted through copper wires to be received and manipulated by appliances connected to the circuit, electromagnetic currents pulse through the body's mineral ion bridges, transferring electron energy to cellular and tissue operations.

During cellular reactions, tiny electromagnetic waveforms work to define which reaction will occur when. The specific assembly of minerals provides the basis for the molecular combinations that create the appropriate electromagnetic interference patterns.

Illustrating our need for ions for proper metabolism, several World Health Organization-sponsored studies have determined that people who drink water with low hardness—with a lack of calcium, magnesium and other ions—there is a greater risk of heart attack (Bernardi et al. 1995).

The respective interference patterns created by the biowaves transferred through an assembly of ion bridges form the instructional signals that turn on and off specific biochemical reactions. Without this instructional signaling system, there would be no operational control over the body's reactions. They would simply begin randomly; and after beginning, they would run indefinitely and likely out of control.

These is on-off state functions are starkly illustrated by the inflammatory pathway. The body responds to an injury with a number of inflammatory repair cells such as plasmin and fibrin to patch up the injury. Blood will usually coalesce around the injury to deliver these and other nutrients required to repair the wound. At some point in the process, signaling molecules will stop the inflammatory process, and initiate a clean out of the area to allow for the next steps of the healing process.

Cortisol is one of these switching conductors. As cortisol levels increase, inflammation is reduced. Pharmaceutical medicine has discovered this link, prompting the success of cortisone-based pharmaceuticals.

Cortisol also so happens to modulate both sodium and potassium concentrations within the body. It also modulates insulin levels and stimulates gastric juices, and stimulates copper-based enzyme functions such as superoxide dismutase. All of these functions are driven by the transmission functions of the cortisol molecule. Cortisol's molecular structure is made up of a combination of carbon, hydrogen and oxygen, just as are many of the body's molecules. It is the unique combination of standing electromagnetic bonds between the hydrogen and oxygen ions that facilitate cortisol's transmission capabilities. The commingled arrangement of its electromagnetic electron cloud waveform interference patterns enables cortisol's unique information structure.

Conductance: Acids and Bases

In traditional chemistry, acids and bases are defined in hydrogen atoms—or proton proportions. An acid is typically described as a substance with an excess of hydrogen atoms ($H+$), which acts as a net proton donor. A base, on the other hand, is considered either a hydroxide ($OH-$) donor or a proton acceptor—a substance often described as having excessive electrons. Net charge is also used to describe these solutions. An acid solution is one with a net positive charge, while a base solution has a net negative charge. An acid is often referred to as *cationic* (with cations) because it has a positive net charge, while a base will have a negative charge and thus is referred to as an *anion*.

We can also describe this in the more suitable context of electromagnetic waveforms. The imbalance between units of positively oriented waveforms and units of negatively oriented waveforms creates the measure of its acidic or basic state. This "orientation" is purported to compose of quantum mechanical elements. We can summarize these as containing multi-dimensional magnetic fields with unique spin directions. As mentioned, every electronic wave is accompanied by a perpendicular magnetic field. This field also relates to the spin orientation and magnetic field direction of the molecule.

A measurement of the level of acidity or alkalinity using a logarithmic scale is called pH. The term pH is derived from the French word for hydrogen power, *pouvoir hydrogene,* which has been abbreviated as simply pH. pH is measured in an inverse log base-10 scale, measuring the proton-donor level by comparing it to a theoretical quantity of hydrogen ions (H+) in a solution. Thus, a pH of 5 would be equivalent to 10^5 H+ *moles* worth of cations in the solution. (A mole is a quantity of substance compared to 12 grams of the six-neutron carbon isotope.) Put another way, a pCl (chlorine) concentration would be the negative log of chlorine ion concentration in a solution, and pK would be the negative log of potassium ions in a solution.

The pH scale is 0 to 14, for 10^{-1} (1) to 10^{-14} (.00000000000001) range. The scale has been set up around the fact that pure water's pH is log-7 or simply pH7. Because pure water forms the basis for so many of life's activities, and because water neutralizes and dilutes so many reactions, water became the standard reference and neutral point between an acid and a base. In other words, a substance having greater hydrogen ion concentration characteristics than water will be considered a base, while a substance containing less H+ concentration characteristics than water is considered an acid.

Of course, a solution concentration may well be lower than log-14 or higher than log-1, but this is the scale set up based upon the typical ranges observed in nature. Using this scale, any substance measuring a pH of 7 would be considered a neutral substance, though it still has a significant number of H+ ions. In humans, a pH level in the range of 6.4 is considered a healthy state because this state is slightly more acidic than water, enabling alkaline ionic current flow through the body. Better put, a 6.4 pH offers the appropriate currency of energy flow because there are enough negatively oriented waveforms present for the passage of positively oriented waveforms. The earthly minerals like potassium, calcium, magnesium and others are typically positively oriented—or alkaline in nature.

The proof to these points is provided by conventional science: pH is simplified in conventional chemistry as the level of proton donor capability. Yet we know from emission measurements that the higher the electron orbit, the higher the energy emission. Energy release is measured by waveform emission characteristics such as frequency. If we remove the concept of electron particles from the equation, and replace with this the understanding of wave mechanics, we can then realize that the charge is *traveling through* a particular medium, and the pH of the substance simply quantifies the type of waveforms able to be conducted through that medium. This is why pH meters are voltage meters.

This concept of current traveling through a medium is understood when we consider how an electric charge can be maintained by a battery. A lead battery is set up to perform two reactions (stated conventionally): One reaction oxidizes lead—in a solution of sulfuric acid—to lead sulfate. During this reaction, energy is given off as electrons are emitted, along with hydrogen protons. The other reaction is a reduction, which converts lead dioxide to lead sulfate. This also releases energy, but this is accomplished as hydrogen protons and electrons are being absorbed to create the lead sulfate. Meanwhile, two types of lead plates attract and adhere to the resulting lead sulfates. The positive plates are filled with lead dioxide to drive the oxidation side, while the negative plates are made of lead to drive the reduction side of the battery. These two processes combined are called *electrolysis*—the utilization of ions to conduct current through a particular medium.

We note in this discussion the obvious: Batteries—between their positive and negative poles—exchange an electrical current. This current is used in an automobile to start the engine, after which a generator will create enough electromagnetic energy to recharge the battery. This event reverses the changes to the lead, lead dioxide and sulfuric acid. We must also note that the initial flow of electricity out of the battery is not a spontaneous reaction, nor is the recharging of the battery. Both of these processes have been designed and assembled by humans with the conscious intention to draw a flow of electricity for a specific purpose: To start our automobile for example. If our car were not in use for a while, the battery would gradually lose its charge, requiring a charge.

As we examine the currency properties of the living body, we recognize the same general features of the battery. The living body performs a number of reactions, some oxidizing and some reducing. In these reactions, energy is often converted from one type to another—a conversion of electromagnetic bonding energy into different forms of kinetic energy such as movement via muscle cells. The exact utilization of the energy is steered by consciousness, which steers usage.

For example, the principal energy conversion of glucose and oxygen into the energies mentioned is a complex oxidative reaction called the Krebs cycle. This Krebs cycle will utilize the waveform bonds of ADP to ATP to generate a transport mechanism, which results in kinetic energy, heat, and ion release. The body also has similar energy conversion mechanisms such as the NADP transport system. These are only two of the billions of ionic conversion systems working within the human physiology.

All metabolism operates on this waveform conversion process. Our sensory nerves all conduct impulses through waveform ionic exchanges. Taste is driven by the acid or alkaline nature of our foods. Acidic solutions taste sour while alkaline solutions taste bitter. As we taste food, waveform characteristics set off a chain of ionic signals through the nervous system. Our taste buds, retinal cells, olfactory bulbs and tactile nerve endings all have similar waveform sensing electrodes with ionic gateways. The different types of waveforms emitted by physical matter simply stimulate these gateways, setting off an ionic charge relay within the body's sensory nervous systems.

We know that different substances will invoke entirely different responses in the body depending upon that substance's constituents and biomolecular structures. Some biomolecules create euphoria with drug-like qualities, while some, like caffeine, increase the heartbeat and stimulate the nervous system.

The effects of these constituents are produced through their molecular interaction with the body's biochemistry. While the transmission of nerve impulses can be seen as an ionic situation—invoking principles of acid-alkaline properties, they are ultimately atomic waveform reactions processed through ionic exchanges of electrons.

These responses can be transferred directly from the biomolecule or through a medium. We can use electricity as an example. A person can be shocked by touching an electrical wire or touching a pole connected to the electrical wire. The transfer of that electricity is called conductance and the pole is called a conductor.

The world is full of conductors. The question in homeopathy is whether water is an adequate conductor for conducting the electrical information contained in homeopathic remedies that are diluted using water.

This depends. It depends upon the substance and its molecular nature, and the solutes within the water besides the water, as well as the water's container. For example, if a person was sitting in a bathtub and an electrical appliance—a conductor of electricity—was put in the water, the person would likely be electrocuted, even if the appliance didn't touch the person. Why? Because the water helped conduct the electricity.

This conductance takes place because of the ability of ions to conduct electrons. The $H+$ ions within the water, plus other ions such as $Ca+$ (calcium) and $Mg+$ (magnesium) serve to transfer electrons and their information, just as these ions serve to conduct electromagnetic information (waveforms) through the body's nervous system.

Let's discuss the pathways of electromagnetic information through the body further as we continue to prove homeopathy and why it only works sometimes.

Chapter Four
Biowave Pathways

Just as a series of waves over a pond of water can transmit the information about a rock thrown onto its surface, waves that travel through our bodies transmit information. These waveforms can be summarized as macro waves in the form of pulses of different sorts, and atomic and subatomic waves that travel through the ionic pathways of our nerves. Let's discuss both of these types of biowaves.

In other words, a heartbeat is a pulsing waveform. Sound is transmitted through waveforms. Vision is transmitted through waveforms. Sleep cycles are waveforms. Moods and hormones also utilize waveforms. Every part of our physiology is connected to pulses, cycles and waveforms large and small.

Of Waves and Men

Over the past 150 years, researchers have tried to understand the electrical nature of physiology. The electric quality of the body was hard to deny even in the early days of electricity exploration. Gradually the apparatus for this probing were refined. Though crudely applied, Dr. Hans Berger is credited to be the first researcher to use the *electroencephalogram* (or EEG) to record brainwaves in the early 1920s. These efforts gradually gave brainwave testing credibility in psychological research. Today the EEG is utilized for medical diagnostics, psychological testing, biofeedback testing and polygraph detection.

Several types of brainwaves, each with unique frequencies, were discovered using EEG testing. Further testing using the later-discovered *magnetoencephalograph* indicated that a variety of subtle magnetic pulses also pulse through the body. First used by Dr. David Cohen in 1968, the MEG picked up another dimension of magnetic polarity among waveform transmission. MEG technology was further developed using superconductors. This equipment has been referred to as *superconducting quantum interference devices* (or SQUID).

The multitude of EEG and MEG studies over the years has confirmed the existence of several major brainwave pulses, ranging from one to sixty cycles per second. Our neurons pulse with waveforms with frequency bandwidths that correspond to particular moods, stress levels, and physiological status. As we focus on the complexities of daily life, our brains reflect and emit shorter-frequency *alpha* or *beta* brainwaves. A relaxing mood tends to accompany the deeper *delta* or even the more meditative *theta* waves. The greater the stress, the higher frequencies tend to get. Just as higher-pitched sounds tend to indicate intensity or urgency, higher frequency brainwaves reflect a mind hustling to keep up with life's details. Because initial EEG and MEG research predominantly focused upon the brain, these waves were tagged as *brain*waves. Actually, we find these waves resonating throughout the body. They tend to be more predominant among the central nervous system and the brain because the brain and spinal cord tend to be the main collection foci for these waves. As will be detailed further, the central nervous system provides freeways for high-speed wave transit.

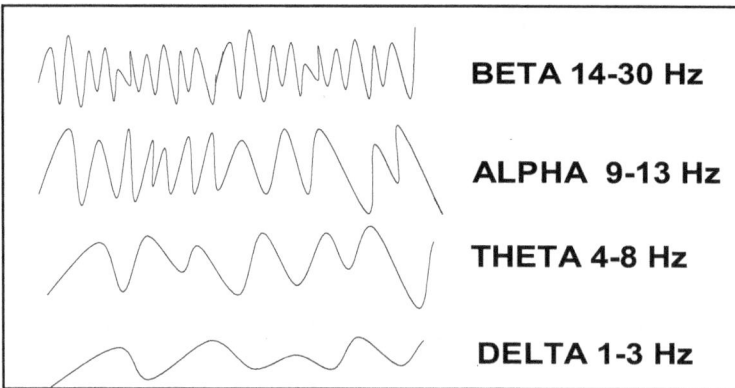

BETA 14-30 Hz

ALPHA 9-13 Hz

THETA 4-8 Hz

DELTA 1-3 Hz

Researchers have divided the millions of possible brainwave combinations into five general ranges. Alpha waves are the typical dominant cycle during dream states and light meditation. The alpha waves are oscillations with between eight and thirteen cycles per second (same as hertz). Beta brainwaves are dominant during normal waking consciousness, and range from fourteen to thirty cycles per second.

Theta waves range from four to seven cycles per second and dominate during normal sleep and meditation. On the lower frequency side are the delta waves, which range from less than one cycle per second to about three cycles per second. These slow waves tend to be dominating during the deepest sleep and meditation states.

On the other side of the spectrum, some of the fastest rhythms recorded in the brain are the gamma waves. The high-energy gamma waveforms typically dominate during periods of advanced problem solving or critical thinking. They oscillate at between thirty and sixty cycles per second. Over the past decade, researchers have discovered the existence of even shorter-wavelength and faster brainwaves. Ranging from sixty to two hundred cycles per second or more, these high-speed waves are referred to as *high gamma waves.* The high gamma waves are thought to accompany critical thought processes and brain functions.

Multiple brainwave types occur simultaneously in our body. One type will often predominate, however. Just as multiple tuning forks will align to one dominate tone, the body will typically tune— harmonically—to the predominant waveform driven from the pervading consciousness.

A recent neuroscience study—done jointly by researchers from the University of California at Berkeley and the University of California at San Francisco (Sanders *et al.* 2006)—has concluded that it is likely these brainwaves are conduits for signaling between the various regions of the brain. Dr. Robert Knight, professor of neuroscience at the University of California at Berkeley, and a director of the research observed that some regions of the brain emitted waves, others reflected waves, and still others modulated waves. Meanwhile, a confluence of these waves corresponded with particular activities, indicating different brain centers were using brainwaves as a sort of information exchange system.

As these respected researchers correlated the type of wave with the part of the brain involved in some functions and thought processes, they began to see longer-wavelength theta waves synchronizing or *coupling* with shorter-wavelength gamma waves. They considered this coupling as part of a hierarchical signaling process. Regions of coordinated neurons produce resonant coherent wave patterns, which provide the means for one group of neurons to communicate with another group. Synchronizing waveforms between neurons appear to coordinate firing patterns. The brainwave synchronization provides a process for ranking between brain regions in operational order. Theta waves appear to provide an executive control mechanism, which bridge the operations of various neuron groups.

Using epileptic subjects, the researchers found consistent relationships between cognition and the occurrence of coherent theta and gamma waves. These two types of waves provide a locked resonation process. As cognitive processes change, one wave from one region first couples with, then transitions into the next type of waveform. A congruent harmonic becomes apparent between these brainwave transitions.

Biofeedback therapy has focused on the relationship between stress and brainwave types for a number of decades. Biofeedback research has confirmed that stress directly influences brainwave activity and vice versa. Researchers have tested brainwave activity with patients in a number of different circumstances. Stressful conditions are linked to higher beta wave levels and lower alpha and theta wave levels. Consequently, a person who feels more relaxed and less stressed will produce more alpha and theta waveforms.

Many of us are aware that certain sounds influence relaxation. Most of us have experienced greater relaxation as we listen to soothing music or the songs of birds for example. Melinda Maxfield, PhD (2006) determined that slowly beating a drum at 4.5 beats per second readily brings about a state of theta brainwave activity. In 2006, Stanford University's Center for Computer Research in Music and Acoustics held a symposium with a purpose of *"interdisciplinary dialogue on the hypothesis that brainwaves entrain to rhythmic auditory stimuli, a phenomenon known as auditory driving."* This symposium brought together some of the nation's leading sound researchers. Many discussed the implications of auditory driving as it relates to our mental and physical wellbeing. The implications of the research, reflected by the consensus at the symposium, were that we are merely at the tip of the iceberg of this research.

The applications of brainwave entrainment through auditory driving are numerous. Successful auditory driving and brainwave entrainment treatments have contributed to resolving psychological trauma, chronic pain, stress, and weakened immune systems. Research comparing normal subjects with schizophrenic subjects (Vierling-Claasen *et al.* 2008) has illustrated how gamma and beta waves interface and guide cognitive processes. Normal subjects will tune to a 40 Hz wave in response to either 20 or 40 Hz driving frequencies. Schizophrenic subjects will typically respond with 20 Hz waveforms. The study's authors comment that these results illustrate *"how biophysical mechanisms can impact cognitive function."* This research confirms that brainwaves provide a mechanism for signaling specific information throughout the physical anatomy.

Biofeedback testing has further demonstrated that with practice and proper feedback access, human subjects can consciously change their brainwave levels. As a stress-reduction technique for example, a person can decrease their beta wave activity and increase their alpha and theta activity. The procedure entails the subject sitting down in front of a computer screen visually displaying rates from an electroencephalograph, photoplethysmograph (PPG—heart rate and blood flow), and/or possibly an electromyograph (EMG—muscle tension) to read waveform activity feeding back from different body parts connected to a variety of electrodes. Electrodes may be placed around the head, typically either on the scalp or in some cases around the cerebral cortex. Skin electrodes may also be applied to the arm, and PPG electrodes may be connected to the chest. The computer will monitor the waveform output of these different locations—displaying the results on a graphic display screen for the subject and therapist to monitor.

Most of us will generate brainwave signals reflecting our mental or emotional state—be it anxious, focused, relaxed, tired, angry or asleep. A good biofeedback machine will register several of these waves and their relative strengths around the body. Using a good biofeedback machine, most people can gradually learn to significantly lower or increase their alpha and theta wave strengths. For a few people, there will be an almost immediate ability to influence their waves as soon as the monitoring begins.

For most of us, it will take a bit of practice—a number of sessions usually—to be able to effectively modulate our brainwaves. Researchers have found that most everyone is able to modulate their brainwaves at one point or other. Researchers have yet to understand why there is such a variance among people's ability to control their brainwaves.

Nonetheless, once people do learn to change their brainwaves using the biofeedback, they can usually transition successfully into being able to adjust their brainwaves without the biofeedback equipment. Bringing about a relaxed mental state through visualizing relaxing situations or hearing relaxing sounds are probably the most effective techniques used for this result. Auditory driving with rhythmic sounds has been increasingly used in biofeedback therapy.

Biofeedback therapy illustrates that our brainwaves are expressions of the role of consciousness within the body. An alteration of brainwaves from primarily beta to theta waves will almost invariably result in a lower heart rate, a slower, deeper rate of breathing, and a lowering of blood pressure. Conversely, a lower heart rate, and slower breathing—as long as there is no mental disruption—will also tend to induce a theta brainwave state. We thus have an intersection between consciousness and the cascade of brainwaves with physiological states.

Physicians specializing in the central nervous system have observed another wave associated with the circulating spinal fluid: Aptly named *cerebrospinal fluid pulse waves* (or CSF waves). The data have suggested this wave is composed of five different harmonic waves, ranging in pressure from .25-1 mm Hg range, and averaging .72 mm Hg (Nakamura *et al.* 1997). This is a pressure wave. In comparison, the standard atmospheric pressure at sea level is equal to 760 mm Hg. It has not been completely ascertained as to the exact source of the CSF waves. One theory says that the pulse waves are due to the pressure gradient between arteries supplying the spinal cord and the spinal fluid. Another says they are based upon brain pulses sent through the spine's subarachnoid spaces. Many osteopaths, chiropractors, and cranial practitioners believe the cerebrospinal fluid pulses are due to the tiny movements of the cranial bones during breathing. Some research has linked breathing with these pulse waveforms. Correlations with ventricle pressure have also been made.

An interesting connection is made when CSF pulses are measured for wavelength: Beta-frequency waves seem to dominate the CSF pulse. Further EEG testing in controlled environments has demonstrated an interference relationship between the CSF pulses and the neural biowaves exhibited during memory retrieval and cognition. It seems these CSF waves play an important role in the orchestration of brainwave interference patterns.

From the research we can also understand that each cell produces a unique collection of coherent electromagnetic emissions. Because each type of cell function has been connected with different types of emissions, it is safe to say coherent emissions by groups of brain and central nervous system cells should yield resonating patterns through constructive interference. The collection of weaker emissions should yield larger biowaves, just as thousands of stadium fans may each make unique sounds, but their confluence together creates a single sound of the crowd. Most of us have heard someone mimicking the single sound of a large stadium crowd full of cheering and jeering fans.

As subtle waveforms traveling in from our sense organs interface with internal biowaves feeding back from around the body, they combine to form a compounding of interference patterns reflecting our body's inner and outer environment. This is accomplished because these biowaves interfere in different ways with each different waveform. The collection of interference patterns create a combined picture that resonates within our brain's cortices—predominated by the prefrontal cortex. The combined collection of interference patterns provides our unique perception of physical reality.

Neural Conduction

Information waveform transmissions travel from neuron to neuron as they travel through the nervous system. Neurons stretched end to end make up the nerves—and the nerves are the pipelines for neural transmission.

Waveform transmissions pass between neighboring neural cell bodies through arms called *dendrites*. The dendrites of neighboring neurons do not touch, however. Rather, between them exists a space called the *synaptic cleft* within a region called the *synapse*. This region contains a special fluid called the *neurotransmitter fluid*. The chemistry of this fluid provides the medium for the specific waveform signals that travel between neurons.

CNS neurons can range in dendrite and synapse count. Large neurons might have several thousand while others have significantly less. Through these synapses, each neuron may be firing up to 100,000 electromagnetic pulse inputs into this fluid at one time.

This tiny sea of neurotransmitter fluid contains various biochemical components, most of which are ionic in nature. These ions combine with the protein neurotransmitters to create a medium that can buffer, accelerate or malign transmissions. The overall conducting ability of the neurotransmitter fluid is considered its electromagnetic *synaptic potential*.

The neurotransmitter fluid chemistry facilitates particular waves of different frequencies, wavelengths and amplitudes. At the same time, the fluid chemistry provides filtering mechanisms to buffer and screen out some transmission elements. Depending upon its particular makeup at the time, the fluid will provide a combination of *excitatory potential* and *inhibitory potential*. This balance serves to escort or conduct waveform information from one nerve to another, while at the same time dampening or filtering these waveforms to prevent overload and over-stimulation.

This process might well be compared to the process of transistors and resistors we see in integrated circuits. Neurotransmitters are tremendous semiconductors. Their precise molecular structures allow them to buffer and/or amplify waveform transmissions within a particular spectrum.

Two examples of active neurotransmitters are acetylcholine and adrenaline (or epinephrine). These two biomolecules conduct and/ or magnify waveforms that relate to autonomic function and physical response. Acetylcholine will accelerate instructions to muscle fibers to contract, while adrenaline will amplify internal conditions that perpetuate the 'fight or flight' response: Causing a quickening of heart rate and blood flow, immediate motor muscle response, visual acuity, and so on. These two biochemicals are interactive throughout the body. They impact the functioning of digestion, the secretion of mucus, defecation, the immune system, and many other processes around the body. They occupy the neurotransmitter fluid chemistry, but they also interact with processes outside the confines of the synaptic fluid. For example, acetylcholine also stimulates skeletal muscle cells directly. This means the body's autonomic response programming is facilitated through these chemicals, much as a key might facilitate the unlocking of the front door and our passage into the house.

Neurotransmitters and hormones have similar actions in the body, and some hormones are also neurotransmitters. By definition, a neurotransmitter is released by a nerve cell into the synapse, while a hormone is produced by an endocrine gland. For example, when epinephrine is secreted by the adrenal gland, it is a hormone. When it is secreted by the synapse it is a neurotransmitter. Most hormone secretions of the body follow a chain of command. Their secretions are stimulated by other secreted conductors, produced in turn by the pituitary gland. The pituitary gland is the master gland stimulating most of the various hormones. Neurotransmitters, on the other hand, are produced through waveform-nerve reception. While hormones will stimulate a variety of responses in cells throughout the body, neurotransmitters are typically associated with the effects of the nerves.

At the same time, both hormones and neurotransmitters are waveform conductors. They both facilitate the transmission of electromagnetically-generated information from location to location around the body. The pituitary gland is considered the master gland for hormone productivity. The pituitary is about the size of a cherry. It is located behind the eyes in a depression of the sphenoid bone, just behind where the optic nerves cross. It is also lying within the region of the sixth *chakra*.

The pituitary produces master hormones that directly stimulate the body, such as growth hormone (GH), vasopressin, oxytocin and others. The pituitary gland connects to the hypothalamus by the *infudibulum,* a stalk of portal veins and nerves tracts. It is through this stalk that the pituitary gland's activities are regulated by the hypothalamus. The hypothalamus sends *releasing hormones* to the pituitary. These stimulate the releases of the pituitary.

The hormone's chemistry provides a conductor for the body's instructional signals. Hormones are in essence tiny crystals that resonate particular types of waveforms. These resonations are passed on to cells and organs by stimulating the gateways of tiny receptors that sit on the surface of cell membranes. We'll discuss this interaction between ligands and receptors in more detail shortly.

We must be careful not to confuse chemicals with waves, however. Waves are informational, and conduct *through* chemicals. Their interference patterns can be stored within biochemicals in the form of standing waves between atoms. This is why biomolecules have unique properties. Biochemicals serve primarily as echo chambers, reflecting the informational waveforms being transmitted around the body. We might compare this to hearing a radio playing a song broadcast from a distant station. The radio does not contain the song, nor is it the source of the radiowaves that are being broadcast to millions of radios from the same radio station. The radio does not contain the singer either. Rather, the radio is simply a conducting vehicle, which temporary crystallizes and transforms the radiowaves into the speaker sounds that we can hear. In the same way, biochemicals reacting throughout the body during metabolism are merely vehicles of wave conduction. Waves and their informational interference patterns are being broadcast in multiple bandwidths as they are released and move through the body.

Neurotransmitter and hormone conduction also might be compared to opening our eyes under water. Were we to dive into a river during a rain storm and attempt to open our eyes and look through its murky, muddy waters, we would not see much. We would be lucky to see our hand in front of our face underneath the muddy brown waters. That same river during a warm summer day might be so clear that we could see the bottom ten feet down. The difference between seeing within the two rivers is due to the muddy river mud being stirred up by the rain and stormy weather. It is not that our vision has gotten worse.

In the same way, an imbalanced chemistry among the neurotransmitter fluid and/or hormones within the bloodstream will alter the transmissions passing from neuron to neuron. Some chemicals will interfere in the waveform transmissions. Others will facilitate them, while still others may subdue or distort the transmissions.

Case in point: When we drink alcohol, the alcohol will affect the chemistry of the synaptic junction—the neurotransmitter fluid—in such a way that distorts the electromagnetic signals that travel from one neuron to another. This produces an altered synaptic state that affects how nerve cells control motor functions. The motor cells may receive slow or even inaccurate signals. The same ethanol neurochemistry will distort sense and feedback signals as they are sent to the brain. The distortion can cause disorientation, coordination impairment, irrational behavior and mood swings: A potentially disastrous combination we often refer to as being drunk.

The key role of the neurotransmitter is to create a potential for the electromagnetic transmission. This creates a bridge of sorts for the waveforms to transverse. The type of neurotransmitter also dictates which type of channel gateway will be opened on the post-synaptic nerve—the receiving nerve. The type of ion channel will typically dictate what kind of information will be transduced through the linkage of neurons.

One of the more interesting players in neurotransmitter biochemistry is GABA, which stands for *gamma-aminobutyric acid.* GABA is considered an inhibitory neurotransmitter in that it slightly slows down wave conduction. This actually has a positive effect upon the synaptic transmissions, allowing nerve signals to pass through without as much distortion. As a result, GABA is known for producing feelings of relaxation and alertness. Research has indicated that various mood disorders such as depression, anxiety and even insomnia are related to the body having lower GABA levels within neurotransmitter fluids. Epileptics typically have insufficient amounts of this neurotransmitter as well. Many of the popular anti-depressant pharmaceuticals increase GABA levels. It should be noted, however, that these drugs also produce various side effects as well.

Healthy amounts of GABA in the neurotransmitter fluid are also associated with an increase in alpha brainwaves. L-theanine (a GABA precursor) directly was given to thirteen subjects in one study (Abdou 2006). Electroencephalography examinations were conducted, and each subject given L-theanine had heightened levels of alpha waves and reduced beta waves. Remember that beta waves are associated with nervousness and anxiety while alpha waves accompany increased concentration.

Dr. Abdou's research also demonstrated the effect chemical neurotransmitters have upon the biocommunication of fear around the body. Two groups of eight volunteers were divided into a non-GABA (placebo) group and a GABA group. Both groups were monitored for IgA immunoglobulin levels following the crossing of a suspension bridge. Because IgA levels tend to shut down during anxious or fearful moments as the adrenal gland prepares for 'fight or flight,' this test illustrated GABA's effects upon fear-based immune response. The GABA group had normal IgA levels while the non-GABA group experienced significantly lower IgA levels. It was thus concluded that GABA levels are associated with reducing inappropriate fear responses as well as facilitating alpha waves.

As we assess this last trial, we can conclude that GABA's effect upon the neurotransmitter fluid allowed the subjects to realistically assess the dangers involved. Using the senses to realistically assess the strength of the bridge and the likelihood of the bridge actually collapsing would be considered a clear-headed response. On the other hand, a heightened fear of falling simply by looking down (acrophobia) would not be considered a realistic assessment of the situation, simply because the bridge could be easily crossed and obviously was strong enough to handle all of the walkers.

A normalized neurotransmitter environment at the synapse (including GABA) allows for a clearer broadcasting of waveform information through the neural pathways. Just as clear water allows us to see the bottom of a stream, normalized neurotransmitter fluid produces less resistance and distortion along the conducting synapses placed along the transmission pipelines of the neural network.

Tubulin Transference

During the 1970s, Dr. Stewart Hamerhoff from the University of Arizona, and Dr. Kunio Yasue and Dr. Mari Jibu from the Okayama University began researching the pathway of transmission between neural cells. One of the mysteries they probed in independent research was how anesthesia agents such as chloroform and nitrous oxide could disable the consciousness of a patient. Through their respective research, they independently discovered that conscious activity within the body had to do with a curious matrix of twisted spiral filaments they called *tubulins*. These tubulins are arranged into networked pathways that wind through the neural cells in three-dimensional protein spirals called *microtubules*. The research showed that these microtubules are conducting tracts for electromagnetic transmission. Microtubules make up a previously unseen network for subtle waveform biocommunication throughout the neural net (Hameroff 1974; Hameroff 1982; Hameroff *et al.* 1984; Hameroff 1987; Hameroff and Penrose 1996).

The nerve tracts are pathways for lower-frequency reflexive biowaves, while the microtubules broadcast higher-frequency, complex information waves. As the larger waveforms are processed and transmitted through dendrites, they conduct through the neurotransmitters between the synapses. As they are conducted through this medium, the waveforms meet with other waveforms traveling within the neural network. This convergence creates coherent interference patterns. The resonating results of these interference patterns are 'stepped up' to higher frequencies. These high frequency waveforms contain more information, and they create holographic wave patterns. These hologram patterns are ultimately reflected (or mirrored) onto the 'screens' of the cortices. Once on the screens, these holograms interact with others to create a organized view of the body and the world around us. The inner self interacts with these cortices through the frontal cortex and pre-frontal cortex to view this holographic 'picture.'

Within these microtubules also travel the various subtle biowaves that conduct the emotional responses of the self through the body. The discovery of these microtubule pathways confirms much of the ancient wisdom of the *nadis* and *meridians,* which we will discuss later in detail. The ancients described these channels as pathways for the flow of living energy.

We might compare the microtubular process of projecting wave interference patterns onto the mind to the recording of a musical composition in a modern studio. The studio producer will record the guitar onto one track, the piano onto another track, the drums onto another and the voice onto another track. The producer may even overlay background singers' voices onto other tracks. Then using these various individual sounds, the producer will assemble all the tracks together at particular sound levels to form the entire piece of music. This is often referred to as a *composition*. Each track makes up a piece of the total song. To listen to each track alone without the other tracks will sound weird. In much the same way, the mind captures the various waveform frequencies coming through the microtubular network, neural net and biochemical conducting system—combining them to form unified holographic images of the outside world.

One of the basic principles of holography is that each part mirrors the entire image. This is accomplished through a splitting of waves as they interfere, creating a multitude of waves, each containing all the information via the composition of waveforms. Using waveform interference, the mind orchestrates holographic assembly in both directions. The mind reflects its images semiconducted through particular neurons. The mind also stimulates effector neurons to act reflectively by transmitting the emotional responses of the self.

Each cortex assembles biowaves from different locations. The mind projects the whole image, drawn from the various cortex images. This collection of images is broadcast through crystallized neuron pathways. Each cortex consists of a grouping of crystalline neurons with common genetic structures, ion channel systems and microtubule networks. This gives each cortex the ability to combine with others to create an broader waveform interference pattern.

Cell Reception

Otto Loewi's research illustrated the involvement of biochemistry with metabolic signaling mechanisms. Biochemical information pathways have since been clearly established. Different biochemicals conduct different waveforms because of their unique subatomic bonding orbitals. These orbitals (or energy states) are either excited or stabilized by waveforms being conducted through their medium.

Ever since Dr. Morgan Hunt discovered a protein existing within the cell membrane—part in and part out, researchers have been convinced that inter-cell signaling requires that a ligand (e.g., hormone or neurotransmitter) must "physically" touch a receptor.

Receptors are cell membrane switches understood to receive ligand instructions. Once received, the instructions are translated to the cell's nucleus and/or organelles for activation. For this reason, they've been called *transmembrane protein receptors.*

Dr. Hunt's protein ligand system was called the *notch* transport system. Notch information biocommunication has since been observed among cardiac cells, neurons, bone cells (osteocytes), glandular cells and many others, progressing and stimulating some of their most critical functions.

Intercellular communication is often referred to as *paracrine* activity—signals being translated from one nearby cell to another. In comparison, *intracrines* are considered the cellular conductors within the cell, while *intercrines* are cell-to-cell conductors. Note in this respect that *endocrines* are biochemical conductors produced by specific glands, which are circulated around the body. The question is whether conduction requires a "physical" chemical binding between the ligand and its particular receptor.

Two cells are also thought to have what is considered a direct nucleus-to-nucleus interaction. This occurs through a type of direct-nucleus receptor called a *connexin protein.* When six of these proteins come together within a group, they form a pore or tube within the membrane called a *gap junction.* This allows cells to exchange genetic instructions, or one cell to inject instructions into another cell.

Many receptors lie on the surface of the cell membrane. Most are connected to ion channels between the cell membrane. These provide a transduction channel for the information to pass from the receptor to within the cell. Many neurotransmitters and hormones utilize this pathway to transmit their information. The assumption is that the ligand (hormone or neurotransmitter) *binds* with the receptor on a chemical basis, creating an electrical signal, which is transmitted through the ion channel.

These assumptions come from seeing ligands in the area of physical responses. Since they are in the vicinity, they must be involved in a binding reaction, right? It has been justly assumed that these neurochemical molecules must be intimately involved in the dissemination of metabolic signals. However, the notion that a chemical binding is required in all cases and among all endocrine transmissions appears unlikely, given the evidence we will present here.

A physical molecular connection between hormones and receptors on each and every cell membrane—even with some cells communicating with paracrines—would require circulation time for the master hypothalamic hormones, pituitary hormones and endocrine gland hormone pathways to execute simultaneously. It would require enough hormones to be secreted fully into the bloodstream, and physically be pumped from the endocrine glands—sometimes halfway around the body—to chemically and physically touch the appropriate receptor on *every* cell involved in the metabolic change.

Let us consider this scenario carefully. A receptor is a protein with an electromagnetic affinity. This requires either a polarity match, or even a constructive combination of spin or angular momentum between the ligand and receptor. In the human body, it is estimated there is one protein molecule for every 10,000 molecules in and around the cells of the body. Furthermore, there are about 200 trillion cells in the human body, and billions if not trillions of them are activated immediately in fearful or stressful response. Every cell in the toes must be activated immediately to break into an immediate run for example. According to the physical ligand-receptor theory, not only does each hormone molecule have to connect with each and every cell membrane, but each hormone must also locate an open, active receptor on every cell membrane.

Observation and *in vitro* testing has shown receptors to have four basic scenarios: They can be *agonized,* or stimulated. They can be *partially agonized* of partly stimulated. They can be *inversely agonized,* and their response lowered. They can also be *antagonized*, whereby they are blocked by a molecule and thereby not be stimulated. So we ask: How is it these hormones can intelligently weave through every tiny capillary and dense maze of tissue systems to bump into the right receptor on every needed cell instantaneously?

Now if we perceived parts of our body being activated first and then other parts, corresponding to the circulatory routes these hormones or neurotransmitters take, we might be able to agree with this hypothesis. Consider circulatory restrictions such as atherosclerosis and other artery diseases restricting blood flow. In addition, consider that many tissue cells are reached only through tiny microcapillaries—some barely large enough to be able to allow a single red blood cell through at a time within the diameter of the lumen (the opening). If a response required the blood to deliver a hormone molecule to a receptor on every cell within a particular tissue system before that tissue system could respond, we would really be in trouble if we needed to run from an attacker.

We could only imagine the situation where we were frightened by a tiger in the woods, only to find that our upper hamstrings were ready to take off but our toes were not—leaving us stuck while the tiger pounced. Rather, the toes, hamstrings, knees and every skeletal muscle cell, along with the eyes, lungs, brain, and vocal cords all respond at the same moment as we scream and run instantaneously.

The body's process of stimulating metabolic activity has been a mystery to researchers for thousands of years. In modern research, the process of discovery has been to identify hormone presence using radiography with dye markers to trace the flow of chemicals. This physical 'snap-shot' process is combined with harvesting and analyzing organ chemistry with spectroscopic analysis. Via these two methods, researchers figure that since the hormone/ligands are in the proximity of the response, they must be physically setting off the response of each and every cell. This is often confirmed with the techniques pioneered by Loewi to provide the conclusion. While conferring biochemical presence, finding biochemicals in the region offers no conclusive mechanism. We might compare this to finding a gun near a murder victim. We can assume the gun was involved, but this fact alone does not tell us who shot the murder victim.

For example, we know the thyroid gland is one of the central endocrine drivers of metabolism. Researchers have linked cellular metabolic rates and thermogenesis to the presence of thyroid hormones thyroxine and triiodothyronine. These are also referred to as T4 and T3, respectively. The chemical makeup of these conductors are not that exciting—a combination of the amino acid tyrosine and iodine. However, these rather simple molecular structures T4 and T3 somehow charge trillions of cells throughout the body—increasing the speed and output of their various metabolic processes. Without enough of either T4 or T3 (T3 is considered to be the more active of the two, but T3 is derived from T4) the body begins to cool down. A feeling of fatigue will overwhelm a thyroid hormone-deficient body. Suddenly the most basic tasks become difficult in TSH (thyroid stimulating hormone), T3 or T4 deficiencies. The thyroid also produces calcitonin, which works with parathyroid hormone to balance bone calcium levels.

Once the blood contains enough thyroid hormones, the body becomes almost suddenly energized. This is evidenced by the oral intake of synthetic and analogous thyroid hormones. How again do all those trillions of cells become energized from a pill or two? Again, the theory of cell reception requires that each cell has a set of little chemical receptor 'locks' on its cell membrane, and these ligand chemicals provide the 'keys.' Thus, each cell receptor must be physically touched and unlocked with those chemical ligands. Are there enough moles of chemicals in one or two pills to circulate through the blood system and basal membrane to reach every cell's receptors and energize them? Or perhaps the paracrine system provides a mechanism for filling the gap for cells the chemicals do not physically bind to?

This problem is complicated by the fact that thyroid hormones are hydrophobic—they are not water-friendly. They are not water-soluble. Since the blood, the cells, and their basal surroundings are mostly water, this makes their journey to every cell difficult. Perhaps thyroid hormones require thyroxine-binding globulins, transthyrein and albumins for adequate circulation. It is thought that these may provide a carrier mechanism to each cell. Somehow, these chemical conductors T3 and T4 manage to instantly and simultaneously make their way around the body to stimulate and energize each cell. In other words, the neck does not warm up first, and then the arms warm up, and so on. All the body parts will become energized simultaneously with some exception for diseased tissue systems.

The cell membrane is composed of a variety of lipids—cholesterol, phospholipids and sphingolipids—specialized proteins and glycoproteins. The lipids making up most cell membranes are structurally double-layered and arranged to prevent unwanted molecules from passing through the membrane. The lipid wall is also hydrophobic—keeping water from penetrating the surface without passing through the cell membrane's complex ion channels.

Some cell membranes—particularly in nerve cells—are *myelin*. Others are *inner mitochondrial* in nature. Mitochondrial inner membranes are made up of electron transport proteins, while a myelin membrane will be composed primarily of plasma with less protein. The lipid cell membrane is negatively charged. This sets up an ionic gradient between the inside and the outside of the cell membrane. Crossing the cell membrane is not a physical experience for most molecules—it is primarily an electromagnetic crossing.

Water and nutrients are escorted through the membrane through ionic diffusion. This is complicated by the various proteins that electromagnetically identify substances as they pass. Mineral ions pass through the cell membrane via *ionic transport chains*. Ionic transport chains made from protein are similar to ion channels except they allow entry to key nutrients and minerals needed in the cell—particularly sodium, potassium and calcium but also many trace elements.

These ions provide just the right electromagnetic environment to set up channels for ionic instructional signals to pass through the cell membrane into the cytoplasm, where they can stimulate RNA, mitochondria and other organelles into action. Thus, the cell membrane's ionic transport mechanisms escort appropriate nutrients in and out of cell, while receptors receive and transmit the signals of hormones like thyroid hormones, insulin, and acetylcholine through ion channels into the cell.

Some might contend that some biochemical conductors are delivered through tissue spaces and ion channels. Yes, certainly there are basal channels that provide access. Still we must remember that the adrenal gland is a very small gland in the abdominal region of the body. The thyroid gland is a tiny gland in the neck. To assume that cortisol, epinephrine, acetylcholine, and thyroid hormones must jettison from these tiny organs to every cell—even in fingers and toes—to stimulate the correct cellular and tissue responses should these appendages come under attack is a stretch. Certainly, a strictly physical chemical delivery system would result in a lot more missing fingers and toes than we generally see.

It is interesting that we can accept that informational signals can travel instantly throughout the body via the nervous system. The nervous system can stimulate a particular skeletal muscle system to activate instantly. The ability of all the support systems to come into play, however, is the result of these biochemical informational messenger systems. A perfect example is vasopressin's ability to concentrate urine in the kidneys and constrict artery walls.

Environmental drivers of hormones include light, temperature, gravity, the changing seasons, and cellular metabolism. Internal drivers, however, stem from emotional consciousness. Hormones are complex body chemicals, made of either glycoproteins or steroids. Among other functions, hormones turn on cellular switches for many metabolic functions:

Growth hormones encourage cellular growth. Thyroid hormones regulate cellular metabolism speed and temperature regulation. Follicle stimulating hormones and luteinizing hormones stimulate reproductive mechanisms. Insulin stimulates the clearing and attachment of glucose into cells for energy production. Vasopressin decreases urine volume, constricts blood vessel walls and stimulates certain memory functions. Cortisol counteracts insulin, inhibits immune system processes such as inflammation and lymphocyte function, stimulates increased circulation and blood pressure, helps regulate potassium/sodium balance, stimulates stomach acids, and increases glucogenesis to name a few.

These are just a few of the hundreds of signaling hormones that make up the complex waveform broadcasting system working within the body. Hormones are directly and indirectly involved guiding all of the physical body's various mechanisms. Hormones turn on and shut off genetic switches in particular cells, typically through stimulating the transmembrane receptors. Hormones work primarily within pathways often referred to as *cascades.* As in the 'domino-effect,' a cascade is the progressive stimulation of one activity, which in turn stimulates another. These cascades fire at tremendous speeds, as ligand-receptor triggers initiate pathways of stimulating mechanisms.

An example of a cascading signaling system is the emotional response to feedback received from the sensory system and transmitted through the neurons to the brain. The pre-programmed sympathetic response (the reflex arc) is typically accompanied by conscious reception of the sensation via the limbic system. The focal point of this stimulation is the thalamus, which acts as a waveform signal translator and decoder. Waveform-transmitting neurons deep within the thalamus are engaged, stimulating waves that combine with others to form an interference pattern—also referred to as a neural mapping. As these waveform interference patterns are decoded, some are reflected back to the cerebral cortex.

Here an exchange of waveform patterns takes place. A relay of information is conducted between the cerebral cortex and the thalamus, reflecting the information back onto the prefrontal cortex. The information is responded to, followed by a return of pulses that stimulate the hypothalamus gland to secrete biochemicals. These biochemical conductors either stimulate endocrine or cellular function directly, or stimulate the pituitary gland to in turn secrete biochemical conductors that precisely activate endocrine glands and physical response.

The hypothalamus, located at the base of the brain under the thalamus, encapsulates part of the third ventricle. The body's autonomic responses are processed here, some of which stimulate the pituitary gland to release key master hormones. These master hormones signal responses that control the critical phase cycles of metabolism, body core temperature, appetite, thirst and so on.

The hypothalamus responds to waveform inputs from the brain centers and limbic system. These brain centers provide the platforms for conscious interaction with waveform signaling. Waveform interference patterns are created from the various sensory nerve transmissions and response neurotransmitter biochemicals. These interactive interference patterns form the basis for information. This facilitates perspective, and allows a sorting process to prioritize the information within the limbic system. Stresses on the body such as infection and immune response also feed into the limbic system for response. For these waveforms, the hypothalamus activates immediate response cascades using the limbic system's programming.

The hypothalamus and limbic system thus respond to a wide range of stimuli, and construct biochemical responses by activating an orchestrated flow of biochemical conductors to stimulate particular physical responses around the body. Dispatched conductors include dopamine, melatonin, somatostatin and others.

The hypothalamic hormones are sent through the hypophyseal capillary beds before they are delivered to the pituitary gland. Once arriving at the pituitary, these biochemical conductors instruct the pituitary gland to secrete specific 'master' hormones. These in turn stimulate particular endocrine glands around the body to produce yet another level of biochemical conductors. These instructional biochemicals include growth hormones, adrenocorticotropic hormones, luteinizing hormones, follicle-stimulating hormones, prolactins, estrogens, testosterone, thyroid stimulating hormones; as well as neurotransmitter-hormones like adrenaline, serotonin, acetylcholine and others.

Amazingly, the subsidiary endocrine glands and tissue centers receive the master hormone signals, and react instantly by initiating the release of even more specific informational biochemical conductors. These are hormones that precisely and directly affect the body's cellular metabolism, organ function and tissue mechanisms. As we all have experienced, the signals stimulate action at tremendous speeds—perhaps at speeds at or above the speed of light. So not only does the limbic system and master glands respond instantly to sensory stimuli, but the entire cascading system responds instantaneously with biochemical messenger cascades that broadcast precise instructions throughout our body's physiology.

Adrenocorticotropic hormone or ACTH is a good example. ACTH is produced by the anterior pituitary gland. Its function is to stimulate the adrenal cortex to release cortisol, and to a lesser degree androgens such as testosterone. The adrenal cortex also produces aldosterone, which stimulates the retention of urine and heightened blood pressure, involved in the renin/angiotensin cycle. The adrenal medulla is also stimulated by sympathetic nerves into producing epinephrine and norepinephrine. Epinephrine is considered a fight-or-flight hormone because it stimulates glycogen and fat breakdown while increasing the heart rate. It dilates the pupils and stimulates awareness. Epinephrine also constricts some blood vessels while dilating others. A gated pathway through the liver using inositol and liver enzymes activates glucose release to help coordinate this. Epinephrine's selective combination of constriction in particular blood vessels effectively diverts blood and nutrients from unnecessary tissues to those deemed necessary for a well-coordinated fight-or-flight response. How does a chemical—a combination of hydrogen, carbon, oxygen and nitrogen—produce this sort of complex selectivity? How does it select which way to divert circulation? How does it know which muscles will be needed? Can a simple chemical structure make these sorts of selections—instantly?

Medical researchers believe this is driven by epinephrine's ability to stimulate multiple receptors, most notably the alpha-1 and beta-2 receptors. The alpha-1 tends to stimulate a liver signaling process affecting insulin, while the beta-2 tends to stimulate the process of converting glycogen to glucose. However, this simplistic version of the process can hardly explain how this hormone can instantly gear the body up for fight or flight mode while concurrently coordinating which tissue groups are fed and which tissue groups are starved.

The pituitary gland also produces follicle-stimulating hormone, which stimulates the ovarian follicle to produce estrogen in women. It also stimulates the testes to produce sperm in men. Estrogens are complex because they will assist in the development of female sex organs and female characteristics like breasts, while they also stimulate the uterine environment by expanding the endometrium at the early part of the menstrual cycle. Indeed, the rhythmic cycles of menstruation and ovulation, and of pre- peri- and post-menopause tell us that estrogens also have complex signaling pathways within various tissue mechanisms—some significantly affecting moods and nerve activity. Testosterone is also complex, as its levels relate not just to prostate health in men, but also to general vitality and overall health among both men and women.

Although modern medical science has assumed a physical proximity particle-molecule receptor binding mechanism for hormone effects within the body, it is a rather academic debate because at the same time, science is thoroughly aware that there is no touching within the subatomic atmosphere of atoms and molecules. Quantum mechanics and the law of uncertainty tell us that subatomic units are particle-waves, which rotate around the nucleus at dramatic relative distances. As atoms merge to become molecules, a sharing of particle-wave orbitals takes place. These orbitals do not have the ability to come into physical contact with each other within the molecule. So even in the paradigm of a ligand bonding with physical proximity to a receptor to create a new molecule, there is only a sharing of electromagnetic energy states (orbitals) involved, which are of course waveform in nature.

Logically, while we can say that close proximity orbital binding can and does occur with some signaling, the nature of the electromagnetic exchange of information logically should not require physical proximity to transfer the signal. We might compare this with two people standing next to each other exchanging information. They conduct this exchange through speaking. The nature of speaking is such that the two people could easily stand further away from each other and still exchange the information through speaking. They may have to speak a little louder, but the passing of the information would suffer no deficiency between standing next to each other and standing several feet apart.

The biochemical signaling process comes without the merit of observation, albeit indirect. Scientists cannot open up a human intercellular process and analyze the process to determine the exact mode of biocommunication. However, lab researchers can isolate a complex metabolic process requiring a signaling event, and run a chemical analysis on the whole region to see what chemical changes occurred. Before and after chemical analyses (typically via centrifuge followed by mass spectrometry, or possibly electron microscope) will illustrate a chemical change within the region. A change in the composition would infer that the biocommunication coincided with the ligand-receptor exchange. However, this does require an initial assumption that the biocommunication process is indeed biochemical-driven.

We cannot deny confirmed research indicating that chemical reactions in some cases coincide with biocommunication. The question that arises, however, is whether the chemical reaction causes the biocommunication event or the biocommunication event causes the chemical reaction? It is altogether possible that one of the byproducts of the biocommunication transmission was a chemical reaction. Chemical changes often coincide with waveform transmissions. The microwaving of food will likely create a chemical change in the food, for example. The sun's rays often spark composition reactions in soil and water as well. In fact, most electromagnetic waveform transmissions result in chemical reactions of some sort, because the waveforms interfere with the electromagnetic bonds within molecules of the substance being struck, creating a chemical response.

This basic question of which comes first might be compared to seeing some blood in a hungry shark's tank and assuming the blood made the shark hungry. It is quite possible (and probably more likely) that the shark was hungry before the water was bloody. It is more likely that the shark's hunger drove him to eat, making the tank bloody from the fish he ate. This is also logical, noting shark behavior.

This is not such a fantastic supposition. Every type of communication signal we receive externally is transmitted via waveforms. The most basic signaling event, vision, is produced via an electromagnetic reception of the visible spectrum. When we look at a star billions of light years away, we are seeing waveform transmissions that may have traveled for several days or even years before reaching our eyes. Hearing is also a waveform-stimulated process, as our inner ears convert air pressure waves to electromagnetic pulses. If the body conducts its most basic communication events via waveform signaling, why should we assume cells should not share those capabilities? Do we feel our cells are any less technical than the rest of our bodies?

This does not necessitate us completely abandoning the *lock-and-key* mechanisms theorized between ligands and receptors. Waveform communications can also be compared to a lock-and-key mechanism. The concept of the receptor simply has to be expanded to include waveform communications. It is also altogether possible that ligands can stimulate biocommunication through the lock-an-key biochemical basis in addition to remote biocommunication signaling.

We might justly compare this mechanism with our ability to turn on and off a television. We can either walk up to the television and turn it off by pressing the on-off button "manually," or we can use the remote control to achieve the same purpose. In the same way, hormones may make biochemical contract or utilize waveform transmissions to stimulate receptors. Furthermore, just as we can walk around our living room with our remote and control our television volume and channel, hormone-signaling molecules can move around the body and stimulate multiple cells into action simultaneously. Just as we are more assured of accurate channel changing when our remote is within close proximity of the television, the body is assured of more accurate responses among the cells when the signaling hormones are within close proximity of the cells and their receptors. It is for this reason that conductors are dispatched. Information exchange can begin instantly using radio signaling between these ligands and their receptors.

It is this information exchange through which diluted electromagnetic informational waveforms can be conducted, reaching the most intrinsic parts of our body: the cells.

Extroverted Waves

These mechanisms were proven by over two decades of research headed up by Jacques Benveniste, M.D. and several other research teams. Dr. Benveniste was one of the foremost experts in the study of ligand-receptor mechanisms within the immune system for many years. He was the research director for the French National Institute for Health and Medical Research (INSERM) for a number of years. Dr. Benveniste's career was very distinguished. Several years earlier, he was credited with the discovery of the platelet-activating factor.

It was during his rigorous immune system research on the action of basophils that Dr. Benveniste and his research technician Elisabeth Davenas accidentally discovered that an allergic response in solution took place even though the tested allergen was effectively diluted out of the solution. Because the allergen was responded to without an apparent molecular basis (as the substance was diluted out), Dr. Benveniste began a search for what actually caused the immune response.

This discovery led to a four-year study on the immunoglobulin IgE response. The research included joint trials and confirmations with five laboratories in four countries. The combined studies using independent laboratory teams concluded that even at dilutions of 10^{120} (one part to ten parts with one hundred and twenty zeros behind it), and no probability of available molecules, the same immunoglobulin immune responses would occur as with significant concentrations. After confirming this variously, Dr. Benveniste and his team proposed that water somehow acts as a carrier for immune system signal transmission.

After eliminating alternative causes for transmission conduction, Dr. Benveniste and his research associates began to focus on the potential for a radio signaling process of some type. After much experimentation, the right technology and equipment led to the understanding that cells respond to low-frequency electromagnetic waves. Remarkably, certain biochemical conductors like acetylcholine produce unique electromagnetic waveforms. The question was now whether these waveforms played a role in the immunoglobulin communication.

Dr. Benveniste eventually developed sensitive audio equipment to record the frequencies of these biochemicals. In the early 1990s, using his digital sound equipment with computerized technology, Benveniste and his associates recorded thousands of these low-frequency waves from various biochemicals. Amazingly, by playing back these recordings in the midst of cells and tissues, the recorded frequencies were able to stimulate the exact same responses the biochemicals had stimulated. After several years of testing, Benveniste and his associates built up quite a library of biochemical waveform recordings. Frequencies of established biochemical conductors such as heparin, ovalbumin, acetylcholine and dextran were digitized and recorded. Unbelievably, these digital recording files were then put on CD and mailed—or even emailed—to other labs. The other lab would play back the recordings onto various cell tissues—producing the same responses that the physical biochemicals stimulated within the tissues!

This proposition more accurately fits with the body's ability to bridge consciousness with external stimuli. An advanced signaling process using low- and extra-low frequency electromagnetic radiation creates a signaling system to elicit instantaneous responses simultaneously from billions of cells, just as radio broadcasts will bridge a single radio disc jockey with millions of remote listeners simultaneously.

This model also supports the observation of some ligands coming into close proximity with cells in certain regions. These ligands may require close proximity to their receptors in order to elicit a response. Others, however, are designed to elicit responses from further distances. This might again be compared to the radio-to-radiofrequencies used for communications. A CB-band, walkie-talkie system, remote telephone, or television remote may have a relatively short range of reception, depending upon the power of the signal. Therefore, remote telephones that transmit with greater power can be used at greater distances. Radio station broadcasting is also based upon the strength of the waveform signals. For this reason, some radio stations can be heard at much greater distances than others can. In contrast, other radiofrequencies, such as shortwave or ham radios, can transmit over thousands of miles, even at lower power.

We can apply this same signal strength issue to the intracellular biocommunication process. Different hormones or ligands within the body have different purposes. Therefore, they each broadcast with different signal strengths, and at different frequencies. Just as we choose different types of communication devices for different communication priorities, the type of electromagnetic conductor and signal strength used in the body would relate to the need and timing required.

Consider for example our use of modern communications. For some communications, we are likely to use email. For these, we will not usually expect a response for several hours or even days. In a more urgent situation, however, we will likely pick up the phone and call the other person. In this case, we are looking for a more immediate response.

As we examine signaling broadcasting and reception within the body, the cell's transmembrane receptors must *resonate* with the particular frequency emitted by the ligand. This follows the logic of any radio broadcast. Radios utilize not only a receiver but also a tuner, so the radio can synchronize with the broadcast's frequency. This is also a form of resonation. As we turn the tuner on a radio to find the right station, we are locating a point where the radio's receiver is resonating with the waveforms of the broadcasting station's signals. This process was developed using the radio crystal to receive and semiconduct particular waveforms into particular electronic pulses. In the case of the body, the crystals being used for semiconducting are the biochemical structures of hormones and neurotransmitters.

Arranged to these crystalline-like structures are programmed waveform signals being broadcast through the channel pathways of synapses and receptors. As we trace this programming process back further, we find the various brain cortices like the prefrontal cortex at the apex of these arcs—at the seat of consciousness. We might compare this to a song we hear playing on the radio being traced back to a particular radio station broadcast, and eventually back to the musician who originally wrote and performed the song.

Indeed, when we consider every response and movement within the physical body, we are seeing a relayed broadcasting process. These broadcasting pathways stimulate physical activity through the network of endocrine glands, the bloodstream, the nervous system, the basal membranes, transmembrane receptors and of course an army of semiconducting hormones and neurotransmitters. Every beat of our heart and every hunger pang or skeletal muscle twitch is the result of one of these conducted signaling processes. Waveform broadcasts relay information from one biochemical conductor to another. We can thus compare the transmembrane protein receptors to antennae, the neurotransmitter/hormone broadcasting systems to radio stations, and the paracrine and microtubule systems to integrated circuitry.

Biochemical conductors are not dumbwaiters. They each have

unique informational fingerprinting and translation processes. They translate signals specific to the particular body and situation. In other words, each signal is unique to a circumstance, emotion, event, personality, fear, and so on. A person injected with hormones from a donor might have a physiological response generic to that hormone, but the specific signal-response being carried through the donor's hormones will not be translated specifically through the body of the recipient. The signal is the specific information that stimulate particular muscles, dilate particular arteries, and so on. We can test this by injecting epinephrine donated from one person into another person. The injected person's tissues might still be stimulated in a non-specific way, depending upon the location of the injection and the physical state of the injected subject. However, the injection will not stimulate the precise emotional response occurring in the body and person the hormones were extracted from. This is observable. The injected person simply will not engage in the exact same physiological responses.

The injection of vaccines has the same affect. Each body receiving the injection will respond slightly differently to the vaccine. The injection will stimulate to different degrees, the body's own immunoglobulins to fight the same antigen. Furthermore, none of the responses will match the response of the organism source of the vaccine.

Consider for a moment the translation of a United Nations speech given by a foreign diplomat into a number of foreign languages concurrently. The translating technology (and/or live interpreters) works to translate each word and each phrase from the speaker's language into these other languages. This allows each UN representative the opportunity to hear the speech in his or her native language simultaneously. It was simply translated in real-time into their respective languages.

As a particular waveform is sent via one part of the body to another, the signal is also being translated in real-time into the various functions necessary for the body. When the hypothalamus sends hormonal signals to the pituitary, they are encoded with the needed response for that event. They are also accompanied by brainwave and nerve cell signaling for additional support information. The pituitary translates this combined signal into a multitude of responses to each part of the body. These are broadcast out for processing to each endocrine gland through secreted hormones. Each endocrine organ receives this translated signal, and each one of these organs translates the signal into more specific biochemical signals in the form of hormones.

This broadcasting and translation system is specific and intelligent. If the translation system at the United Nations incorrectly translated any of the words spoken by the speaker, the speech could be grossly misinterpreted. This could be dangerous. It could theoretically start a war. Therefore, the speech must be translated using an intelligent and impartial translating system.

The signals sent through the endocrine system must also be intelligent. Imagine our endocrine system sending out the same signal regardless of whether we were being chased by a tiger, or were in danger of a head-on car collision. We simply could not react to these two situations with an identical physiological response.

Specific and complex signals are being broadcast from the intelligent centers of the neural network, whether on a purely sympathetic process or autonomic bandwidth. These signals travel within biowaves just as our radio and television communications travel within broadcast radiowaves. The body's waveform broadcasts utilize crystallized amplification mechanisms called hormones to set the stage for the response. Each endocrine organ—or relay station—receives the signals and translates them into a more specific waveform broadcast. This more specific broadcast is meant to stimulate activity with increased specificity for a particular organ or tissue system. As the signal is translated at the endocrine organ, it is broadcast throughout the body, using the hormone molecule-crystals to regulate, amplify, boost or even restrict the signal in some way. This enables a transmission to resonate with and appropriately instruct specific cells or tissue systems.

The use of these receptors and ligands are quite analogous to the functions of semiconductors and resisters among electrical circuits. Resistors and semiconductors—depending upon their positioning and makeup—will slow, redirect and in general modulate the flow of electrical pulses while providing an insulation process. This dampening affect allows the semiconductor or resistor to prevent the pulse from overloading the appliance or shocking its user.

The signaling biochemicals of the body—the hormones and neurotransmitters—must damper, modulate and sometimes even reverse the instructional flow in order for the signals to be properly and precisely engaged. We want to *just* outrun the tiger without killing the body with a heart attack, for example.

The broadcast signals of these relayed signals come with a *continuous flow* of waveform sequences. This continuous flow allows the same semiconductors to broadcast a response to a changing situation. For example, we might need to increase our running speed to stay in front of the tiger. This changing need is translated through the same semiconductors. The endocrine system does not produce one type of epinephrine molecule for five miles an hour, and another type for 10 miles an hour. The same molecule is used, but the biowaves being conduced *through* those molecules change in response to the changing situation.

These biowaves resonate with specialized receptors on the cell membranes. The receptors on the cell membranes then *translate* and *reflect* those continuous signals though the cytoplasm to mitochondria, RNA, and other organelles of the cell, depending upon the signal. These biowaves impart *specific* instructions to stimulate or modulate certain activities. These instructions serve to coordinate each cell's metabolic activity with the needs of the situation and the needs of the rest of the body.

In the case of T3, the information is sent to the cell's ribosomes— responsible for increasing the rate of ATP transport chain processing—which directly increases the metabolic processes. In the case of insulin, the signaling initiates the preparation of micropores to absorb glucose for energy use, together with a stimulation of mitochondria. This will also be signaled to other cells—such as liver cells that convert glycogen and adipose cells to store up fatty acids from glycogen.

The receptors on the cell membranes are the smart receivers for this intelligent signaling system. It might be comparable to having a satellite dish set up on a house. The dish is designed to pick up particular signals from particular satellites, and not others. The size of the dish and its positioning is established to pick up the specific waveforms emitting from that particular satellite. In the same way, particular receptors on the cell membrane are tuned to particular waveform signals sent from specific biochemicals. Whether those biochemicals are in close proximity or at a distance, their reception can be instantaneous.

Biophoton Information

Molecular homeopathic information transference ultimately involves pulses that are not only waveforms—they are akin to light. Biophotons, in fact.

In 1958, Harvard's Dr. Woody Hastings and Dr. Paul Mangelsdorf illustrated how the marine species *Gonyaulax polyedra* (now named *Lingulodinium polyedrum*) lit up the night's ocean timed to the sun's path. Exposing the tiny plant to various light pulses at different times, Dr. Hastings concluded that some internal biological mechanism within the organism must be responding to the sun, switching on and off its illuminating appearance and quite possibly reflecting the sun's light. Over the next decade, various other organisms—including humans—were observed for their biological response to light.

This research began a focused hunt to corner the body's biological connection to light. Researchers assumed that plants and animals possessed cell-switching mechanisms sensitive to light.

In 1972, University of Chicago professor and researcher Dr. Robert

Moore discovered the existence of two small clusters of neurons deep within the hypothalamus. These pinhead-sized clusters of about 10,000 nerve cells were named *suprachiasmatic nuclei* (or SCN) cells. It was discovered that SCN cells are implicated in the body's response to light along with the body's biological clock.

Over the next few years, Dr. Moore, together with Dr. Nicholas Lenn and Dr. Bruce Beebe, confirmed that the body's SCN cells responded specifically to the reception of electromagnetic radiation in the visible part of the spectrum. SCN cells were found to be the conducting means that initiated the body's responses to the rhythms of the sun and the passage of light within the retina and optic nerve (Lenn *et al.* 1977).

For the next two decades, Dr. Moore and many other researchers, including Dr. Charles Weitz, Dr. David Welsch, and Dr. Eric Herzog, investigated these SCN cells. They found that without the SCN cells' synchronization to the sun, an animal's body rhythms would collapse into chaotic patterns.

Initially, SCN cells were observed within the hypothalamus. This rendered the assumption that the body's clock was located within the hypothalamus as well. Furthermore, SCN cells connect the hypothalamus with the activities of the pineal gland—a small conical structure lying above the hind side of the third ventricle. The pineal gland receives waveform impulses directly from the optic nerves.

SCN cells are implicated in the secretion of most if not all the major hormones and neurotransmitters within the body. Their switching system appears to be related to the mechanisms of double-neuron oscillation guided by a combination of light and genetic expression (Ilonomov *et al.* 1994, Fukada 2002).

Further research has concluded that SCN cells are not only responsive to light. They also respond to selected mRNA and prostaglandin molecules. It was also found that every cell seems to have its own independent clock genes, and groups of cells synchronize their clocks to a common setting. The genomes of

SCN cells indicate that they provide this synchronization facility (Buijs *et al.* 2006).

In 2005, Dr. H. Okamura from the Kobe University School of Medicine confirmed that SCN clock cell genes are located throughout most of the body's major tissue and organ systems. Apparently, the genetic expressions of SCN cell oscillations are coupled with the independent clock genes in these locations. This coupling (or resonating) of genetic expressions appears to synchronize the pacing of the SCN-stimulated activities within the cell.

A larger mystery is how the SCN cells and clock genes communicate throughout the body. In 2004, Dr. David Welsh and a team of researchers observed individual fibroblasts under various conditions. Fibroblasts are cells that will differentiate into connective tissue cells, bone cells and other types of cells. It turns out that fibroblasts also contain self-regulating circadian clockwork genes. These apparently synchronize their differentiation with the genetic clocks inside SCN cells.

Cave studies like Kleitman (1963), Siffre (1972), and Miles *et al.* (1977) have indicated that the human body's daily revolution without the resetting mechanism of daylight is about 24.9 hours. This exact period has been debated to some degree, but many studies have confirmed this range.

In a study done by Folkard in 1996, a woman was isolated for twenty-five days without daily light cues. While her temperature cycle was close to twenty-four hours long, her sleep cycles were closer to thirty hours. This study indicated that over time, the clock tends to stretch out without any sun. It also indicates some individuality among responses to a lack of daily sun waves. Without the daily resetting mechanism of the sun, we might be going to bed later and later each night, and after a few days, we might be doing all-nighters and sleeping during the daytime.

Consistently, the studies on the body clock illustrate how predictably the body's clockworks mechanisms reset with sunlight.

For example, Dr. Czeisler performed studies (1989) with the Naval Health Research Center on Trident nuclear submarine crewmembers. Sub operation schedules required crew to attempt to maintain an 18-hour body clock. Dr. Czeisler's results found this just was not possible. The onboard lights were simply too weak to entrain their body clocks to that schedule. Dr. Czeisler and others had previously established that bright light from between 7,000 and 13,000 lux (daylight) was necessary to produce such a dramatic resetting of the body clock (Boivin et al. 1996).

The human body does respond to lower intensities of light, however. In another study, Dr. Czeisler and Boivin (1998) studied eight healthy men with eight control subjects. They found that a mere 180 lux of light (typical office lighting ranges from 200-400 lux) had the ability to shift the circadian body clock and increase body core temperature. In another test, Dr. Czeisler found that 100 lux of indoor light has about half the alerting response as 9100 lux of outdoor light (Cajochen et al. 2000). In a study of twelve adults, Dr. Czeisler and his associates (Gronfier et al. 2007) found that 100 lux is sufficient to slightly shift the clock, but 25 lux was not enough to shift or reset the body's clock.

Body core temperature, or thermoregulation, appears to be a little less sensitive to the body's reception of light as other rhythms are (St Hilaire et al. 2007). Studies of people tested in isolation without light have confirmed that if the body is deprived of light, the body clock will stubbornly maintain thermoregulation cycles long after other cycles fall off.

After a couple of weeks in *temporal isolation* chambers—meaning with only artificial light and no time signals—subjects will sleep highly irregular hours. Some days a subject might sleep up to 19 hours a day, while other days the sleep length might be as few as four hours. Interestingly, on days with as little as four hours sleep, subjects did not recognize that they had too little sleep. They might even remain awake for as many as 30 hours in a row without apparent sleepiness. Furthermore, these subjects' body temperature cycles—together with their melatonin and cortisol cycles—would remain constant despite drastic swings in sleep and waking hours.

Circulating melatonin levels in the blood have been shown to increase into the evening, proportionate to the level of darkness. Melatonin is a hormone/neurotransmitter that helps us fall asleep. Melatonin alternates with cortisol to time our sleeping and waking cycles.

Deficient melatonin levels have also been linked to lowered immunity and heightened risk of cancer and other diseases. A number of pro-inflammatory cytokines are produced when the body is not sleeping enough or is operating on an irregular cycle. Pro-inflammatory interleukin-6 is one of these, and its release correlates with irregular sleep patterns. Another pro-inflammatory trigger, *tumor necrosis factor* (or TNF), is observed higher in persons with inadequate or irregular sleep cycles. Heightened levels of these cytokines have been particularly evident during daytime sleepiness episodes and low levels of nighttime melatonin (Vgontzas *et al.* 2005).

Light and its absence are key triggers for a number of hormone/neurotransmitters. Dopamine and serotonin levels are also related to the reception of sunlight. Light stimulates the pineal gland. The pineal gland in turn stimulates the hypothalamus. The hypothalamus releases neurotransmitters that stimulate the anterior pituitary with releasing hormones. These releasing hormones stimulate the pituitary to release master hormones that drive the endocrine system. For example, ACTH hormones stimulate the adrenal gland to release glucocorticoids. The pituitary's release of TSH hormone stimulates the thyroid to produce secondary hormones T3 and T4, which help maintain metabolic balance. All of these and more are due to the reception (or absence) of the electromagnetic wavelengths of sunlight into the optic nerve.

Our bodies also produce light. In the early 1970s, German researcher Dr. Fritz-Albert Popp was focusing on cancer cell treatment at the University of Marburg. In one particular trial, he discovered weak emissions coming from living cells and multiplying tumor cells at wavelengths of 260-800 nanometers. Fascinated,

Popp and his associates confirmed this phenomenon over repeated assays. Over the years, Dr. Popp conducted many studies and wrote many scientific papers on the topic. He called these weak emissions *biophotons* because of their resemblance to the waveform properties of light radiation. As for his cancer research, Dr. Popp was able to correlate greater biophoton emission levels in expanded cancer cell growth, and lower emissions during slower growth. His tests also indicated that anti-carcinogenic therapies had the effect of lowering emission levels during tumor reduction and remission (Popp 1976, 2003; Chang *et al.* 2002).

Dr. Popp, Dr. Chang and fellow researchers (1976, 1997, 2000) found that different frequencies were emitted from healthy cells as compared with diseased cells. He also found that cells positively responded to specific frequencies of light by increasing repair mechanisms. Especially productive were emissions from other cells. There appeared to be low-level radiative communications occurring between cells in response to cell damage.

The strange new ultra-weak radiation produced by cells was termed bioluminescence. Research by Gisler *et al.* in 1983 and Dobrowolski *et al.* in 1987 confirmed Dr. Popp's observations of distinctive bioluminescence effect among healthy and cancer cells.

Dr. Popp's research confirmed that every living organism emits unique frequencies (Popp and Chang 2000); just as each body has a unique fingerprint. The use of identification methods soon led to the description of *cellular fingerprints*—using signature frequencies and amplitudes to differentiate one from another. This concept correlates with differentiated DNA sequencing among cells as demonstrated by researchers like O'Brien *et al.* (1980) and Thacker *et al.* (1988).

This effect was confirmed variously using different types of cells. Dr. Popp's equipment was also able to distinguish conventionally grown tomatoes from organically grown tomatoes. Their ultraweak emissions were measured using another device he developed called the *photon detector*. In 1991, Dr. Barbara Chwirot and Dr. Popp co-authored a report confirming light-induced luminescence during mitosis among yeast cells. His biophoton device was able to predict the relative germination rate of barley seeds prior to sprouting as well. Apparently, biophoton emissions are increased during cellular growth and reproduction (Lambing 1992).

Research led by Professor Franco Musumeci at the Institute of Physics of Catania University in the early 1990s confirmed the existence of these weak emissions. Professor Musumeci studied cancer tissue systems and confirmed these ultraweak waveforms among growing tumor lines (Grasso *et al.* 1991). He and his associates also compared normal tissues with cancer tissues, confirming consistent variances between the two (Grasso *et al.* 1992). In 1994, Professor Musumeci and his associates analyzed food for biophoton emission, finding higher emission levels in freshly picked food. Older, storage-bound food had significantly lower emission levels. While early-picked tomatoes might have had the same red color as ripe-picked tomatoes, they were distinguished by lower biophoton emissions (Triglia *et al.* 1998).

Professor Musumeci's research also focused upon yeast growth and soybean germination: Measuring weak photon emissions during growth and sprouting. In his yeast growth studies, he discovered a consistent increase in photon emission levels with increased yeast growth. His soybean germination studies yielded some very interesting results as well. Both active soybeans and devitalized soybeans were tested together, and their photon levels were measured over time and against mass increase (growth). Consistently, the active germinating seeds displayed higher sustained photon emission levels than the devitalized ones. The devitalized soybean seeds had higher initial emission levels however. These decreased over time, while the vital germinating soybeans had increasing emission levels through germination until they leveled off as they matured (Grasso *et al.* 1991).

Cohen and Popp (1997) eventually conducted human trials, testing 200 subjects for biophoton emissions over a period of several years. These trials showed consistent emission levels among the test subjects. Some tests measured levels of a particular subject daily over an extended period. In one of Cohen and Popp's human trials, human biophoton emission was measured daily for several months. These longer-term measurements demonstrated correlations between biophoton emission and human biowaves. Rhythms estimated at 14 days, one month, three months, and nine months were evidenced by rising and falling emission level rates.

These human biophoton trials also revealed a number of other whole-body trends. These include left-right symmetry among biophoton emissions throughout the body. This symmetry was found to become disturbed in diseased states. Various biophoton channels appeared to be functional within the body, appearing to transfer information between different anatomical regions. They found these corresponded closely with acupuncture *meridians*.

Cohen and Popp proposed that these biophoton measurements could be useful as non-invasive diagnostic techniques. Emission levels were studied before, during, and after the application of skin therapy on psoriasis patients, for example. This confirmed that biophoton emissions tend to rise with therapy and an improvement of symptoms.

Other research also correlated biophoton emission with the human immune response. It was determined that during immune activity or wound healing, blood will reflect higher biophoton levels. Biophoton levels increase with greater neutrophil levels, which also happen to be active redox conductors. The blood is naturally extremely sensitive to immune threats, and biophoton levels appear to reflect the rise with immune cell response (Klima *et al.* 1987).

Other studies have demonstrated that fibroblasts (cells that participate in injury repair) have greater photon emission levels following mitosis. This provides additional confirmation that the body's healing and immune responses yield greater photon emission levels (Niggli 2003).

Biophoton measurements have also been closely studied by a number of other researchers from other disciplines. Among them, bioluminescence was observed by Edwards *et al.* in 1989 using electrotherapeutics. This research again confirmed a connection between acupuncture *meridians* and biophoton emissions.

Between 1986 and 1991, Dr. Humio Inaba, a professor at the Research Institute of Electrical Communication at Tohoku University, led a research project focused on these ultraweak emissions. Dr. Inaba's work utilized a single-photon counting device with an amplification system to enable photon-counting images with narrow photon ranges approximating single waveforms. His research demonstrated that these biophotons occur coincidentally with biochemical reactions within cells. The possibility that this effect was a response to external light was also eliminated. Although external radiation has been shown to prompt a delayed photon response within the body, these ultraweak biophoton emissions were unique and independent. Using his equipment, Dr. Inaba's research also measured similar biophoton emissions in the germinating seeds of various plants, soybeans, spinach chloroplasts, sea urchin eggs, and mammalian nuclei (Inaba 1991).

In 2003, Dr. Michael Lipkind noted higher photon emissions from cell cultures infected with viruses when compared with healthy cell controls. Virus-infected cells not only had higher but also more peculiar ranges than the more standardized ranges coming from healthy cells. The peculiarity of the virus emissions also closely correlated with the virus' replication cycles. These results closely corresponded with the tumor-cell growth studies done by Professor Popp.

In a study by Dr. Chwirot and associates published in 2003, colon lesion cells were measured for biophoton activity after their surgical removal from diseased patients. The biophoton levels significantly differed in colon lesion cells as compared with healthy colon mucosal cells. This has led some to suggest that photon emission testing could be an effective tool in diagnosing colon cancers and lesions.

Studies conducted by Russian researchers V.P. Kaznachejew and L.P Michailowa have confirmed and quantified the transmission and reception of these ultra-weak biowaves within the body. These results show that organs also produce and receive ultra-weak light emissions, and translate this information into metabolic processes (Schumacher 2005).

Further biophoton investigations have determined that greater toxic loads in living cells result in greater photon emission. As toxin levels or stressors increase, emission levels increase. This has been confirmed in other studies of plant responses to stressors. Higher lipoxygenase and peroxidase levels in plants have correlated with higher emission levels.

Biophoton research indicates that although each cell and each individual appears to emit unique waveforms, a significant level of coherence is observed between photon emissions of various cells. More significantly, coherence is observed as these emissions are broken down into their respective spectra. Coherent biowaves create informational interference patterns—either destructive (reducing) or constructive (expanding). The coherency factor became relevant to Dr. Popp and his fellow researchers as it provided a rational holistic model for information transmission within the body (Popp and Yan 2002; Li 1981; Popp 2003).

Communication signaling systems indicating biophoton activity were demonstrated with *dinoflaggellates* by Chang and Popp in 1994. A dinoflaggellate is a single cell organism that typically lives in the ocean or fresh waters of the world. Many plankton species are dinoflaggellates. Though single-celled, they have tremendous complexity, yielding cellulose armor plates for defense, and the ability to change structural shape to give them tremendous propulsion for escape. They also convert sunlight to nutritional energy. Dinoflaggellates thus provide the foundation for the nutrient content of the marine habitat. They also emit bioluminescence.

Most of us have seen the nighttime phosphorescent sparkling of the ocean's surface during plankton blooms. This bioluminescence is a biophoton event, occurring at a wavelength perceivable by human retinal cells. When *Lingulodinium polyedrum* blooms in red tide events, the billions of dinoflagellates will turn the seashore waters phosphorescent blue. It is quite an awesome scene.

Biologists now understand that these single cell dinoflagellates are communicating on a grander level during these bioluminescence events. These communications are referred to as *quorum sensing*. Quorum sensing is created when small organisms biocommunicate a general consensus between each other to effect an action on a mass population basis. Pathogenic microorganisms also have this capability within the body. This is why common yeasts like *Candida albicans* can exist in small colonies within the body without any detriment, but once they their populations grow, they can overwhelm the immune system. Not unlike what is seen among dinoflagellates, *Candida* microorganisms coordinate with waveform signaling to expand their colonies to take advantage of times of weakened immunity within the host.

While cells are not independent living organisms, quorum sensing illustrates the extent that electromagnetic signaling mechanisms occur within and around us. Every cell within our body is involved in electromagnetic signaling. These mechanisms provide the basis for synchronization among our metabolic processes. Biophoton signaling systems provide only one dimension of this. Others include neurotransmitters, hormones, ion channels, brainwaves and nerve conduction. We can conclude that the basic signaling systems of the body are multi-layered and multi-dimensional. Together, they provide a network and smart map that answers the mystery of how every cell in the body seems to know its precise place and function among so many other cells.

Most of us have observed how easily the reception of a radio station can be interrupted by an intruding hillside or building. Because electromagnetic radiation is dependent upon its medium and lack of destructive interference, it is quite easy to empirically establish that the introduction of synthetic electromagnetic radiation should certainly interfere—at least subtly—with the body's orchestrated and synchronized flow of hormones, neurotransmitters, biophotons, brainwaves, neurons, and so on. As we've shown, the interruption of these should effect metabolism, reproduction, digestion, and so many other processes within the body. Depending, of course, on the extent of the interference.

Homeopathic Pathways

Can a homeopathic remedy travel through the informational pathways of the body? This depends upon the molecular nature of the remedy and whether the remainder of the remedy after the dilution still contains the molecular information of the original substance.

By simple observation we know that biomolecule substances can produce physiological changes through consumption. Any medication illustrates this. The question in homeopathy is whether the molecular information from a particular substance can make it through numerous dilutions to the tune of thousands to one.

For this very reason, Dr. Samuel Hahnemann's methodologies for succussion and dilution did not use water alone, but rather utilized what he considered were neutral foundations for allowing the nature of the substance to continue, such as water, milk and glass containers.

What Hahnemann didn't realize is that these three substances are not neutral: They are each conductors. They may appear to be relatively neutral, but they each will conduct electromagnetic information. This is why water and milk are good solvents:. A variety of substances can be dissolved in either because their constituents will bond with the various constituents of particular solutes to make a solution.

Take milk. Various powders can be dissolved in milk. This is why chocolate and other flavored milks are so popular: Because these flavors can so easily be mixed with milk.

Water is the same way. So many substances can be dissolved in water to make many flavored drinks, cleansers and so on. Water is a great solvent.

Glass is not known as being a good solvent and this is why glass—

composed of sand—is molecularly well-balanced, and thus does not readily dissolve.

But glass maintains another characteristic. It can be adhered to. Adhesion can occur between molecules when their bonds become electromagnetically joined together by electron exchange—a chemical bond—or they are simply pulled together by the poles of their respective molecules.

This latter form of adherence is often produced by a force we now call Van der Waals forces. This is a polar attraction between two molecules. Molecules in the glass and molecules dissolved in milk or water can become adhered to the molecules of the glass.

This is seen easily on a daily basis. If we were to leave milk or other substance in a glass for a couple of days, and then wash the glass out, we would likely smell the milk in the glass for some time, even after the glass was seemingly cleaned of the milk or other substance. Why can we still smell it? Because some of the molecules of the substance have adhered to the sides of the glass. Even a good soap and water washing will not release the forces of this adhesion completely. Over time and multiple washings, the glass will become clear of the smell.

Even then, there will likely remain atomic remnants of the substance on the surface of the glass for some time—depending upon the washing method.

This is what soap is used for. To release the adhesion of substances on the surface of our dishes. But even the best soap will not necessarily release adhesion of molecules that have undergone lengthy adhesion—even possibly creating some chemical bonding.

Chapter Five
Pulses of Bioinformation
Homuncular Metabolism

If we look at a very small wave break onto the sand or in our bathtub, we can make an interesting observation: *The tiniest wave looks exactly like a big wave.* This tiny wave has precisely the same waveform characteristics of even the largest monster wave. While it might have a different frequency, wavelength, and amplitude, the proportions between these measurements will be the same. This is the same principle of a harmonic—a proportionate reflection of a fundamental basis.

We might call this effect *waveform relativity.* To be more precise we might call this phenomenon *harmonic holography.*

This relative holographic effect is observed throughout nature. As we look around us, we see patterns of replication and duplication with size and proportion relativity. As we scale from the smallest to the largest, we see unified yet individual structure. We see multiple atomic structures cooperatively interacting to form molecular structures. We see multiple molecules interacting to form cellular structures. We see multiple cellular structures interacting to form organ and tissue structures. We see multiple organ and tissue structures interacting to form organism structures. We see multiple organism structures interacting to form family structures. We see multiple family structures interacting to form colonies, cities, villages, or tribes. We see multiple cities, villages, or tribes interacting to form nations. We see multiple nations interacting to form societies. We see multiple societies interacting with the environment as part of a living planet. We see multiple planets interacting to form galaxies. We see multiple galaxies interacting to form universes.

Many researchers may refer to this effect as *homuncular functionality.* This refers to the operations of sub-systems harmonizing with the purpose of a grander system—each part working with congruity and synchronization to the overall purpose of the larger system. We see in the largest and the smallest plants and animals this

synchronized sub-system effect, tying together the larger
ecosystems of the planet and even the universe with the smallest
molecular activity. On a structural functionality, we see waves,
crystals, spirals and their various interference patterns all forming
homunculi with replicated architecture and motion throughout the
natural universe.

Harmonic, holographic, and homuncular concepts have pervaded
the ancient sciences of the Greeks, as found among the works of
Pythagoras, Socrates, Aristotle, Hippocrates, and others. We also
find these concepts documented among the works of ancient China
(Tao, Buddhism), the ancient Vedas of India, the Egyptians, and
various other cultures over the centuries. The term and theory of
holography was formally put forth by Dennis Gabor in 1947 in an
effort to improve electron microscope resolution. Gabor's general
assumption was that a waveform crest would contain the complete
information on the source of the waveform. His concept provoked
the term from Greek meaning *holos* for "whole" and *gramma* for
"message." In its current use, holography uses light (later laser) to
separate an image into its third dimension with depth-of-field. This
is a process called *wave front reconstruction*. The ability of light to
present the parallax view—a view with a dimensional perspective—
was contrived by splitting a light beam into two parts, each traveling
to the object with different paths. The two beams arrive at a
photographic plate from two angles—one referencing the object
and the other reflecting the object. As they arrive, they create an
interference pattern, which unveils a combined view with depth
from two different perspectives.

A *homuncular hologram* then would exist when each of the parts, when
separated, still reflect the whole. Often when we hear the word
"hologram" we think of the space ships of a certain futuristic
television show that use laser holograms reflecting a person or
multi-dimensional object in its reproductive entirety. This is
considered holographic in one respect because it reflects a three-
dimensional physical shape or person into another theatre. This is
not a true hologram however, because the anatomy or physiology of

the subject is not carried through this reflection—only the exterior shell is.

Photon Holography

Dr. Gabor's light holography images were crude estimations or modelings of true holography. True holography requires the interference of multiple coherent beams. An interference pattern produced by two laser beams can partially accomplish this same feat by reflecting the laser sub-parts into components of the whole image. Following the laser's invention (or discovery) in 1960, its use to reflect the wholeness of an image through coherent light beam splitting was accomplished through the efforts of Emmett Leith and Juris Upatnieks at the University of Michigan in 1962. Their laser applications produced realistic 3-D images with holographic clarity because the two beams interacted with coherence. While this is considered an image modeling rather than a full hologram, the ability of a laser to produce a hologram image illustrates this ability within nature. Since most if not all of nature's rhythmicity is coherent in one respect or another, holography is naturally resident throughout the physical world.

An outer image reflection can be holographic if each section of the image is reflects the entire form. In a real hologram, the image is duplicated throughout the smaller parts. To this is added the function ability and physiology of the whole reflected in each part. This is the case in nature. While we may not perceive the reflection of the image nor the physiology as perfect in the natural world, there are reasons for variances. Without variances in nature, there is no room for the conscious elements to make choices and learn lessons. A strict hologram with no flexibility would simply be a machine.

To picture this holographic effect in nature we could toss two rocks into a still pond a few feet from each other. As we watch the waves of concentric circles collide with each other, we notice a rather unusual event. As the waves from the first toss collide with the waves from the second rock toss, the resulting circular waves reflect the combination of both rock tosses: If there were conformity among the rock tosses—say the rocks were of the exact same weight and tossed simultaneously, we would see one type of interference pattern. If they were rocks of different sizes tossed at different times, the interference pattern would be altogether different. In both cases, the interference pattern reflects and retains the history of the two tosses.

One of the most obvious indications of nature's holography is the sheer breadth and size of the database of mathematical formulas accurately reflecting many of the specifications of nature's functionality. When we consider that one simple formula—such as mass-equals-force-times-acceleration ($F=ma$)—can be applied to physical movement in so many different applications—large and small, we can see the mathematical holographic. How could nature reflect this same simple property specification through all matter when it comes to mass, force and acceleration? *Bernoulli's principle of fluid*—another example—relates fluid pressure with velocity. This formula will apply to a large amount of water moving through a large pipe or channel, or a small amount of water moving through a small water pipe. It can also be applied to air and other gases and liquids. The pressure and velocities will relate every time with the same formula, but with a slight variance to allow uniqueness. This is because the elements and activities of nature transmit holographic reflection.

Genetic Holography

The ideal case for homuncular holography is made with DNA. Each cell within the body contains a blueprint of the body's entire structure. The typical location of DNA is within the nucleus of each cell. Within this nucleus, DNA imparts instructional messaging throughout the cell using a process called transcription. This process requires RNA to copy the coding of DNA onto its own strand. Once copied, the RNA can execute or instruct the coding instructions of DNA by assembling specific proteins such as enzymes or hormones, which perform specific functions according to the cell's defined duties.

Each DNA molecule inside of each cell also reflects the entire body's structure and function. Each cell's particular function is differentiated by a repression of sections of genetic code not applicable to that cell. Even though repressed, those non-essential codons are still present in every nucleus of the trillions of cells of the body—giving each cell a reflection of the genetic code for the entire body. As biologists have broken down the process of fertilization via *mitosis* and *meiosis,* they have observed that genetic information is assembled together and shared between the sperm and the ovum. During the initial fertilization stages, the embryonic *blastocyst* duplicates a complete set of DNA into each initial cell as though each cell will perform all the functions of the entire body. Each cell has all the instructions for the eventual efforts of all the various cells.

Somehow, through a process biologists and medical researchers do not quite understand, the process of cellular differentiation will define and determine each cell's activity. This creates specialized cells within the body. Some cells become liver cells while others become bone cells, each with their specific function. Each cell has its own "brain" or nucleus, from whence it instructs the rest of the cell in its functioning. While each cell contains the blueprint for the entire body's structure—and therefore can synchronize its activities with the entire body—each cell has a predetermined specialty. Thus while the parts reflect the whole, the parts also engage in unique activities contributing to the whole function.

As we investigate this further, we can see that our bodies, this planet, and most of the organisms on it operate in the same manner: Each part contains a seed of the whole, while each part contributes in a special way to accomplish the functioning principles of the whole. For this reason, most of us have at some point imagined an atom to be a tiny universe and the tiny ant farm to be a tiny city. This is because each cell; each molecule; each atom around us is a homuncular holographic reflection of the entire universe. Certainly our tendency to envision this is natural.

Another interesting thing we find with the human body is that it is host to trillions of separate living biological microorganisms. These tiny living organisms live primarily in our intestinal tract, but they also live around all of our orifices, in our bloodstream, in our urinary tracts, between our toes—and in just about any organ or tissue system. They include various yeasts, molds, and bacteria. Many of these tiny living organisms are *probiotic,* in that they contribute to the health of the body. Many however—and depending upon the state of the body—are pathogenic.

The body is the host of both these pathogenic and probiotic species. Most of these microorganisms live within colonies, in different organ systems or areas. Most live in the digestive tract. They cooperate and work as teams. Within their colonies, some perform different functions, just as people work in different occupations. Some help digestion by breaking down food to aid nutrient absorption. Many battle with competitive microorganisms. Pathogenic intestinal bacteria typically interfere in digestion and poison our system with endotoxins (their waste products). Probiotic microorganisms often secrete antibiotics to kill their enemies, which are typically also our body's enemies. Probiotics are thus considered a key element of our immune system. Many health experts have concluded that probiotics make up a good 60% of our body's immune function.

The body is homuncularly holographic with respect to the earth. The body, like the earth, is a host. The earth harbors many organisms just as the body does. Some of these organisms are helpful to the planet, while other organisms—notably much of the human race—are pathogenic to the earth. Just as pathogenic bacteria poison our bodies with endotoxin waste materials, human toxic waste is poisoning the earth.

Natural Rhythm

Over the centuries, humankind has been observing that our activities and the activities of other organisms within our environment seem to be organized with rhythm. Not one beat or rhythm mind you. Rather, many concurrent rhythms that seem to inter-relate and correlate with each other. The relationships between the various beats or rhythms of the universe have been studied by many prominent scientists over thousands of years. The prevailing conclusion is that the body and its environment are somehow acting within a synchronic relationship.

The appearance of rhythmic behavior within the human physiology is evident from both an external and internal view. Certainly, anatomical characterizations of the physical body present a means to measure and observe the outward structural mapping of the body, just as an architectural drawing of a building allows us to know the dimensions of every room in a building. The weakness of the architectural drawing is that it will not tell us how each of the rooms are being used and who may be living within them. In the same way, our anatomical characterizations of the human body, despite their visual endowment, may present the structural nature of the physiology but hardly the depth of its metabolic functions. The inner workings of the body still primarily confound modern physicians, and thus require a view with a whole other perspective.

As Da Vinci and others have illustrated among nature, should we unfold and measure every living organism's physical development, we observe growth following a unique design. Virtually every occurrence in the natural world follows these same designs. Among these include the *Fibonacci sequence*, which maps out to the *golden rectangle*, the *golden mean* and the *golden spiral* as measured multi-dimensionally.

The Fibonacci sequence, 0, 1, 2, 3, 5, 8, 13, 21, 34, 55.... is observed throughout nature. A *Fibonacci number* is found by adding the two preceding Fibonacci numbers together: 1+2=3, 2+3=5, 3+5=8.... Observed by Italian Leonardo Pisano Fibonacci in the thirteenth century while tracing a family tree of rabbits, the *Fibonacci sequence* is recognized as the fundamental progression throughout nature. Its accounting is observed among every living organism, from shape and growth to genetic heredity. For example, the outward projection of branches and leaves from trees and plant stalks assemble precise Fibonacci fractions: one-half in grasses, lime and elm; one-third in sedges, beech, hazel and blackberry; two-fifths in roses, oak, cherry, apple and holly; three-eighths in bananas, poplar, willow and pear; five-thirteenths in leeks, almond and pussy willow; and eight-twenty-firsts in pine cones and cactus. Some plants are aligned in a related sequence, called the *Lucas sequence,* named after nineteenth century Frenchman Edouard Lucas. Like Fibonacci numbers, Lucas numbers are also assembled by adding two consecutive numbers to get the third. However, the Lucas sequence begins with two and one rather than zero: 1+2=3, 1+3=4, 3+4=7, 7+4=11, and so on, to arrive at 1, 2, 3, 4, 7, 11, 18....

When Fibonacci measurements are arranged into polygons, they form rectangles. One of these rectangles is laid against a square of the next Fibonacci number to become the famous *golden rectangle* or *Phi.* The golden rectangle is made from two adjacent 1x1 squares to become a 1x2 Fibonacci rectangle. This can be laid against a 2x2 square to become a 2x3 Fibonacci rectangle. Laid against a 3x3 square, it becomes a 3x5 Fibonacci rectangle and so on. The Fibonacci rectangle is observed throughout nature, including the outer and inner regions of plant, animal and human organisms and their appendages.

Another pattern observed throughout nature is the spiral. The *golden spiral* is most prominent, determined as an array of concentrically outward *golden sections* with dimensions of 1:1.618. The golden spiral is seen repeatedly throughout the natural world. It is seen in the nautilus shell. It is seen in the sections of tortoise shells and fingerprints. It is seen among the tops of plant florets like cauliflower and broccoli, and among cell and nerve patterns.

The Fibonacci sequence is functionally a *harmonic sequence.* A harmonic sequence repeats a pattern of pacing of either an integer or a ratio of integers. An example of a harmonic sequence would be 5, 10, 15, 20, 25, which has a fundamental integer change of five. This type of sequence produces a wave harmonic. Fibonacci and Lucas sequences are progressive harmonics because the fundamental pace is progressively being updated by the previous two factors of the sequence. We might then refer to the typical music harmonic as a *static harmonic,* and the sequencing in nature as a *living harmonic,* as it engages consciousness.

The harmonic series also provides a specific waveform. A repeating cycle can be broken down and charted over a two dimensional horizontal plane, which converts to the sine wave. Sine waves are the waveforms of light, sound, radiowaves, cosmic rays, gamma rays, the infrared spectrum, the ultraviolet spectrum, and even ocean waves. Over a hundred years ago, French physicist Jean Fourier discovered that almost every physical motion could be broken down into sinusoidal components. This demonstrated his famous mathematic *Fourier series.*

We also see these sinusoidal, helical and spiraling dimensions within all the human body's physiology. From top to bottom, the body illustrates this golden design. Should we look at the top of a human head from above we will see an unmistakable swirling of the hair inward from a location in the area of the occipital fontanel—in the neighborhood as the infant's 'soft spot.' This spiraling appearance is seen throughout the hairs of the body. We can see an inward spiraling of hair growth in key anatomical areas such as the pubis, chin, the back, the belly button and elsewhere. For this reason, shaving typically requires several different angles to accommodate the spiraling nature of hair growth.

A quick review of our fingerprints will display a unique spiraling effect. The osteocytes within our bony structures are also arranged helically, as are many of our nerves and cells. The iris is arranged helically. The ear is arranged in a spiraling fashion, strikingly similar to a dissected wave or weather system. The cochlear inner ear is also spiraled, each bend and curve working to translate air pressure waves into electromagnetic pulses that reflect sound onto the audio cortex. A cross-section of the disks of our spine, if viewed from above, also reveals a noticeable spiraling helix as the vertebra become gradually narrower.

Leonardo Da Vinci exhaustively measured the various appendages of the body. He compared them with other parts and the body as a whole. Da Vinci's famous *Vitruvian Man* illustrates a human body within the context of a circle, with the arms and legs each rotating around the circumference of the circle with the belly button marking its center point. Da Vinci also measured length of hands, feet, arms, fingers, and so on, and found that the length and width of these body parts were all congruent when compared relationally. For example, Da Vinci observed that the arm from the wrist is four times the length of the hand from fingertips to wrist. He also established that at three years old a human male almost precisely half his full-grown height, among many other amazing relativities within the human organism.

Da Vinci also noted the symmetry among movement and metabolism. He once wrote that, "The same cause which stirs the humours in every species of animal body and by which every injury is repaired, also moves the waters from the utmost depth of the sea to the greatest heights."

In 1590, Thomas Harriot proposed that the *equiangular spiral,* or *spira mirabilis* could be observed from the side view (with the thumb wrapped under the finger) of the clenched fist. This observation was also described by Descartes and later elaborated on mathematically by Jakob Bernoulli. It was described as the logarithmic spiral. This spiral was noted as strikingly similar to the spiraling nature of the nautilus and the swirling of water, well before many other natural helices and spirals were found among nature by other scientists. For centuries, the medical profession assumed this fist-spiral relationship was correct. The specific measurements between the digits of the fingers and thumb supported the precise measurement of *Phi* (about 1.62—the golden section or golden rectangle). This assumption became the subject of heated debate amongst the medical profession.

The debate has continued to the modern era. A more recent motion analysis by Gupta *et al.* (1998) confirmed experimentally that the fingers' motion path towards fisting follows the equiangular spiral. A later study of the bones of the hand done by Andrew Mark, M.D. and associates in the 2003 *Journal of Hand Surgery* took standardized x-rays from 100 healthy volunteers and found a low correlation to a precise *Phi* measurement within the fisted spiral. At the same time, the authors of this study also concluded that the rotation of the metacarpophalangeal joint to the center of rotation of the interphalangeal joints should still yield the Fibonacci relationship. The center of rotation for each digit pivots though the space between the joints. They concluded that discrepancies could occur between the functional and absolute bone lengths.

In other words, there are unique differences in the development and movement of each body. These are related to individual habits and function. Just as no two fingerprints, ears or retinas are alike between different human bodies; there are subtle individual variances between the various body proportions, depending upon use and medical history. We are not making a case for the body being a machine here. The body has a particular design, but it is also designed to reflect the individual consciousness and history of each individual. This points to the body's metabolism being a flexible yet elegant interplay between nature's design and individual consciousness.

Magnetic Resonance

Advancements in physics during the nineteenth century led to the realization that electricity is not a single waveform. Rather, it is a dual waveform, consisting of an electronic pulse and a magnetic field. Gradually we have also come to the realization that the ionic cellular mechanisms of the body also have this dual waveform nature. Like the electric current, the mechanisms of the body are both electronic and magnetic. As electronic biochemical reactions cascade through our bodies with transport mechanisms, we are also generating magnetic fields. These magnetic fields are dispatched through our local environment with real-time results. Some fields are by-products of electronic processes, while others are specifically magnetic, affecting metabolism directly. The anatomical effects of magnetism are not readily addressed by modern medical science. This is odd, noting the extensive use of diagnosis using magnetic resonance technologies. Magnetic resonance (MRI) utilizes radiative polarity to visual the body's anatomy. Just as electrical currents moving through appliances generate magnetic fields, the various currents running through the body's ionic mechanisms utilize magnetic fields. As physics found over a century ago, magnetism influences electronics and vice-versa.

Scientists have long suspected electromagnetism stimulates response among living organisms. The Greeks, in particular Hippocrates, are thought to have applied the magnetic lodestone as a healing therapy. The lodestone was also apparently used by the ancient Egyptians, as Cleopatra is said to have wore lodestone on her forehead around 2000 B.C. The ancient Ayurvedic medicine of the 2000-3500 B.C. Indus Valley applied *siktavati*, or "instruments of stone" in their therapies, and early Tibetan monks applied bar magnets in their training.

Two thousand years after Hippocrates, William Gilbert, the physician to Queen Elizabeth I, demonstrated a number of logical arguments on magnetism and life in his treatise *De Magnete*. Gilbert believed that the earth was a magnet, and that magnetic forces were somehow tuned to the forces of life. Another great physician to adopt magnetic forces was German physician Franz Mesmer. Mesmer professed that living organisms transmitted a subtle aethereal current crudely translated as "animal magnetism," which could influence biology and provide healing benefit. Due to his being investigated and condemned by a King Louis XVI commission (thought to be encouraged by the jealousy of other physicians for his healing successes); Mesmer's work was abandoned by medicine for many centuries.

The eighteenth and nineteenth centuries brought a renewed focus upon electricity and the living organism. The work of physician Luigi Galvani on electrical nerve conduction eventually led to disappointment when it was found that two dissimilar metals were required for electrical activity ("Volta's pile"). Galvani's nerve "animal electricity" proposal had to be abandoned, and electromagnetism was indelibly dissected from medicine for another century.

The connection between life and magnetism became evident

following the publication of the successful research of Finnish scientist Karl Selim Lemström during the late nineteenth and early twentieth centuries. Lemström, an expert on polar and electromagnetic forces, found a connection between tree rings and solar geomagnetic storm activity. He also conducted experiments on plant growth using overhead electrical wires with poles set into the soil. The plants surrounded by electromagnetism grew almost 50% more than similar plants without the electromagnetic wiring environment—which we now know conducts magnetic fields.

Horticultural magnetic research has continued over the past century with consistent results. James Lee Scriber's electromagnetic butterbean trials resulted in twenty-two foot tall plants. Italian Bindo Riccioni treated seeds with capacitors, resulting in 37 percent greater yields. Tests in the Soviet Union during the 1960s also treated seeds with electromagnetic currents. Green mass yields went up to 15 percent higher for corn, up to 15 percent higher for oats and barley, up to 13 percent higher for peas and up to 10 percent higher for buckwheat.

The concept of magnetism within human physiology rose again as a late nineteenth century Julius Bernstein proposed that nerve impulses transferred through polarization. This *membrane polarization* model became the basis for the later conclusive research of Otto Loewi in the early 1920s, which led to his 1936 Nobel Prize for synaptic transmission. Loewi's experiment—which apparently came to him during a dream—was to extract two frog hearts and retain them in a bath of saline. Some of the solution surrounding the faster heartbeat was extracted and put into the bath of the other heart. This made the other heart beat faster, providing the evidence of the biochemical synaptic transmission.

The polarity exchange between ions and biochemicals is unmistakably magnetic. Magnetism is after all, a polarity issue of ions or atoms aligning in one direction or another. The irrefutable link between magnetism and biological response has been confirmed by study and clinical application during the last half of the twentieth century, as the existence of ion channels has been clarified.

Furthermore, the link between intention and magnetism has become evident. This was illustrated by Dr. Grad's research at Canada's McGill University in the late 1950s and early 1960s, when growth rates of barley sprouts were stimulated by the focused intentions of particularly gifted individuals. Further studies indicated these growth rate effects were similar to the influence magnetism has on plant growth.

The central subject of these investigations was a Hungarian refugee named Oskar Estebany. Mr. Estabany appeared to be able to exert extraordinary intentional effects through his touch. A number of tests confirmed that magnetism was involved in Mr. Estebany's abilities. In one, Dr. Justa Smith at the Rosary Hill College (1973) compared Mr. Estebany's ability to increase enzyme reaction rates with those of magnetic field emissions. After Mr. Estebany affected increased reactivity among enzyme reaction rates, Dr. Smith applied magnetic fields and compared the rates. It turned out that the increased growth caused by Mr. Estebany precisely matched that caused by a 13,000 gauss magnetic field.

Dr. Smith had spent a number of years studying these effects prior to and after her tests with Mr. Estebany. She authored a book on the topic (1969) called *Effect of Magnetic Fields on Enzyme Reactivity*. While this research was considered radical at that time, other scientists soon confirmed her findings. In the 1990s, a flurry of research was published from around the world showing magnetic fields in the 2,500-10,000 gauss range affecting reaction rates of various enzymatic reactions. By 1996, more than fifty different enzyme reactions were found to be influenced by magnetic fields. In two linked studies by University of Utah's Charles Grissom, (1993, 1996), single-beam UV-to-visible spectrum and rapid-scanning spectrophotometers with electromagnets built in were applied to two different cobalamine (B12) enzymes. One enzyme (ethanolamine ammonia lyase) had significantly different reaction rates in response to magnetic fields, while the other enzyme (methylmalonyl CoA mutase) had no apparent response. It could thus be concluded that some biochemical processes are sensitive to magnetic field influence and others are not. This effect is still mysterious, but it has become increasingly evident that within the body lie precise flows of magnetic fields.

There have been a number of controlled studies showing that key body tissues respond to magnetic stimulation. Amassian *et al.* (1989) stimulated the motor cortex with a focal magnetic coil, which rendered movement to paralyzed appendages. Maccabee *et al.* (1991) stimulated almost the entire nervous system with a magnetic coil. This particular stimulation instigated responses from the distal peripheral nerve, the nerve root, the cranial nerve, the motor cortex, the premotor cortex, the frontal motor areas related to speech, and other nerve centers.

Dr. Howard Friedman and Dr. Robert Becker studied human behavior and magnetic fields in the early 1960s. They found *extremely low frequencies* (ELF) such as .1 or .2 Hz affected volunteer reaction times (Becker 1985). This paralleled work by Dr. Norbert Weiner and Dr. James Hamer with low-intensity fields, seen as "driving" waveforms already existing in the body. Spaniard Dr. Jose Delgado's research illustrated that low intensity ELF magnetic fields could influence sleep and manic behavior among monkeys. Furthermore, a substantial amount of evidence demonstrates that magnetic fields generated from powerlines and transformers can modulate physiology, noting these and the effects of electromagnetics on plants. Research linking cancer and powerlines has been controversial. Still, enough evidence enables a conclusion that magnetic fields can alter certain physiological processes.

The magnetic nature of the body is revealed through *nuclear magnetic resonance* (NMR). Its application of *magnetic resonance imaging* (MRI) is now one of the more useful diagnostic machines used in medicine when a true cross-sectional analysis of the body is required. The NMR scan is performed on the human body by surrounding the body with strong magnetic fields. These fields polarize the hydrogen ($H+$) proton ions in water (as the body is mostly water). As these ions' north poles align, they emit a particular frequency.

Radio beams positioned around the body (tuned to this frequency) give detectors a cross-sectional scan of the body via these polarized ions. The body is guided underneath magnetic fields ranging from about 5000 to 20,000 gauss (the earth's magnetic field is about .5 gauss). As the altered polarity of the hydrogen protons become excited with radio signals, a computer calculates the water content differences to form an image of the body. Were it not for the magnetic nature of the body, these three-dimensional images would not be possible.

Over the past few years, researchers are increasingly discovering commercial applications for the tiny ion channels within cell membranes. The magnetic reactivity of these *microchannels* (or *micropores*) has enabled technicians to alter the flow through these channels with certain *nanoparticles* (Wee *et al.* 2005). Exerting magnetic influence on these channels—and even etching new channels onto single-celled living organisms—allows the technician to utilize cell structures as microprocessors, drug testers or tiny manufacturing systems. Various functional nanoparticles are under development, and many are in use today in an attempt to exploit nature's magnetic ion channels. Some ethical concerns have voiced on the use of nanobots. What might these magnetized miniature robots become after several generations of evolved intention?

Biocommunication

In 1966, Cleve Backster, a former CIA employee and licensed polygraph examiner, began experimenting with polygraph equipment connected to plants. His first plant was a dracaena cane plant. After connecting the polygraph's electrodes, he immediately began to notice that its *galvanic skin response* readings appeared not so different from human examination charts. What surprised Dr. Backster was that the plant's exam also registered emotional responses of fear. Furthermore, these responses were highest during moments where an intention to harm the plant came to mind. The simple thoughts of considering how the plant would be harmed produced a precise fear response in the plant (Backster, 2003).

The prospect of a plant responding to a threatening intention was certainly incredible to Dr. Backster—then an owner of a polygraph school and research laboratory. Following this incident, Dr. Backster spent the next thirty years carefully conducting controlled experiments to study conscious mechanisms within plants, eggs, and then human cells. Dr. Backster published two scientific papers on the subject, along with a number of popular magazine articles. He also wrote a book on the topic (*Primary Perception,* 2003) and consulted on a number of other titles.

Dr. Backster also appeared on television, radio, and several university lecture series. Dr. Backster carefully conducted hundreds of experiments on emotional intention, devising automated research equipment to remove extraneous influences. Many of these studies were reviewed by well-known scientists, and some even took part in the research. His results were clear, and many were replicated by other scientists—although this also proved to be difficult to the spontaneity required by consciousness research. Dr. Backster discovered that plants were not the only living organism to sense intention. Through exhaustive tests using various subjects and perspectives, he found that human leukocytes separated from their host and kept *in vitro* somehow had the ability to sense and respond to emotions of fear and excitement that occurred within their host *remotely*. Furthermore and amazingly, he found this effect can occurs at a distance of up to fifty miles.

Anyone who has taken a polygraph will report that the examination is complex and requires some technical training in physiology and psychology. A polygraph examiner is thus typically expert in physical-emotion expression. The equipment utilizes primarily galvanized skin response (GSR) and electrocardiography equipment to monitor the physical reflections of specific emotions. What polygraph examination techniques have taught scientists over the years is that the skin, heart and many other parts of the body will reveal heightened emotions with particular physical responses. One of the most noticeable physical responses results from the emotion of fear. Lie detection has thus become recognized as a verifiable science after over thousands of polygraph examinations and hundreds of studies. Even with the occasional variance in specific results, there is undeniable evidence that the body reflects heightened emotional response. Polygraph research has revealed that some people have the ability to cheat the polygraph, assuming they understand how to control certain emotional and physical responses. Here again, this underscores the connection between intention and physical response. Whether cheating the polygraph or not, intention is being expressed through the various responses of the body.

The human polygraph examination focuses upon our fear of detection. The fear of harm through discovery is the typical emotion being tested. This is also controlled in Dr. Backster's research on plants, eggs and human cells. Because the fear of detection is closely related to the fear of harm, the physiological results of the two emotions are practically identical.

One of the dramatic findings of Dr. Backster's research with plants was that once a person consistently begins caring for a plant, that plant becomes emotionally connected to that person. Dr. Backster discovered that even when the person has traveled miles away from this plant, emotionally charged circumstances occurring in the life of the person would affect the plant. In other words, the plant becomes emotionally tied to the person taking care of them. This sort of emotion is typically referred to as *empathy*.

In vitro cells separated from a human responded very similarly in Dr. Backster's research, but only with their host. Living cells being incubated and electroded with the equipment responded to heightened emotional activity of their former host, even when the host was located rooms or even miles away from the cells. This indicated the separated cells somehow had the ability to receive remote communication transmissions from the host. How is it that cells have this ability? Furthermore, Dr. Backster's research demonstrated that the cells were able to prioritize their responses specifically for their host, even amongst emotional controls set up to distract the response.

Dr. Backster's research controls were thoroughly vetted by a number of scientists. Still, it is regarded as controversial, and has been difficult to duplicate in some cases. Nonetheless, communications between a remote ex-host is not altogether different from the cell's known ability to instantly receive instructions from the brain and other remote locations in the body—located many feet away, amongst trillions of other cells. Medical researchers recognize that the body's nervous systems and various biochemicals such as neurotransmitters and hormones help carry messages from one location of the body to another. This begs the question of how billions of cells can be orchestrated to commit a particular action *instantly* upon the intention of the person? Yes, nerves are certainly high-speed, but every cell in the body is not specifically innervated. So how do all the cells instantly respond to intention?

Every cell making up a living organism is a waveform receiver. Each cell has the ability to receive instructional waveforms just as any radio can receive a local broadcast. In addition, groups of cells can align and organize to receive and respond to specific types of waveforms. Actually, the living organism as a whole is a multi-spectrum waveform sensor. Groups of cells called the senses have organized around receiving specific types of waveforms. We can perceive waves in the visible spectrum with the eyes, infrared radiation with the skin, air pressure waves with the ears, and subtle electromagnetic waveforms with the tongue and nose. These are only a few of the multitude of waveforms that are received and translated throughout the body. This is compounded by the fact that the cells also conduct various waveforms via ion channels and receptors.

The body's cells pick up waveforms beyond our current technologies. This is the only explanation for plants and cells to be able to receive precise information from remote locations. Dr. Backster's research illustrated these waveforms were transmitted through insulated and even metal walls.

Waveform communications outside our range of recognition is not a new paradigm to science. The past few hundred years of research have continuously revealed previously unperceivable waveforms.

The eyes have the ability to perceive a variety of waveforms previously considered outside the visible wavelengths. Wavelengths shorter than violet such as ultraviolet, x-rays, and gamma rays have been observed visually under extraordinary circumstances such as a darkened room penetrated with radiation leakage. Both x-rays and gamma rays have been observed on occasion with the naked eye, as a yellow-green glow. Meanwhile, some have identified nuclear leakage in flashes of blue. As the rods of the eyes sensitize for night vision they also become sensitive to other waveforms. Longer and less damaging radiowaves have also been received by humans in extraordinary circumstances. Hearing radio stations through dental fillings, bridgework, and even bobby pins has been an odd but well-documented occurrence.

The body's cells translate radiowaves into electrical brain impulses just as a radio crystal translates radiowaves into electronic pulses. The senses illustrate this well. Once received through the antenna mechanisms of the eyes, ears, nose, tongue and so on—the crystalline structure of nerve cell molecules convert these waveforms to electronic pulses in the same manner. Individual cells have these same antenna systems. The ability of radiowaves influencing single cells and single-cell living organisms is well documented. In 1958, for example, *The New England Institute for Medical Research* published articles documenting that radiowaves could influence red blood cell movement and bacteria motion. Murchie (1978) observed amebas, euglenas, and paramecia aligning their movement with radiating field lines of five to forty megacycle radiowaves. Many other studies have documented similar effects.

The reception and translation of ultraviolet radiation by skin cells is obvious and well understood. The sun's ultraviolet B waveforms stimulate the production of vitamin D_3 when wavelengths of 270-290 nanometers enter the epidermal layer. The *conrotatory electrocyclic reaction* cycles 7-dehydrocholesterol to pre-vitamin D, and eventually to 1,25 dihydroxyvitamin D, or 25-OHD. During this cycle, melanin production is stimulated to provide a filtering and buffering mechanism for additional rays from the sun. Vitamin D is an essential nutrient to the human body. It is important for immunity, cardiovascular health, nerve health and bones and teeth health. Our primary source is through the sun, although a limited number of foods contain small amounts as well.

For many decades, researchers have been studying the effects of light upon other human cells. We all know about photosynthesis— where plant cells utilize light, water and carbon dioxide to produce starches, sugars and oxygen. The molecular structure of chlorophyll acts as a semiconducting crystal, absorbing some ultraviolet waveforms from the sun while reflecting others. With these absorbed waveforms, the unique biochemical reaction of photosynthesis is stimulated among special chloroplasts— specialized proteins embedded inside chlorophyll.

This process illustrates the intimate connection between waveform conversion and living organisms. The complex transformation of light waveforms to plant nutrition is a conversion related to the intention to survive—a conscious act. This intention creates the impetus for energy transformation. We see a similar transformation process occurring through the human cellular production of energy from oxygen and glucose. Cellular energy production occurs through a waveform transition process called *electron transport* (reminiscent of the characterization of electricity as electron movement). ATP and NADPH are created and water is split, releasing oxygen. Part of this process uses an interesting exchange of phosphorus ions called *phosphorylation*. This process is one of transporting waveform energy through a transport chain to create an NADP+ molecule, after which an additional transformation takes place through a process of *redox* to create an energized NADPH. Some theorized that the continuing process of ATP conversion and glucose takes place without UV. Further research has revealed that light is at least indirectly involved, as it stimulates the production of some of the enzymes used as catalysts.

In the 1920s, a Russian scientist Alexander Gurwitsch picked up a weak photoemission from living tissue. The emissions appeared stronger during mitosis, so he termed these UV-range wavelength rhythms *mitogenetic rays*. The presence of living radiation emitted from dividing cells was confirmed shortly thereafter by some German researchers. Even still, their conclusions were overshadowed by doubts from skeptics. Nonetheless, ongoing biochemical experiments have continued to confirm a link between cellular division and radiation.

The topic did not gain much additional research attention until after World War II. Research teams from Italy, Germany and Britain independently worked on the living photon research. Each confirmed waveform observations from living cells, which they named variously. One name stuck: *low-level luminescence ultraweak chemiluminescence*. The prevailing opinion was that the radiation originated from the oxidation of free radicals.

In the early 1970s German researcher Dr. Fritz-Albert Popp was focusing on cancer cell treatment at the University of Marburg. In one particular trial, he discovered weak emissions coming from both living cells and multiplying tumor cells at wavelengths of 260-800 nanometers. Fascinated, Popp and his associates confirmed this phenomenon over repeated assays over the years. He published many scientific papers and wrote a number of books on the topic. He called these weak emissions *biophotons* because of their resemblance to the waveform properties of light radiation. As for his cancer research, Dr. Popp was able to correlate greater emission levels in expanded cancer cell growth, and lower emissions during slower growth. His tests also indicated anti-carcinogenic therapies had the effect of lowering emission levels, indicating a reduction of tumor growth (Popp 1976, 2003; Chang *et al.* 2002).

Dr. Popp, Dr. Chang and fellow researchers (1976, 1997, 2000) found particular frequencies and waveforms among healthy and diseased cells: Cancerous cells emitted certain frequencies and healthy cells emitted certain frequencies. He also found that cells responded to specific frequencies of light by repairing themselves. Especially productive were responsive emissions from other cells.

There appeared to be low-level communications occurring between cells in response to cell damage. Research by Gisler *et al.* in 1983 and Dobrowolski *et al.* in 1987 confirmed this luminescence effect among cancer cells.

Cells each emit unique waveforms, and each living organism emits unique waveforms. Dr. Popp's research confirmed that every living organism emits unique frequencies (Popp and Chang 2000); just as each body has a unique fingerprint. The use of identification methods soon led to the description of *cellular fingerprints*—using signature frequencies and amplitudes to differentiate one from another. This concept correlates with differentiated DNA sequencing among cells as demonstrated by researchers like O'Brien *et al.* (1980) and Thacker *et al.* (1988).

This effect was confirmed variously using different types of cells. Dr. Popp's equipment was also able to distinguish conventionally grown tomatoes from organically grown tomatoes. Their ultraweak emissions were measured using another device he developed called the *photon detector*. In 1991, Dr. Barbara Chwirot and Dr. Popp co-authored a report confirming light-induced luminescence during mitosis among yeast cells. His biophoton device was able to predict the relative germination rate of barley seeds prior to sprouting as well. Apparently, biophoton emissions are connected to cellular communication (Lambing 1992).

Research led by Professor Franco Musumeci at the Institute of Physics of Catania University in the early 1990s confirmed the existence of these weak emissions. Professor Musumeci studied cancer tissue systems and confirmed these ultraweak waveforms among growing tumor lines (Grasso *et al.* 1991). He and his associates (Grasso *et al.* 1992) also compared normal tissues with cancer tissues, confirming consistent variances between the two. In 1994, Professor Musumeci and his associates analyzed food for biophoton emission, finding higher emission levels in freshly picked food. Older, storage-bound food had significantly lower emission levels. While early-picked tomatoes might have had the same red color as ripe-picked tomatoes, they were distinguished by lower biophoton emissions (Triglia *et al.* 1998).

Professor Musumeci's research also focused upon yeast growth and soybean germination: Measuring weak photon emissions during while they grew and sprouted. In his yeast growth studies, he discovered a consistent increase in photon emission levels with increased yeast growth. His soybean germination studies yielded some very interesting results as well. Both active soybeans and devitalized soybeans were tested together, and their photon levels were measured over time and against mass increase (growth). Consistently, the active germinating seeds displayed higher sustained photon emission levels than the devitalized ones. The devitalized soybean seeds had higher initial emission levels however. These decreased over time, while the vital germinating soybeans had increasing emission levels through germination until they leveled off as they matured (Grasso *et al.* 1991).

Cohen and Popp (1997) also conducted human trials, testing 200 subjects for biophoton emissions over a period of several years. These trials showed consistent emission levels among the test subjects. Some tests measured levels of a particular subject daily over an extended period. In one of Cohen and Popp's human trials, human biophoton emission was measured daily for several months. These longer-term measurements demonstrated correlations between biophoton emission and human biowaves. Rhythms estimated at 14 days, one month, three months, and nine months were evidenced by rising and falling emission level rates.

These human biophoton trials also revealed a number of other whole-body trends. These include left-right symmetry among biophoton emissions throughout the body. This symmetry was found to become disturbed in diseased states. Various biophoton channels appeared to be functional within the body, appearing to transfer information between different anatomical regions. They found these corresponded closely with acupuncture meridians.

Cohen and Popp proposed that these biophoton measurements could be useful as non-invasive diagnostic techniques. Emission levels were studied before, during, and after application of skin therapy on psoriasis patients, for example. This confirmed that emissions tend to rise with therapy and an improvement of symptoms.

Other research also correlated biophoton emission with the human immune response. It was determined that during immune activity or wound healing, blood will reflect higher biophoton levels. Biophoton levels increase with greater neutrophil levels, which also happen to be active redox messengers. The blood is naturally extremely sensitive to immune threats, and biophoton levels appear to reflect the rise with immune cell response (Klima *et al.* 1987).

Other studies demonstrated that fibroblasts (cells that participate in injury repair) have greater photon emission levels following mitosis. This provides additional confirmation that the body's healing and immune responses yield greater photon emission levels (Niggli 2003).

Biophoton measurements have also been closely studied by a number of other researchers from other disciplines. Among them, bioluminescence was observed by Edwards *et al.* in 1989 using electrotherapeutics. This research again confirmed a connection between acupuncture meridians and biophoton emissions.

Between 1986 and 1991 Dr. Humio Inaba, a professor at the Research Institute of Electrical Communication at Tohoku University, led a research project focused on these ultraweak photon emissions. Dr. Inaba's work utilized a single-photon counting device with an amplification system to enable photon-counting images with narrow photon ranges approximating single waveforms. His research demonstrated that these biophotons occur coincidentally with biochemical reactions within cells. The possibility that this effect was a response to external light was also eliminated. Although external radiation has been shown to prompt a delayed photon response within the body, these ultraweak biophoton emissions were unique and independent. Using his equipment, Dr. Inaba's research also measured similar biophoton emissions in the germinating seeds of various plants, soybeans, spinach chloroplasts, sea urchin eggs, and mammalian nuclei (Inaba

1991).

In 2003, Dr. Michael Lipkind noted higher photon emissions from cell cultures infected with viruses when compared with healthy cell controls. Virus-infected cells not only had higher but also more peculiar ranges than the more standardized ranges coming from healthy cells. The peculiarity of the virus emissions also closely correlated with the virus replication cycles. These results closely corresponded with the tumor-cell growth studies done by Professor Popp.

In a study by Dr. Chwirot and associates published in 2003, colon lesion cells were measured for biophoton activity after removal with surgery from diseased patients. The biophoton levels significantly differed in colon lesion cells as compared with healthy colon mucosal cells. This has led some to suggest that photon emission testing could be an effective tool in diagnosing colon cancers and lesions.

Further biophoton investigations determined that greater toxic loads in living cells resulted in greater photon emission. As the toxin levels or stressors increased, the emission levels increased. This was confirmed in other studies of plant responses to stressors. Higher lipoxygenase and peroxidase levels in plants correlated with higher emission levels.

Human cell membranes interact intimately with ions such as sodium, potassium and other electron-transporting mechanisms like ATPase. The electro-chemical aspects of ions led to our early discoveries of electricity and its magnetic field qualities. This is because ions are electromagnetic messengers. Ions are activated with pulsed electromagnetic fields. This provides a means to carry and exchange waveform information. As the ionic waveform messaging interacts with other waveform messages from other sources, an interference pattern results, creating a complex information mapping system.

Ion channels have been observed transferring chemical charges and communicating processes such as glucose utilization and immune response between cell membranes and intercellular tissues. These electro-chemical pathways have been correlated with biophoton emissions, illustrating the reality that information-messaging systems exist on more than a chemical basis. Biophoton research indicates that although each cell and each individual appears to emit unique waveforms, a significant level of coherence is observed between photon emissions of various cells. More significantly, coherence is observed as these emissions are broken down into their respective spectra. Coherent waveforms create informational interference patterns—either destructive (reducing) or constructive (expanding). The coherency factor became relevant to Dr. Popp and his fellow researchers as it provided a rational holistic model for information transmission within the body (Popp and Yan 2002; Li 1981; Popp 2003).

In other words, bioemissions are bound together into substantial messages by a common, coherent thread: *Conscious intention.*

Communication messaging systems correlating biophoton activity were demonstrated with *dinoflaggellates* by Chang and Popp in 1994. A dinoflaggellate is a single cell organism that typically lives in the ocean or fresh waters of the world. Many plankton species are dinoflaggellates. Though single-celled, they have tremendous complexity, yielding cellulose armor plates for defense, and the ability to change structural shape to give them tremendous propulsion for escape. They also convert sunlight to nutritional energy. Dinoflaggellates thus provide the foundation for the nutrient content of the marine habitat. They also emit bioluminescence.

Most of us have heard about or experienced the nighttime phosphorescent sparkling of the ocean's surface during plankton blooms. This bioluminescence is a biophoton event, occurring at a wavelength perceivable by human retinal cells. When *lingulodinium polydrum* blooms in red tide events, for example, the billions of dinoflagellates will turn the seashore waters phosphorescent blue. It is quite an awesome scene.

Biologists now reason that dinoflagellates are communicating on a grander level during these bioluminescence events. These communications are referred to as *quorum sensing*. Quorum sensing is created when small organisms communicate a general consciousness to make a mass change when they have significant enough numbers. Pathogenic microorganisms also have this capability within the body. This is why common yeasts like *Candida albicans* can exist in the body without any detriment, but once they grow to certain populations, they can overwhelm other populations of symbiotics or probiotics, and burden the body with various symptoms. Not unlike what is seen among the dinoflagellates, *Candida* microorganisms coordinate with waveform messaging to expand their colonies to take advantage of times of weakened immunity within the host.

Gradually we are learning just how smart other organisms large and small are. Marine researchers have realized for example that sharks actually have keen senses and the ability to 'see' their prey by picking up subtle waveforms. In addition to a keen sense of smell and rather good eyesight, the shark has a series of *electroreceptors* positioned within lateral line channels throughout the shark's head, running down the length of the body into the tail. Many fish and even amphibians also have lateral line organs, allowing the fish to sense various waveforms from the surrounding water environment. In sharks, these lateral line channels are implanted with sensors that allow a shark to pick up subtle electromagnetic pulses of life in its environment. This allows sharks to recognize targets or enemies hiding within the sand or in murky waters. These electroreceptors can also sense motion from extreme distances. The shark can identify the splashing of a seal pup up to two miles away, for example. Through these sensory ampules, a shark can also sense fear or panic among other organisms. What is the shark sensing with these electroreceptors? These are the organism's combined biophoton emissions—waveforms reflecting conscious emotions—given off by the unlucky living organism.

These various waveform processes illustrate the connection between cellular biophoton emissions and message reception. Ion channel transport systems existing within and around each of our cells combine with our DNA's molecular bonding structures to crystallize instructional messaging. Together these systems provide the basis for cellular communication and broadcasting mechanisms. This biophoton messaging system also provides the mechanisms for the holographic display of brain waveforms during vision, hearing and other sense perception, as will be covered in depth later.

Cellular division and replication is the culmination of these biophoton messaging systems. The specific traits of the cell—its genetic blueprint of the body's metabolism—are communicated during this process. The higher levels of photon emissions picked up by researchers during replication illustrate this effect. We can conclude that the basic messaging systems of the body are multi-layered and complex. They provide for a smart mapping network of waveforms, wholly unobservable in cadaver dissection.

As we survey the empirical evidence, we arrive at the reality that along with specialized metabolic functions, each cell is a communication device. Each cell is designed to both receive and transmit information. This exchange of information occurs between cells and the outside environment, between one cell and another, and between each cell and the body's various messaging systems stemming from its master guidance systems.

Ion Pathways

Cells might be compared to smart radio-driven generators with multi-layered reception and transmission communication systems. As physiologists have delved deeper into the activities of the estimated trillion cells in the human body, they have continued to see increasingly deeper levels of biocommunication activity amongst the electrolyte ions within and around the cell. Increasingly, we are finding that ion channels provide a window into this complex network of conscious information messaging.

The ion channel is an informational device because it establishes an on-off state in the form of an open or closed gateway. Actually, the gateway of most ion channels is even a bit more complex. Research has indicated that one of three possible states is produced within the typical ion channel gateway: deactivation, activation or inactivation. Both a deactivated state and an inactivated state are closed, while an activated state is open. The difference between the two closed states is that a deactivated gate is blocked by an opposing open gate, while the inactive gate is simply closed in process after activation. In other words, the latter produces a rhythmic opening and closing adherent to voltage potential changes.

One of the most prominent potential conductors in the body is the sodium ion. Sodium ions negotiate electromagnetic waveforms efficiently. *Sodium channels* thus lie within cell membranes of the most active cells in the body, including muscle and nerve cells. These protein complexes are activated by the voltage potential changes provided by sodium ions as they cycle through their biochemical processes. In response to ionic state changes, many sodium channels will generate a change in electric potential inside the cell by conducting sodium ions through the cell membrane. By changing the cell's electrical potential, the cell's inner polarity and reactive potential with various nutrients and biochemicals will change. This will stimulate particular types of biological processes within the cell. Among sodium channels are various subunit types—specialized for a particular cellular activity, organ or tissue system.

Potassium channels exist in almost every cell in the body. They are involved in regulating the secretion and reception of various types of hormones. Potassium channels also lie primarily within the cell membrane. Much like the sodium channels, they provide voltage gates through which potassium ion charges can travel. Potassium channels are activated by various means with specific response ranges. A newly discovered type of potassium channel system is the double-pore system, quite extraordinary compared to the mostly single pore system of other known ionic channels. This double-pore potassium channel is thought to be a complex regulator in vascular cells—it stimulates tone and flexibility to the artery walls.

Calcium channels provide another type of voltage circuit. Calcium ion channels are found among various specialized cells in brain, organ, and nerve systems. The calcium gateways have been linked with an informational depolarization process. This turns on and off the release of various neurotransmitters and hormones. Like the sodium and potassium channels, calcium channels have various subunit types. These will often produce specific results within specialized cells.

Chloride channels appear to be related to regulating the cell's nutritional contents. No less than thirteen different types of chloride channels have been discovered. Each type regulates different nutrients and informational functions within different types of cells.

These are merely the tip of the iceberg. There are trillions of waveform channels throughout the body. Information flows through each and every one constantly. Other types of voltage potential channels have been isolated by research over recent years. *Cation channels* are activated through a combination of ions. They predominate within sperm cells. Cation-selective double pore channels provide both inward and outward voltage potential changes. *Rhodopsin channels* are activated open through the reception of light. *Transient receptor potential channels*—also called TRPs—have so far been observed among fruit flies. Many scientists suspect these also within humans. TRPs are channels that respond to photoelectric waveforms. There are a number of different types of TRPs with various functions. Another type of voltage channel is the *cyclic nucleotide channel.* These are thought to regulate the entry of various ions and nucleotides, which drive energy use and cellular clockworks activity. The heart's pacemaker neurons function extensively with cyclic nucleotide channels, for example. To the billions of channels of the types mentioned above, we can add the cAMP and IP3 channels, and many others.

There are about 80 known macro and trace minerals in the body. As nutritional research into macro minerals has continued, we have gradually come to understand that every mineral plays an important role. Should the human body be lacking in any of these elements, imbalances in metabolism begin to occur. Some of the more prevalent macro minerals include, among others, calcium, potassium, magnesium, sodium and phosphorus. These are called macro because they exist in larger quantities in the body. These minerals contribute to the ionic informational activities of the vast legions of catalysts, proteins, enzymes, cell walls, artery walls, and so many other structural elements of the body's anatomy. They also facilitate communications between cells by providing gateway messaging mechanisms.

All the trace and macro minerals are vital to metabolism. The balance between both macro and trace elements is one of the key governing factors in maintaining physiological balance. Zinc, for example, was long considered not that critical to health. Some thought that zinc was poisonous. Recent research has found that this trace element is a key factor for at least one hundred enzyme and immune system processes. Zinc is a participant in immune function, growth, wound repair, DNA production and enzyme reaction. Without zinc, the body will function in a depressed immune state. Immunity will drop. Foods will taste bland. Today zinc is considered a critical mineral.

It might be surprising that other important trace elements include fluorine, cadmium, copper, chlorine and even uranium are also utilized by the body, albeit in minute quantities. In larger quantities, these elements can be toxic. They are nonetheless essential for many metabolic functions. They are each involved directly or indirectly in innumerable enzyme functions, protein sequencing, immune cell composition and many other functions. Without a consistent source of trace elements, our body's metabolic operations quickly become handicapped.

Each mineral ion provides a specific polarity and covalence for sub-atomic bonding. Each also provides a unique facility for waveform conductance. Conducting ions provide a bridge for information transmission throughout the body. Mineral-conducting waveforms converge through a variety of ion bridges and channels into interference patterns. From these interference patterns, instructional messages emerge. This might be compared to putting a hand in front of a projector screen. The hand blocks part of the light, allowing the opportunity to communicate through various hand gestures. These hand gestures can communicate an idea or shape. The interference between the hand and the light enable the communication. A mineral might be compared to the hand, with each type of mineral and mineral combination providing a different shape. Just as standard 110 household current can be manipulated by the appliance and transformed into specific functions, minerals provide an ion bridge to energy transfer and biomolecules with mineral combinations provide translating devices.

Interference patterns created from viewing different visual spectrum waveforms through the retina and optic nerve also provide good illustrations. Each light and color reflection waveform seemingly has no meaning alone. When waveforms converge within an interference pattern, however, they create information packages. During cellular reactions, tiny electromagnetic waveforms work to define which reaction will occur when. The specific assembly of minerals provides the basis for the molecular combinations that create the appropriate electromagnetic interference patterns.

The respective interference patterns created by the waveforms transferred through an assembly of minerals and ions form the instructional messages that turn on and off specific biochemical reactions. Without this instructional messaging system, there would be no operational control over the body's reactions. They would simply begin randomly and after beginning, they would run indefinitely, out of control.

This is on-off state is starkly illustrated by the inflammatory pathway. The body responds to an injury with a number of inflammatory repair cells such as plasmin and fibrin to patch up the injury. Blood will usually coalesce around the injury to deliver these and other nutrients required to repair the wound. At some point in the process, signaling molecules will stop the inflammatory process, and initiate a clean out of the area to allow for the next steps of the healing process. Cortisol has been seen as involved as one of the key switching messengers. As cortisol levels increase, inflammation is reduced. Pharmaceutical medicine has discovered this link, prompting today's mass prescription of cortisone-based pharmaceuticals. The switching message communicated by cortisol is transmitted via the electromagnetic molecular structure of cortisol. Without cortisol, the inflammatory process would run out of control.

Cortisol also modulates both sodium and potassium concentrations within the body. It also modulates insulin levels and stimulates gastric juices, and stimulates copper-based enzyme functions such as superoxide dismutase. All of these functions are driven by the messenger functions of the cortisol molecule. Cortisol's molecular structure is made up of a combination of carbon, hydrogen and oxygen, just as are many of the body's molecules. It is the unique combination of electromagnetic bonds between the hydrogen and oxygen ions that facilitate cortisol's multifarious abilities. The commingled arrangement of their electromagnetic waveform interference patterns enables its unique messaging.

In traditional chemistry, acids and bases are defined in hydrogen atoms—or proton proportions. An acid is typically described as a substance with an excess of hydrogen atoms ($H+$), which acts as a net proton donor. A base, on the other hand, is considered either a hydroxide ($OH-$) donor or a proton acceptor—a substance often described as having excessive electrons. Net charge is also used to describe these solutions. An acid solution is one with a net positive charge, while a base solution has a net negative charge. An acid is often referred to as *cationic* (with cations) because it has a positive net charge, while a base will have a negative charge and thus is referred to as an *anion*.

We can also describe this in the more suitable context of electromagnetic waveforms. The imbalance between units of positively oriented waveforms and units of negatively oriented waveforms creates the measure of its acidic or basic state. This "orientation" is purported to compose of quantum mechanical elements. We can summarize these as containing multi-dimensional magnetic fields with unique spin directions. As mentioned, every electronic wave is accompanied by a perpendicular magnetic field. This field also relates to the spin orientation and magnetic field direction of the molecule.

A measurement of the level of acidity or alkalinity using a logarithmic scale is called pH. The term pH is derived from the French word for hydrogen power, *pouvoir hydrogene,* which has been abbreviated as simply pH. pH is measured in an inverse log base-10 scale, measuring the proton-donor level by comparing it to a theoretical quantity of hydrogen ions (H+) in a solution. Thus, a pH of 5 would be equivalent to 10^5 H+ *moles* worth of cations in the solution. (A mole is a quantity of substance compared to 12 grams of the six-neutron carbon isotope.) Put another way, a pCl (chlorine) concentration would be the negative log of chlorine ion concentration in a solution, and pK would be the negative log of potassium ions in a solution.

The pH scale is 0 to 14, for 10^{-1} (1) to 10^{-14} (.00000000000001) range. The scale has been set up around the fact that pure water's pH is log-7 or simply pH7. Because pure water forms the basis for so many of life's activities, and because water neutralizes and dilutes so many reactions, water became the standard reference and neutral point between an acid and a base. In other words, a substance having greater hydrogen ion concentration characteristics than water will be considered a base, while a substance containing less H+ concentration characteristics than water is considered an acid.

Of course, a solution concentration may well be lower than log-14 or higher than log-1, but this is the scale set up based upon the typical ranges observed in nature. Using this scale, any substance measuring a pH of 7 would be considered a neutral substance, though it still has a significant number of H+ ions. In humans, a pH level in the range of 6.4 is considered a healthy state because this state is slightly more acidic than water, enabling alkaline ionic current flow through the body. Better put, a 6.4 pH offers the appropriate currency of energy flow because there are enough negatively oriented waveforms present for the passage of positively oriented messaging waveforms. The earthly minerals like potassium, calcium, magnesium and others are typically positively oriented—or alkaline in nature. They thus carry the messaging (and thus nutritional) waveforms transmitted through our living earth.

The proof to these points is provided by conventional science: pH is simplified in conventional chemistry as the level of proton donor capability. Yet we know from emission measurements that the higher the electron orbit, the higher the energy emission. Energy release is measured by waveform emission characteristics such as frequency. If we remove the concept of electron particles from the equation, and replace with this the understanding of wave mechanics, we can then realize that the charge (or message) is *traveling through* a particular medium, and the pH of the substance simply measures the type of messaging able to move through that medium. This is why pH meters are voltage meters.

This concept of current traveling through a medium is understood when we consider how an electric charge can be maintained by a battery. A lead battery is set up to perform two reactions (stated conventionally): One reaction oxidizes lead—in a solution of sulfuric acid—to lead sulfate. During this reaction, energy is given off as electrons are emitted, along with hydrogen protons. The other reaction is a reduction, which converts lead dioxide to lead sulfate. This also releases energy, but this is accomplished as hydrogen protons and electrons are being absorbed to create the lead sulfate. Meanwhile, two types of lead plates attract and adhere to the resulting lead sulfates. The positive plates are filled with lead dioxide to drive the oxidation side, while the negative plates are made of lead to drive the reduction side of the battery. These two processes combine to be called *electrolysis,* which is the utilization of ions to conduct current through a particular medium.

We note in this discussion the obvious: Batteries—between their positive and negative poles—exchange an electrical current. This current is used in an automobile to start the engine, after which a generator will create enough electromagnetic energy to recharge the battery. This event reverses the changes to the lead, lead dioxide and sulfuric acid. We must also note that the initial flow of electricity out of the battery is not a spontaneous reaction, nor is the recharging of the battery. Both of these processes have been designed and assembled by humans with the conscious intention to draw a flow of electricity for a specific purpose: To start our automobile for example. Intent is also needed to keep the battery charged. If our car were not in use for a while, the battery would gradually lose its charge, requiring an intentional charge-up.

As we examine the currency properties of the living body, we recognize the same general features of the battery. The living body performs a number of reactions, some oxidizing and some reducing. In most of these reactions, energy is converted from one type to another—a conversion of electromagnetic bonding energy into different forms of kinetic energy such as movement via muscle cells. The exact utilization of the energy is steered by consciousness, which steers usage. The principal energy conversion of glucose and oxygen into the energies mentioned is a complex oxidative reaction called the Krebs cycle. This Krebs cycle will utilize the waveform bonds of ADP to ATP to generate a transport mechanism, which results in energy and ion release. The body also has similar energy conversion mechanisms such as the NADP transport system. These are only two of the billions of ionic conversion systems working within the human physiology.

All metabolism operates on this waveform conversion process. Our sensory nerves all conduct impulses through waveform ionic exchanges. Taste is driven by the acid or alkaline nature of our foods. Acidic solutions taste sour while alkaline solutions taste bitter. As we taste food, particular waveform orientations set off a chain of ionic messaging through the nervous system. Our taste buds, retinal cells, olfactory bulbs and tactile nerve endings all have similar waveform sensing electrodes with ionic gateways. The different types of waveforms emitted by physical matter simply stimulate these gateways, setting off an ionic charge relay within the body's sensory nervous systems. This relay results in interference patterns within the brain, effectively producing perception.

Biochemical Transmission

Since Loewi's research illustrating the involvement of chemistry in physiological messaging, we have learned a lot about the wave nature of sub-atomic elements, atoms, ions and molecules. Biochemical information pathways have been clearly established. It is evident that within these biochemicals exists a more subtle form of information transmission. This is illustrated by the incredible speed and accuracy of biocommunication within the body. The entire body—all its organs, blood vessels, and other tissue systems—will react instantly to a sensory perception of something potentially harmful. Through an intentionally driven networked biocommunication pathway, the signal of impending danger is broadcast to billions of cells and muscle fibers throughout the body instantaneously— enabling the body to immediately respond to a threat to its survival.

Most researchers are convinced that each hormonal instruction requires that hormone molecules (ligands) must physically touch chemical receptors. This notion was advanced in the early twentieth century by Dr. Morgan Hunt, who discovered a protein existing within the cell membrane—part in and part out. This protein was observed as a switching mechanism, receiving particular ligand instructions, and translating that to the cell's nucleus for activation. This protein was called the *notch gene,* and the notch-transport system of cellular communication has been described as one of the major cell communication pathways that instigated particular metabolic activities and coordination between other cells. Notch information biocommunication was observed among cardiac cells, neurons, bone cells (osteocytes), glandular cells and many others, progressing and stimulating some of their most critical functions. These *transmembrane protein receptors* are purported to require physical contact with a particular ligand, but is often accelerated through a catalyst enzyme process.

It is also assumed that intercellular communication requires physical molecular contact. This is often referred to as *paracrine* activity— messages being translated from one nearby cell to another. In comparison, *intracrines* are considered the cellular messengers within the cell, while *intercrines* are cell-to-cell messengers. Note in this respect that *endocrines* are biochemical messengers produced by specific glands, which are circulated around the body. Each of these messengers is assumed to require a physical chemical interaction between the ligand and its particular receptor.

Two cells are also thought to have what is considered a direct nucleus-to-nucleus interaction. This appears to occur through a type of direct-nucleus receptor called a *connexin protein*. When six of these proteins come together within a group, they form a pore or tube within the membrane called a *gap junction*. This allows cells to exchange genetic instructions, or one cell to inject instructions into another cell.

Many receptors lie on the surface of the cell membrane. Most are connected to ion channels between the cell membrane. These provide a transduction channel for the information to pass from the receptor to within the cell. Many neurotransmitters and hormones utilize this pathway to transmit their information. The assumption is that the ligand (hormone or neurotransmitter) *binds* with the receptor on a chemical basis, creating an electrical signal, which is transmitted through the ion channel.

These assumptions come from observations of ligand biochemicals in the vicinity of physical response. Sometimes new compounds are evident, theoretically indicating a possible binding reaction. It has been justly assumed that these neurochemical molecules must be intimately involved in the dissemination of metabolic messages. However, the notion that physical-chemical touch is required in all cases and among all endocrine transmissions appears unlikely, given the coordinated and instantaneous cell response on a global basis. A physical molecular connection between hormones and receptors on each and every cell membrane—even with some cells communicating with paracrines—would require circulation time for the master hypothalamic hormones, pituitary hormones and endocrine gland hormone pathways to execute simultaneously. It would require enough hormones to be secreted fully into the bloodstream, and physically be pumped from the endocrine glands—sometimes halfway around the body—to chemically and physically touch the appropriate receptor on *every* cell involved in the metabolic change.

Let us consider this scenario carefully. A receptor is a protein with an electromagnetic affinity. This requires either a polarity match, or even a constructive combination of spin or angular momentum between the ligand and receptor. In the human body, it is estimated there is one protein molecule for every 10,000 molecules in and around the cells of the body. Furthermore, there are about 200 trillion cells in the human body, and billions if not trillions of them are activated immediately in fearful or stressful response. Every cell in the toes must be activated immediately to break into an immediate run for example. According to the physical ligand-receptor theory, not only does each hormone molecule have to connect with each and every cell membrane, but each hormone must also locate an open, active receptor on every cell membrane.

Observation and *in vitro* testing has shown receptors to have four basic scenarios: They can be *agonized,* or stimulated. They can be *partially agonized* of partly stimulated. They can be *inversely agonized,* and their response lowered. They can also be *antagonized,* whereby they are blocked by a molecule and thereby not be stimulated. So we ask: How is it these hormones can intelligently weave through every tiny capillary and dense maze of tissue systems to bump into the right receptor without being agonized on every needed cell instantaneously? Now if we perceived parts of our body being activated first and then other parts, corresponding to the circulatory routes these hormones or neurotransmitters take, we might be able to agree with this hypothesis. Consider circulatory restrictions such as atherosclerosis and other artery diseases restricting blood flow. In addition, consider that many tissue cells are reached only through tiny microcapillaries—some barely large enough to be able to allow a single red blood cell through at a time within the diameter of the lumen (the opening). If a response required the blood to deliver a hormone molecule to a receptor on every cell within a particular tissue system before that tissue system could respond, we would really be in trouble if we needed to run from an attacker.

We could only imagine the situation where we were frightened by a tiger in the woods, only to find that our upper hamstrings were ready to take off but our toes were not—leaving us stuck while the tiger pounced. Rather, the toes, hamstrings, knees and every skeletal muscle cell, along with the eyes, lungs, brain, and vocal cords all respond at the same moment as we scream and run instantaneously.

The body's process of stimulating metabolic activity has been a mystery to researchers for thousands of years. In modern research, the process of discovery has been to identify hormone presence using radiography with dye markers to trace the flow of chemicals. This physical 'snap-shot' process is combined with harvesting and analyzing organ chemistry with spectroscopic analysis. Via these two methods, researchers figure that since the hormone/ligands are in the proximity of the response, they must be physically setting off the response of each and every cell. This is often confirmed with the techniques pioneered by Loewi to provide the conclusion. While conferring biochemical presence, finding biochemicals in the region offers no conclusive mechanism. We might compare this to finding a gun near a murder victim. We can assume the gun was involved, but this fact alone does not tell us who shot the murder victim.

For example, we know the thyroid gland is one of the central endocrine drivers of metabolism. Researchers have linked cellular metabolic rates and thermogenesis to the presence of thyroid hormones thyroxine and triiodothyronine. These are also referred to as T4 and T3, respectively. The chemical makeup of these messengers are not that exciting—a combination of the amino acid tyrosine and iodine. However, these rather simple molecular structures T4 and T3 somehow charge trillions of cells throughout the body—increasing the speed and output of their various metabolic processes. Without enough of either T4 or T3 (T3 is considered to be the more active of the two, but T3 is derived from T4) the body begins to cool down. A feeling of fatigue will overwhelm a thyroid hormone-deficient body. Suddenly the most basic tasks become difficult in TSH (thyroid stimulating hormone), T3 or T4 deficiencies. The thyroid also produces calcitonin, which works with parathyroid hormone to balance bone calcium levels.

Once the blood contains enough thyroid hormones it becomes almost suddenly energized. This is evidenced by the oral intake of synthetic and analogous thyroid hormones. How again do all those trillions of cells become energized from a pill or two? Again, the theory of cell reception requires that each cell has a set of little chemical receptor 'locks' on its cell membrane, and these ligand chemicals provide the 'keys.' Thus, each cell receptor must be physically touched and unlocked with those chemical ligands. Are there enough moles of chemicals in one or two pills to circulate through the blood system and basal membrane and reach every cell's receptors to energize them? Or perhaps the paracrine system provides a mechanism for filling the gap for cells the chemicals do not physically bind to?

This problem is complicated by the fact that thyroid hormones are hydrophobic—they are not water-friendly. They are not water-soluble. Since the blood, the cells, and their basal surroundings are mostly water, this makes their journey to every cell difficult. Perhaps thyroid hormones require thyroxine-binding globulins, transthyrein and albumins for adequate circulation. It is thought that these may provide a carrier mechanism to each cell. Somehow, these chemical messengers T3 and T4 manage to instantly and simultaneously make their way around the body to stimulate and energize each cell. In other words, the neck does not warm up first, and then the arms warm up, and so on. All the body parts will become energized simultaneously with some exception for diseased tissue systems.

The cell membrane is composed of a variety of lipids—cholesterol, phospholipids and sphingolipids—specialized proteins and glycoproteins. The lipids making up most cell membranes are structurally double-layered and arranged to prevent unwanted molecules from passing through the membrane. The lipid wall is also hydrophobic—keeping water from penetrating the surface without passing through the cell membrane's complex ion channels.

Some cell membranes—particularly in nerve cells—are *myelin*. Others are *inner mitochondrial* in nature. Mitochondrial inner membranes are made up of electron transport proteins, while a myelin membrane will be composed primarily of plasma with less protein. The lipid cell membrane is negatively charged. This sets up an ionic gradient between the inside and the outside of the cell membrane. Crossing the cell membrane is not a physical experience for most molecules—it is primarily an electromagnetic crossing. Water and nutrients are escorted through the membrane through ionic diffusion. This is complicated by the various proteins that electromagnetically identify substances as they pass. Mineral ions pass through the cell membrane via *ionic transport chains*. Ionic transport chains made from protein are similar to ion channels except they allow entry to key nutrients and minerals needed in the cell—particularly sodium, potassium and calcium but also many trace elements. These ions provide just the right electromagnetic environment to set up channels for ionic instructional messages to pass through the cell membrane into the cytoplasm, where they can stimulate RNA, mitochondria and other organelles into action. Thus, the cell membrane's ionic transport mechanisms escort appropriate nutrients in and out of cell, while receptors receive and transmit the messages of hormones like thyroid hormones, insulin, and acetylcholine through ion channels into the cell.

Some might contend that some biochemical messengers are delivered through tissue spaces and ion channels. Yes, certainly there are basal channels that provide access. Still we must remember the adrenal gland is a very small gland in the abdominal region of the body. The thyroid gland is a tiny gland in the neck. To assume that cortisol, epinephrine, acetylcholine, and thyroid hormones must jettison from these tiny organs to every cell—even in fingers and toes—to stimulate the correct cellular and tissue responses should these appendages come under attack is a stretch. Certainly, a strictly physical chemical delivery system would result in a lot more missing fingers and toes than we generally see.

It is interesting that we can accept that informational messages can travel instantly throughout the body via the nervous system. The nervous system can stimulate a particular skeletal muscle system to activate instantly. The ability of all the support systems to come into play, however, is the result of these biochemical informational messenger systems. A perfect example is vasopressin's ability to concentrate urine in the kidneys and constrict artery walls.

Environmental drivers of hormones include light, temperature, gravity, the changing seasons, and cellular metabolism. Internal drivers, however, stem from emotional consciousness. Hormones are complex body chemicals, made of either glycoproteins or steroids. Among other functions, hormones turn on cellular switches for many metabolic functions. Growth hormones encourage cellular growth. Thyroid hormones regulate cellular metabolism speed and temperature regulation. Follicle stimulating hormones and luteinizing hormones stimulate reproductive mechanisms. Insulin stimulates the clearing and attachment of glucose into cells for energy production. Vasopressin stimulates the decreases urine volume, constricts blood vessel walls and stimulates certain memory functions. Cortisol counteracts insulin, inhibits immune system processes such as inflammation and lymphocyte function, stimulates increased circulation and blood pressure, helps regulate potassium/sodium balance, stimulates stomach acids, increases glucogenesis to name a few.

These are just a few of the hundreds of messaging hormones that make up the complex waveform broadcasting system working within the body. Hormones are directly and indirectly involved guiding all of the physical body's various mechanisms. Hormones turn on and shut off genetic switches in particular cells, typically through stimulating the transmembrane receptors. Hormones work primarily within pathways often referred to as *cascades*. As in the 'domino-effect,' a cascade is the progressive stimulation of one activity, which in turn stimulates another. These cascades fire at tremendous speeds, as ligand-receptor triggers initiate pathways of stimulating mechanisms.

An example of a cascading messaging system is the response stimulated by sensory sensation occurring somewhere in the body and transmitted through the neurons to the brain. The pre-programmed sympathetic response (the reflex arc) is typically accompanied by conscious reception of the sensation via the limbic system. The focal point of this stimulation is the thalamus, which acts as a waveform message translator and decoder. Waveform-transmitting neurons deep within the thalamus are engaged, stimulating waves that combine with others to form an interference pattern—also referred to as a neural mapping. As these waveform interference patterns are decoded, some are reflected back to the cerebral cortex. Here an exchange of waveform patterns takes place. A relay of information is conducted between the cerebral cortex and the thalamus, reflecting the information back onto the prefrontal cortex. Here the information is responded to, followed by a return of pulses that stimulate the hypothalamus gland to secrete biochemicals. These biochemical messengers either stimulate endocrine or cellular function directly, or stimulate the pituitary gland to in turn secrete biochemical messengers that precisely activate endocrine glands and physical response.

The hypothalamus, located at the base of the brain under the thalamus, encapsulates part of the third ventricle. The body's autonomic responses are processed here, some of which in turn stimulate the pituitary gland to release key master hormones. These master hormones signal responses that control the critical phase cycles of metabolism, body core temperature, appetite, thirst and so on.

The hypothalamus responds to waveform inputs from the brain centers and limbic system. These brain centers provide the platforms for conscious interaction with waveform messaging. Waveform interference patterns are created from the various sensory nerve transmissions and response neurotransmitter biochemicals. These interactive interference patterns form the basis for information. This facilitates perspective, and allows a sorting process to prioritize the information within the limbic system. Stresses on the body such as infection and immune response also feed into the limbic system for response. For these waveforms, the hypothalamus activates immediate response cascades using the limbic system's programming.

The hypothalamus and limbic system thus respond to a wide range of stimuli, and construct biochemical responses by activating an orchestrated flow of biochemical messengers to stimulate particular physical responses around the body. Dispatched messengers include dopamine, melatonin, somatostatin and others. The hypothalamus also secretes hypothalamic hormones that stimulate the pituitary to produce a number of master endocrine hormones.

The hypothalamic hormones are sent through the hypophyseal capillary beds before they are delivered to the pituitary gland. Once arriving at the pituitary, these biochemical messengers instruct the pituitary gland to secrete specific 'master' hormones. These in turn stimulate particular endocrine glands and regions around the body to produce yet another level of biochemical messengers. These instructional biochemicals include growth hormones, adrenocorticotropic hormones, luteinizing hormones, follicle-stimulating hormones, prolactins, estrogens, testosterone, thyroid stimulating hormones; as well as neurotransmitters like adrenaline, serotonin, acetylcholine and others.

Amazingly, the subsidiary endocrine glands and tissue centers receive the master hormone messages rather instantly, and react instantly by initiating the release of even more specific informational biochemical messengers. These are hormones and neurotransmitters that precisely and directly affect the body's cellular metabolism, organ function and tissue mechanisms. As we all have experienced, the messages stimulate action almost instantly, at tremendous speeds—perhaps at speeds at or above the speed of light. So not only does the limbic system and master glands respond instantly to sensory stimuli, but the entire cascading system responds instantaneously with biochemical messenger cascades that broadcast precise instructions throughout our body's physiology.

Adrenocorticotropic hormone or ACTH is a good example. ACTH is produced by the anterior pituitary gland. Its function is to stimulate the adrenal cortex to release cortisol, and to a lesser degree androgens such as testosterone. The adrenal cortex also produces aldosterone, which stimulates the retention of urine and heightened blood pressure, involved in the renin and angiotensin cycle. The adrenal medulla is also stimulated by sympathetic nerves into producing epinephrine and norepinephrine. Epinephrine is considered a fight-or-flight hormone because it stimulates glycogen and fat breakdown while increasing the heart rate, dilating the pupils and stimulating a number of cognition mechanisms. Epinephrine also stimulates a cascade that constricts some blood vessels while dilating others—namely those feeding needed muscles. An intelligent gating pathway through the liver using inositol and liver enzymes activates glucose release to coordinate with this. Epinephrine's intelligent combination of constriction in vessels effectively diverts blood and nutrients from unnecessary tissues to those deemed necessary for a well-coordinated fight-or-flight response. How does a chemical—a combination of hydrogen, carbon, oxygen and nitrogen—make this sort of distinction? How does it decide which way to divert circulation? How does it know which muscles will be needed? Can a simple chemical make these sorts of judgments—instantly?

Medical researchers believe this is driven by epinephrine's ability to stimulate multiple receptors, most notably the alpha-1 and beta-2 receptors. The alpha-1 tends to stimulate a liver signaling process affecting insulin, while the beta-2 tends to stimulate the process of converting glycogen to glucose. However, this simplistic version of the process can hardly explain how this hormone can instantly gear the body up for fight or flight mode while concurrently coordinating which tissue groups are fed and which tissue groups are starved.

The pituitary gland also produces follicle-stimulating hormone, which stimulates the ovarian follicle to produce estrogen in women. It also stimulates the testes to produce sperm in men. Estrogens are complex because they will assist in the development of female sex organs and female characteristics like breasts, while they also stimulate the uterine environment by expanding the endometrium at the early part of the menstrual cycle. Indeed, the rhythmic cycles of menstruation and ovulation, and of pre- peri- and post-menopause tell us that estrogens also have complex messaging pathways within various tissue mechanisms—some significantly affecting moods and nerve activity. Testosterone is also complex, as its levels relate not just to prostate health in men, but also to general vitality and overall health among both men and women.

Although modern medical science has assumed a physical proximity particle-molecule receptor binding mechanism for hormone effects within the body, it is a rather academic debate because at the same time, science is thoroughly aware that there is no touching within the subatomic atmosphere of atoms and molecules. Quantum mechanics and the law of uncertainty tell us that subatomic units are particle-waves, which rotate around the nucleus at dramatic relative distances. As atoms merge to become molecules, a sharing of particle-wave orbitals takes place. These orbitals do not have the ability to come into physical contact with each other within the molecule. So even in the paradigm of a ligand bonding with physical proximity to a receptor to create a new molecule, there is only a sharing of electromagnetic orbitals involved, which are of course waveform in nature.

Logically, while we can say that close proximity orbital binding can and does occur with some messaging, the nature of the electromagnetic exchange of information logically should not require physical proximity to transfer the message. We might compare this with two people standing next to each other exchanging information. They conduct this exchange through speaking. The nature of speaking is such that the two people could easily stand further away from each other and still exchange the information through speaking. They may have to speak a little louder, but the passing of the information would suffer no deficiency between standing next to each other and standing several feet apart.

The biochemical signaling process comes without the merit of observation, albeit indirect. Scientists cannot open up a human intercellular process and analyze the process to determine the exact mode of biocommunication. However, lab researchers can isolate a complex metabolic process requiring a signaling event, and run a chemical analysis on the whole region to see what chemical changes occurred. Before and after chemical analyses (typically via centrifuge followed by mass spectrometry, or possibly electron microscope) will illustrate a chemical change within the region. A change in the composition would infer that the biocommunication coincided with the ligand-receptor exchange. However, this does require an initial assumption that the biocommunication process is indeed biochemical-driven.

With confirmed research results, we cannot deny there was a chemical reaction that coincided with the biocommunication. The question that arises, however, is whether the chemical reaction caused the biocommunication event or whether the biocommunication event caused the chemical reaction. It is altogether possible that one of the byproducts of the biocommunication transmission was a chemical reaction. Chemical changes often coincide with waveform transmissions. The microwaving of food will likely create a chemical change in the food, for example. The sun's rays often spark composition reactions in soil and water as well. In fact, most electromagnetic waveform transmissions result in chemical reactions of some sort, because the waveforms interfere with the electromagnetic bonds within molecules of the substance being struck, creating a chemical response.

This basic question of which comes first might be compared to seeing some blood in a hungry shark's tank and assuming the blood made the shark hungry. It is quite possible (and probably more likely) that the shark was hungry before the water was bloody. It is more likely that the shark's hunger drove him to eat, making the tank bloody from the fish he ate. This is also logical, noting shark behavior.

This is not such a fantastic supposition. Every type of communication signal we receive externally is transmitted via waveforms. The most basic signaling event, vision, is signaled via visible electromagnetic radiation. When we look at a star billions of light years away, we are seeing waveform transmissions that may have traveled for several days or even years before reaching our eyes. Hearing is also a waveform-stimulated process, as our inner ears convert air pressure waves to electromagnetic pulses. If the body conducts its most basic communication events via waveform signaling, why should we assume cells should not share those capabilities? Do we feel our cells are any less technical than the rest of our bodies?

This does not necessitate us completely abandoning the *lock-and-key* mechanisms theorized between ligands and receptors. Waveform communications can also be compared to a lock-and-key mechanism. The concept of the receptor simply has to be expanded to include waveform communications. It is also altogether possible that ligands can stimulate the biocommunication through the lock-an-key biochemical basis in addition to remote biocommunication signaling.

We might justly compare this mechanism with our ability to turn on and off a television. We can either walk up to the television and turn it off by pressing the on-off button "manually" or we can use the remote control to achieve the same purpose. In the same way, hormones may make biochemical contract or utilize waveform transmissions to stimulate a receptor. Furthermore, just as we can walk around our living room with our remote and control our television volume and channel, hormone-signaling molecules can move around the body and stimulate multiple cells into action simultaneously. Just as we are more assured of accurate channel changing when our remote is within close proximity of the television, the body is assured of more accurate responses among the cells when the signaling hormones are within close proximity of the cells and their receptors. It is for this reason that messengers are dispatched. Information exchange can begin instantly using radio signaling between these ligand messengers and their receptors.

These mechanisms were proven by over two decades of research headed up by Jacques Benveniste, M.D. and several other research teams. Dr. Benveniste was one of the foremost experts in the study of ligand-receptor mechanisms within the immune system for many years. He was the research director for the French National Institute for Health and Medical Research (INSERM) for a number of years. Dr. Benveniste's career was very distinguished. Several years earlier, he was credited with the discovery of the platelet-activating factor.

It was during further immune system research on the action of basophils that Dr. Benveniste and his research technician Elisabeth Davenas accidentally discovered that an allergic response in solution took place even though the tested allergen was effectively diluted out of the solution. Because the allergen was responded to without an apparent molecular basis (as the substance was diluted out), Dr. Benveniste began a search for what actually caused the immune response. This led to a four-year study on immunoglobulin IgE response—research included joint trials and confirmations with five laboratories in four countries. The research concluded that even at dilutions of 10^{120} (one part to ten parts with one hundred and twenty zeros behind it), and no probability of available molecules, the same immunoglobulin immune responses would occur as with significant concentrations. After confirming this variously, Dr. Benveniste and his team proposed that water somehow acts as a carrier for immune messaging. What else was left in the solution to carry the immune response messaging?

After eliminating alternative causes of this phenomenon, Dr. Benveniste and his research associates began to focus on the potential for a radio signaling process of some type. After much experimentation, the right technology and equipment led to the understanding that cells respond to low-frequency electromagnetic waves. Remarkably, certain biochemical messengers like acetylcholine produce unique electromagnetic waveforms. The question was now whether these waveforms played a role in the immunoglobulin communication.

Dr. Benveniste eventually developed sensitive audio equipment to record the frequencies of biochemical messengers. In the early 1990s, using his digital sound equipment with computerized technology, Benveniste and his associates recorded thousands of these low-frequency waves from various biochemicals. Amazingly, by playing back these recordings in the midst of cells and tissues, the recorded frequencies were able to stimulate the exact same responses the biochemicals stimulated. After several years of testing, Benveniste and his associates built up quite a library of biochemical waveform recordings. Frequencies of established biochemical messengers such as heparin, ovalbumin, acetylcholine and dextran were digitized and recorded. Unbelievably, these digital recording files were then be put on CD and mailed—or even emailed—to other labs. The other lab would play back the recordings onto various cell tissues—exciting the same responses the physical biochemicals stimulated.

This proposition more accurately fits with the body's ability to bridge consciousness with external stimuli. An advanced signaling process using low- and extra-low frequency electromagnetic frequencies creates a messaging system to elicit instantaneous responses simultaneously from billions of cells, just as radio broadcasts will bridge radio jockeys with millions of remote listeners simultaneously.

This model also supports the observation of some ligands coming into close proximity with cells in certain regions. These ligands may require close proximity to their receptors in order to elicit a response. Others, however, are designed to elicit responses from further distances. This might again be compared to the radio-to-radio frequencies used for communications. A CB-band, walkie-talkie system, remote telephone, or television remote may have a relatively short range of reception, depending upon the power of the signal. Therefore, remote telephones that transmit with greater power can be used at greater distances. Radio station broadcasting is also based upon the strength of the waveform signals. For this reason, some radio stations can be heard at much greater distances than others can. In contrast, other radio frequencies, such as shortwave or ham radios, can transmit over thousands of miles, even at lower power.

We apply this same variance to the intracellular process. Different hormones or ligands within the body have different purposes. Therefore, they each broadcast with different signal strengths, and at different frequencies. Just as we choose different types of communication systems or devices for different priorities, the type of biochemical messenger and signal strength used would relate to the need and timing required.

As we examine signaling broadcasting and reception, the cell's transmembrane receptors must *resonate* with the particular frequency emitted by the ligand. This follows the logic of any radio broadcast. Radios utilize not only a receiver but also a tuner, so the radio can synchronize with the broadcast's frequency. This is also a form of resonation. As we turn the tuner on a radio to find the right station, we are locating a point where the radio's receiver is resonating with the waveforms of the broadcasting station's signals. This process was developed using the radio crystal to receive and semiconduct particular waveforms into particular electronic pulses, notably a focus of the great early twentieth century inventor, Nicola Tesla.

Within the body, waveform signals and their messengers are programmed for broadcast through the pathways of signaling messengers beginning from the pituitary gland and its master gland the hypothalamus. As we trace this programming process back further, we find the various brain cortices like the prefrontal cortex at the center of these pathways—at the seat of consciousness. We might compare this to a song we hear playing on the radio being traced back to a particular radio station broadcast, and eventually back to the musician who originally wrote and performed the song.

Indeed, when we consider every response and movement within the physical body, we are seeing a relayed broadcasting process. These broadcasting pathways stimulate physical activity through the network of endocrine glands, the bloodstream, the nervous system, the basal membranes, transmembrane receptors and of course an army of signaling hormones and neurotransmitters. Every beat of our heart and every hunger pang or skeletal muscle twitch is the result of such a cascading signal process. Waveform broadcasts relay information from one biochemical type to another. We can thus compare the transmembrane protein receptors to antenna, and the genetic translation sequences as radio semiconductor crystals.

Biochemical messengers are not dumbwaiters. They have their own informational fingerprinting and translation processes as well. They translate messages specific to the particular body and situation. In other words, those messages are unique to that body. A person injected with hormones from a donor might have a physiological response generic to that hormone, but the specific message being carried through the donor's hormones will not be translated specifically through the body of the recipient. The message is the specific information about which muscles need to be stimulated, which arteries should be dilated in one region or another, and so on. We can test this by injecting epinephrine donated from one person into another person. The injected person's tissues might still be stimulated in a non-specific way, depending upon the location of the injection and the physical state of the injected subject. However, the injection will not stimulate the precise emotional response the body it was extracted from was carrying out. This is observable. The injected person simply does not process the same physiological responses.

The injection of vaccines has the same affect. The body receiving the injection will not respond identically with the source from which the antigens were derived. The injection will stimulate the body's own immune system to respond, quite possibly to produce similar immunoglobulins to fight the same antigen. Each body will initiate its own unique immunity messaging system because each body is driven by a unique conscious personality.

Consider for a moment the translation of a United Nations speech given by a foreign diplomat into a number of foreign languages concurrently. The translating technology (and/or live interpreters) works to translate each word and each phrase from the speaker's language into these other languages. This allows each UN representative the opportunity to hear the speech in his or her native language simultaneously. It was simply translated in real-time into their respective languages.

As a particular message is sent via one part of the body to another, the message is also being translated in real-time into the various functions necessary for the body. When the hypothalamus sends its hormonal messages to the pituitary, they are encoded with the needed response for that event, which are accompanied by a nervous signaling to supply additional information. The pituitary translates this combined message into a multitude of responses to each part of the body. These are broadcast out for processing to each endocrine gland through secreted hormones. Each endocrine organ then receives this translated message, and each one of these organs each does the same: They translate the message into specific biochemical signals.

This broadcasting and translation system is specific and intelligent. If the translation system at the United Nations incorrectly translated any of the words spoken by the speaker, the speech could be grossly misinterpreted. This could be dangerous. It could theoretically start a war. Therefore, the speech must be translated using an intelligent and impartial translating system.

The messages sent through the endocrine system must also be intelligent. Imagine our endocrine system sending out the same message regardless of whether we were being chased by a tiger, or say were in danger of a head-on collision driving in a car. We simply could not react to these two situations with an identical physiological response.

Specific and complex messages are being broadcast from the intelligent centers of the neural network, whether on a purely sympathetic process or autonomic bandwidth. These messages travel within waveforms just as our radio and television communications travel within broadcast radiowaves. The body's waveform broadcasts utilize crystallized amplification mechanisms called hormones to set the stage for the response. Each endocrine organ—or relay station—receives the signals and translates them into a more specific waveform broadcast. This more specific broadcast is meant to stimulate activity with increased specificity for a particular organ or tissue system. As the message is translated at the endocrine organ, it is again broadcast throughout the body, using protein crystals to regulate, amplify, boost or even restrict the message in some way. This enables a transmission with the ability to resonate with and appropriately instruct specific cells or tissue systems.

The use of these receptors and ligands are quite analogous to the functions of semiconductors and resisters among electrical circuits. Resistors and semiconductors—depending upon their positioning and makeup—will slow, redirect and in general modulate the flow of electrical pulses while providing an insulation process. This dampening affect allows the semiconductor or resistor to prevent the pulse from overloading the appliance or shocking its user.

The messaging biochemicals of the body—the hormones and neurotransmitters—must damper, modulate and sometimes even reverse the instructional flow in order for the messages to be properly and precisely engaged. We want to *just* outrun the tiger without killing the body with a heart attack, for example.

The broadcast signals of these relayed messages come with unique waveforms and sequences. Proprietary wave sequences will connect on a specifically resonant basis with specialized receptors on the cell membranes. The receptors on the cell membranes then *translate* and *reflect* those signals though the cytoplasm through particular organelles, RNA, DNA, or other proteins—imparting specific instructions to stimulate or modulate certain activities. These instructions serve to coordinate each cell's metabolic activity with the needs of the whole body. In the case of T3, the information is sent to the cell's ribosomes—responsible for increasing the rate of ATP transport chain processing—which directly increases the metabolic processes. In the case of insulin, the signaling initiates the preparation of micropores to absorb glucose for energy use, together with signaling other cells—such as liver cells to convert glycogen and adipose cells to store up fatty acids from glycogen.

The receptors on the cell membranes are the smart receivers for this intelligent messaging system. It might be comparable to having a satellite dish set up on a house. The dish is designed to pick up particular signals from particular satellites, and not others. The size of the dish and its positioning is established to pick up the specific waveforms emitting from that particular satellite. In the same way, particular receptors on the cell membrane are tuned to particular waveform messages sent from specific biochemicals. Whether those biochemicals are in close proximity or at a distance, their reception can be instantaneous.

Brainwaves of Consciousness

Nineteenth century researchers tested animals in an attempt to understand the electrical nature of physiology. The electric quality of the body was hard to deny even in the early days of electricity exploration. Gradually the apparatus for this probing were refined. Though possibly crudely applied earlier, Dr. Hans Berger is credited to be the first researcher to use the *electroencephalogram* (or EEG) to record brainwaves in the early 1920s. These efforts gradually gave brainwave testing credibility in psychological research. Today it is utilized for medical diagnostics, psychological testing, biofeedback testing and polygraph detection.

Several types of brain waves, each with unique frequencies, were discovered using EEG testing. Further testing using the later-discovered *magnetoencephalograph* indicated that a variety of subtle magnetic pulses also pulse through the body. First used by Dr. David Cohen in 1968, the MEG picked up another dimension of magnetic polarity among waveform transmission. MEG technology was further developed using superconductors. This equipment has been referred to as *superconducting quantum interference devices* (or SQUID).

The multitude of EEG and MEG studies over the years has

confirmed the existence of several major brainwave pulses, ranging from one to sixty cycles per second. Our brains pulse to waveforms with frequency bandwidths that correspond to particular moods, stress levels, and physiological status. As we focus on the complexities of daily life, our brains reflect and emit shorter-frequency *alpha* or *beta* brainwaves. A relaxing mood tends to accompany the deeper *delta* or even the more meditative *theta* waves. The greater the stress, the higher frequencies tend to get. Just as higher-pitched sounds tend to indicate intensity or urgency, higher frequency waves reflect a mind hustling to keep up with life's details. Because initial EEG and MEG research predominantly focused upon the brain, these waves were tagged as brainwaves. Actually, we find these waves resonating throughout the body. They tend to be more predominant among the central nervous system and the brain because the brain and spinal cord tends to be the main collection foci for these waves. As will be detailed further, the central nervous system provides freeways for high-speed wave transit.

Researchers have divided the millions of possible brainwave combinations into five general ranges. Alpha waves are typically the dominant cycle during dream states and light meditation. The alpha waves are oscillations with between eight and thirteen cycles per second (same as hertz). Beta brainwaves are dominant during normal waking consciousness, and range from fourteen to thirty cycles per second. Theta waves are considered to be four to seven cycles per second and dominate during normal sleep and meditation. On the lower frequency side are the delta waves, which range from less than one cycle per second to about three cycles per second. These slow waves tend to be dominating during the deepest sleep or deepest meditation states. On the other side of the spectrum, some of the fastest rhythms recorded in the brain are the gamma waves. The high-energy gamma waveforms typically dominate during periods of advanced problem solving or critical thinking. They oscillate at between thirty and sixty cycles per second. Over the past decade, researchers have discovered the existence of even shorter-wavelength and faster brainwaves.

Ranging from sixty to two hundred cycles per second or more, these high-speed waves are referred to as *high gamma waves*. The high gamma waves are thought to accompany critical thought processes and brain functions. Multiple brainwave types occur simultaneously in our body. One type will often predominate, however. Just as multiple tuning forks will align to one dominate tone, the body will typically tune—harmonically—to the predominant waveform driven from a pervading consciousness.

A recent neuroscience study jointly done by the University of California at Berkeley and the University of California at San Francisco (Sanders *et al.* 2006) has concluded that it is likely these brainwaves are conduits for messaging between the various regions of the brain. Dr. Robert Knight, professor of neuroscience at the University of California at Berkeley, and a director of the research observed that some regions of the brain emitted waves, others reflected waves, and still others modulated waves. Meanwhile a particular confluence of these waves corresponded with particular activities, indicating different brain centers were using brainwaves as a sort of information exchange system.

As these respected researchers correlated the type of wave with the part of the brain involved in a particular process correlated with thought patterns, they began to see longer wavelength theta waves synchronizing or *coupling* with shorter wavelength gamma waves. They considered this coupling as part of a hierarchical signaling process. Regions of coordinated neurons produce resonant coherent wave patterns, which provide the means for one neuron (or a group of neurons) to communicate with another (or group). Synchronizing waveforms between neurons appeared to coordinate firing patterns. The brainwave synchronization then appeared to provide a process of ranking between brain regions in operational order. Theta waves appear to provide an executive control mechanism, which bridge the operations of various groups.

Using epileptic subjects, the researchers found consistent relationships between cognition and the occurrence of coherent theta and gamma waves. These two types of waves provide a locked resonation process. As cognitive processes changed, one wave from one region would first couple with, then transition into the next type of waveform. A type of congruent harmonic becomes apparent between these various brainwaves.

Biofeedback therapy has focused on the relationship between stress and brainwave types for a number of decades. Biofeedback research has confirmed that stress directly influences brainwave activity. Researchers have tested brainwave activity with patients in a number of different circumstances. Stressful conditions are linked to higher beta wave levels and lower alpha and theta wave levels. Consequently, a person who feels more relaxed and less stressed will produce more alpha and theta waveforms.

Many of us are aware that certain sounds influence relaxation. Most of us have experienced greater relaxation as we listen to soothing music or the songs of birds for example. Melinda Maxfield, PhD (2006) determined that slowly beating a drum at 4.5 beats per second readily brings about a state of theta brainwave activity. In 2006, Stanford University's Center for Computer Research in Music and Acoustics held a symposium with a purpose of *"interdisciplinary dialogue on the hypothesis that brainwaves entrain to rhythmic auditory stimuli, a phenomenon known as auditory driving."* This symposium brought together some of the nation's leading sound researchers. Many discussed the implications of auditory driving as it relates to our mental and physical wellbeing. The implications of the research, reflected by the consensus of the symposium, were that we are merely at the tip of the iceberg of this research.

The applications of brainwave entrainment through auditory driving are numerous. Successful auditory driving and brainwave entrainment treatments have contributed to resolving psychological trauma, chronic pain, stress, and weakened immune systems. Research comparing normal subjects with schizophrenic subjects (Vierling-Claasen *et al.* 2008) has illustrated how gamma and beta waves interface and guide cognitive processes. Normal subjects will tune to a 40 Hz wave in response to either 20 or 40 Hz driving frequencies. Schizophrenic subjects will typically respond with 20

Hz waveforms. The study's authors comment that these results illustrate *"how biophysical mechanisms can impact cognitive function."* This research confirms that brainwaves provide a mechanism for messaging specific information throughout the physical anatomy.

Biofeedback testing has further demonstrated that with practice and proper feedback access, human subjects can consciously change their brainwave levels. As a stress-reduction technique for example, a person can decrease their beta wave activity and increase their alpha and theta activity. The procedure entails the subject sitting down in front of a computer screen visually displaying rates from an electroencephalograph, photoplethysmograph (PPG—heart rate and blood flow), and/or possibly an electromyograph (EMG—muscle tension) to read waveform activity feeding back from different body parts connected to a variety of electrodes. Electrodes may be placed around the head, typically either on the scalp or in some cases around the cerebral cortex. Skin electrodes may also be applied to the arm, and PPG electrodes may be connected to the chest. The computer will monitor the waveform output of these different locations—displaying the results in a graphic display for the subject and therapist to see.

Most of us will generate brainwave signals reflecting our mental or emotional state—be it anxious, focused, relaxed, tired, angry or asleep. A good biofeedback machine will register several of these waves and their relative strengths around the body. Using a good biofeedback machine, most people can gradually learn to significantly lower or increase their alpha and theta wave strengths. For a few people, there will be an almost immediate ability to influence their waves as soon as the monitoring begins. For most it will take a bit of practice—a number of sessions usually—to be able to effectively modulate ones brainwaves or another other body pulse. Researchers have found that most everyone is able to modulate their waves at one point or other. Researchers have yet to understand why there is such a variance among people's ability to control their brainwaves.

Nonetheless, once people do learn to change their brainwaves using the biofeedback, they can usually transition successfully into being able to adjust their brainwaves without the biofeedback equipment. Bringing about a relaxed mental state through visualizing relaxing situations or hearing relaxing sounds are probably the most successful techniques used for this result. Auditory driving with rhythmic sounds has been increasingly used in biofeedback therapy.

Biofeedback therapy illustrates that our brainwaves are expressions of the role of consciousness within the body. An alteration of brainwaves from primarily beta to theta waves will almost invariably result in a lower heart rate, a slower, deeper rate of breathing, and a lowering of blood pressure. Conversely, a lower heart rate, and slower breathing—as long as there is no mental disruption—will also tend to induce a theta brainwave state. We thus have an intersection between consciousness and the cascade of brainwaves with physiological states.

Physicians specializing in the central nervous system have observed another wave associated with the circulating spinal fluid: Aptly named *cerebrospinal fluid pulse waves* (or CSF waves). The data have suggested this wave is composed of five different harmonic waves, ranging in pressure from .25-1 mm Hg range, and averaging .72 mm Hg (Nakamura *et al.* 1997). This is a pressure-wave. In comparison, the standard atmospheric pressure at sea level is equal to 760 mm Hg. It has not been completely ascertained as to the exact source of the CSF waves. One theory says that the pulse waves are due to the pressure gradient between arteries supplying the spinal cord and the spinal fluid. Another says they are based upon brain pulses sent through the spine's subarachnoid spaces. Many osteopaths, chiropractors, and cranial practitioners believe the cerebrospinal fluid pulses are due to the tiny movements of the cranial bones during breathing. Some research has linked breathing with these pulse waveforms. Correlations with ventricle pressure have also been made.

An interesting connection is made when CSF pulses are measured for wavelength: Beta-frequency waves seem to dominate the CSF pulse. Further EEG testing in controlled environments has demonstrated an interference relationship between the CSF pulses and the neural waveforms exhibited during memory retrieval and cognition. It seems these CSF waves play an important role in the orchestration of brainwave interference patterns.

From biophoton research, we can understand that each cell produces a unique collection of coherent electromagnetic emissions. Because each type of cell function has been connected with different types of biophoton emissions, it is safe to say coherent biophoton emissions by groups of brain and central nervous system cells should yield resonating patterns through constructive interference. The collection of weaker biophoton emissions should yield larger waveforms, just as thousands of stadium fans may each make unique sounds, but their confluence together creates a single sound of the crowd. Most of us have heard someone mimicking the single sound of a large stadium crowd full of cheering and jeering fans—it is not too difficult to do.

As the various subtle waveforms traveling in from our sense organs interface with internal waveforms feeding back from around the body, they combine to form a compounded perception of our body's inner and outer environment. This is accomplished again because these waveforms create multiple interference patterns as they interact. These interference patterns create collective views as they are intermingled with others and transferred onto our brain's cortices—predominated by the prefrontal cortex. The combined collection of interference patterns provides a form of image mapping system to be viewed from a position of consciousness.

The Memory of Water

In the 1990s, Masaru Emoto and an assistant began taking photographs illustrating water crystal formation under different circumstances and influences. He first published these findings in 1999. Emoto's photographic images implied that water crystal formation varied not only to water sources, but also to interactions with music, spoken and even written words. Water exposed to different types of music theoretically formed different crystals: classical music created full symmetrical crystal shapes while hard rock created unsymmetrical and disoriented shapes. Water exposed to different types of words or phrases theoretically formed different crystals: uplifting words theoretically created full, symmetrical crystals while words of hatred or anger theoretically created disoriented shapes (Emoto 2004).

This research became well publicized yet controversial among the scientific community. Some researchers have decried Emoto's reports as lacking the rigor acceptable for peer-review. While the photos themselves create little doubt regarding the variability of ice crystal formation, the question of his research boils down to the extent controls were applied to the process of taking and choosing photographs for publication. Because we now understand that the same water can form a variety of ice crystals shapes, Emoto chose one photo to publish to represent each scenario. Was there any bias in the selection of crystals to publish? This concern has yet to be adequately resolved. Therefore, although Emoto's crystal photograph research is intriguing, and may indicate water's ability to reflect consciousness, Masaru Emoto's research falls short as quotable evidence linking consciousness with crystallization. (The author contacted Mr. Emoto with these questions, and was referred to someone else who did not respond.)

Still there are a number of undeniable characteristics within water that confirm a sort of 'memory' or reflection of consciousness. Water's memory capacity is easily observed should a rock be dropped into a pond. For minutes even hours afterward, the resulting rhythmic waves traveling away from the entrance point of the rock specifically reflect the size of the pebble, its velocity, and even the shape of the rock to some degree. A small rock will create a different rippling than a large rock might. A flat rock will create a different waveform than a round rock might. The size and shape of the ripples will also reflect the velocity of the toss into the water. A harder toss will be reflected quite differently than a light lob might. These ripples will reflect the information about the rock and the throw for some time, affecting various other events occurring within the pond.

We all also know that when water is heated and cooled, it will retain a 'recollection' of that temperature input for a period of time. The hotter the initial flame, the longer the water will remain hot. An electric stove will heat water at a different degree than a gas stove might. Thermal heat from the sun creates still another temperature range. As water is cooled, again it reflects the cooling source. Water cooled with ice will cool differently than water cooled in a refrigerator or even freezer. Though we might expect the result to be proportionate to the temperature the water is exposed to, in reality, different sources have different effects. Those varying effects will also dramatically change the water's characteristics for hours or even days following the changes. Although this 'thermal memory' appears resident among most substances, the presence of water hastens the thermal conduction and retention process, which makes water an efficient thermal conductor. For this reason, food is most often cooked in water as opposed to any other substance. Water is also used in various other thermal conducting mechanisms such as heated floors, baths, and so on. When in need of an instant cooling mechanism, water is also sought after for its ability to immediately conduct cool temperatures. Water quite easily 'remembers' the temperature of its surroundings, easily transporting that memory to other substances.

Water's memory is also observed with regard to water's solubility and surface tension characteristics. When we dissolve a substance into water, the water's specific gravity and surface tension will change, reflecting the properties of the added substance. This solvent will also change the water's boiling and melting points. As the solute is precipitated out of the water, the water will often retain a variance in these characteristics as compared to the original water source. This variance may be caused by the presence of additional hydrogen ions in the water, or by the existence of additional water clustering. However, water's character is altered establishes a sort of memory capacity. While other substances can be used as a solute, water is an efficient solute because of its molecular properties.

As we have touched upon earlier, water's ability to retain memory has been clinically examined through the medical science of homeopathy, beginning with Dr. Samuel Hahnemann's original research with dilutions two centuries ago. While the *'like cures like'* portion of homeopathic therapy is well-accepted by modern medicine (the basis for vaccination among other therapies) the notion that water will retain a distant memory of a substance diluted to the point of theoretically diluting every molecule of the substance away is not acceptable to much of mainstream science today.

As we discussed earlier, research on water memory was advanced greatly by Dr. Jacques Benveniste. Dr. Benveniste, a successful French medical doctor, discovered accidentally in 1984 that white blood cells responded to an allergen in a solution despite there theoretically being no remaining antibody molecules in the solution. This led to hundreds of studies among Dr. Benveniste's team and other research labs, which mostly replicated these results. These results confirm that a water-based solution somehow retains memory after full dilution. Over 300 trials were performed confirming these results.

In 1991, Benveniste developed a system of amplifying molecular signals through sensitive electromagnetic microcoils and transducers. After a few years of application, the process was refined to the point that his research team was able to record molecular emissions into digital form. The molecular signal associated with the digital recordings indicated frequencies in the 0-22 KHz range. Incredibly, the digital recordings could be played back through an amplified transducer in the presence of a particular reactive organ, such as cholinergic activity among harvested pig hearts. His digital playback resulted in the same physiological result the biochemical hormone might have—without the physical biochemical substance present. Dr. Benveniste demonstrated this effect emphatically when he was able to send disks or email recordings to labs in remote locations. In these cases, the playback of the recordings would have the same effect (Benveniste 1997).

As Dr. Benveniste continued his research, he discovered that the effective transmission of the signal had some dependency on the mixing system employed. Without the proper mixing process, the diluted mixture's ability to affect the same result was substantially decreased. On the other hand, proper mixing resulted in a significantly greater effect (22.6 vs. 3.2 coronary flow changes in an acetylcholine dilute, for example) when compared to the solution *prior to mixing* (Benveniste 1999).

The ability of water molecules to retain particular electromagnetic waveform interference patterns is illustrated using these data. As we established earlier, a waveform basis for matter is supported by a century's worth of physics research. We might compare this with voice vibration. In order for voice vibration to be instructive, there must be a precise manipulation of waveforms striking the eardrum, which contain the message of the speaker.

The transmission of sound and visual signals via radiowaves parallels this fundamental process. It also provides an illustration for the ability all waveforms have in carrying specific informational signals.

As we consider a particular area of ocean and its net motion at any particular place and time, we could certainly connect a myriad of atmospheric and tidal events to the current motion and condition of the water. There may have been a large windstorm thousands of miles away that drove some of the waves. There may have been a hurricane storm front, which drove another set of waves from another direction. There may have been a large tidal change due to the moon's orbit, which also influenced the tidal pulses within the ocean's motion.

This holds true for sonar wave composition. There should also be a net effect of the various intelligent transmissions of dolphins and whales as they communicate amongst their own schools. If we take this net effect of all the movement within the ocean, we have the basis for a medium of memory for the reflected rhythms of all these conscious inputs. If we were to have an instrument sensitive enough to pick up all these subtle waves moving through the medium of the ocean from these various sonar waves, we have a confluence not unlike the random number generator and the global consciousness project results from the research of Dr. Schmidt, Dr. Jahn and Princeton's Dr. Nelson as mentioned earlier.

We might also compare this process to the laying down of music tracks at a recording studio. In order to provide a platform for each instrument to be recorded onto one master recording, there must be a process of combining separately recorded music sound tracks. Each track is recorded separately and then mixed together onto one master track. When this master track is played, all instruments are played together. By listening to that one master blended recording, an intelligent studio listener would probably be able to discern the different tracks and instruments recorded separately. This method of mixing reflects a memory device able to blend a number of inputs.

A number of researchers have confirmed water's ability to retain or reflect the touch of a therapeutic practitioner. Dr. Edward Brame, Dr. Douglas Dean, Dr. Bernard Grad, and others have either led or co-authored studies—some confirmed by infrared spectroscopy analysis—that healer-treated water maintained molecular changes reflecting therapeutic touch. In more than one of these, the molecular bond angles had slightly shifted. In others, decreased surface tension of the water confirmed a subtle molecular change. In still others, the rate of growth was effects (Dean 1983; Dean *et al.* 1974; Grad 1964, Grad *et al.* 1984; Schwartz *et al.* 1987).

Emission bombardment effects have been well established by physicists in mass spectrometry research. Because each electron orbit has particular waveform or quantum characteristics, bombarding an atom with radiation of the right frequency will boost certain electrons into lower or higher valence shells, affect the orbit's spin or angular momentum, and/or eject an electron/wave out of the nucleus "orbit" altogether. This effect has been the subject of numerous mass particle accelerator studies, diffraction results, and spectrometry analyses. Brainwaves and body waves are certainly types of radiation as well. There is currently no documented evidence known to this author that would eliminate the ability of these "biological" waveforms to influence electron/wave orbits of molecules touched or otherwise interfered with.

A Liquid Physiology

The makeup of our cells is primarily water. Each cell is also bathed in water. The basal fluid provides an ionic-balance between the water inside the cell and outside the cell membrane. The ionic nature of the water inside the cell membrane is typically charged with negatively charged potassium ions, while the water inside the cell membrane is charged primarily with positively charged sodium ions. This creates what is often called the *sodium/potassium pump*. The sodium/potassium pump provides a dual-balanced mechanism of attraction between the sodium and potassium ions.

This ionic charge difference creates an electromagnetic attraction between the inside and outside surfaces of the cell membrane. This gives the membrane a stable partition. Yet while providing a partition, the ionic gateway channeling contrasting electromagnetic moments provides a vehicle for the exchange of important fluids through the cell membrane. Through tiny channels in the membrane created by spaces between stacked phospholipid molecules come nutrients and water into the cell, escorted by sodium ions. Just within the surface of the membrane is a tiny rhythmic pump network called the *protein pump*. These pumps push the escorting sodium ions that slip through the cell membrane back outside, carrying with them the waste generated by the cell. This entire process is often called *cellular diffusion*. Diffusion allows each cell to bring in nutrition and pass out toxins through the cell membrane, utilizing this ionic attraction and pump process.

As we have discussed previously, there are different types of ion channels throughout the body and within each cell membrane— each of which brings different types of nutrients into the cell. For example, there are specific channels that bring glucose into the cell, often called *glucose receptors*. These channels are connected to specialized gates which are turned on and off by receptors which sit on the surface of the cell membrane. Receptors are switches turned on by special messenger cells like hormones, equipped with ligands that electromagnetically signal the receptor switch. While most ligands are thought to require a touching of biomolecular particles, research is increasingly indicating many ligands communicate from a distance, using rhythmic waveforms.

In the case of channeling glucose into the cell, glucose receptors are switched on by the signaling hormone *insulin*. In the same way, other channels and pumps provide for the flow of the fluids and nutrients that hydrate and nourish our cells. Many researchers theorize molecules line up and move through these conduits one by one when the gateway is open. While this is certainly logical given the size of these tiny channels, this theory is limited by the unproven atomic particle theory. Assuming matter is composed of waveforms, the process of entry would rely upon the specific molecular signals being emitted by the ligands. Input into the cell membrane through receptors and channels appear be similar to light entering into the eyes, or sound entering through the ears: In the case of light, inbound radiation is received and processed through receptors on the retina cells of the eye. In the case of sound, radiation is channeled into the ear canal, stimulating the eardrum *receptor* and signaling through the inner ear transmission system. In each case, waveform emission stimulates the activity, rather than biochemical particles.

A system of sodium and potassium pumps also occurs within nerve cells. In addition to providing channels for the exchange of nutrients and toxins, the nerve cell sodium/potassium pump provides a mechanism of the exchange of information. As electromagnetic pulses traverse the length of the nerve cell, sodium ions are pulled into the nerve cell, while potassium ions are pushed out. Each ion movement instigates the movement of the next ion wave, much like a row of dominos laying down one after another. The electrical conduction through sodium and potassium ions provides the pathway for rhythmic pulses. This mechanism appears to function somewhat similar to the 1s and 0s of computer machine language code. As most of us know, this rather simple computer machine code system of 1s and 0s allows for dramatically complex instructions. The key to the sodium/potassium mechanism is the rhythmic balance established between the potassium and sodium ions. It may go without saying that maintaining this delicate balance between the potassium and calcium ions is the key to healthier cellular function.

pH is the measure of the ionic capabilities of a particular solution. We can thus utilize pH as a tool to determine the ability of our body waters' ability to channel waveform instructions efficiently through the membrane. The body's fluid pH is critical to metabolism because it is through ionic conducting mechanisms that information is transmitted through the cells, organs and other tissue systems. The ionic nature of the body's waters provides the vehicle for the rhythmic flow of consciousness throughout body. Should the ionic balance of the body's fluids not be properly maintained, we will soon discover a number of key metabolic processes being blocked or distorted. Without the proper flow of information conducting through the ion channels of the cell membrane, the cells cannot act harmonically.

We find this condition evident when a person has consumed alcohol or psychotropic drugs. The body's ionic fluids are altered, most notably the neurotransmitter fluid, which provides the medium for the pulses traveling through nerve cell ion channels. As the neurotransmitter fluid chemistry is altered, the information pulses traveling from nerve to nerve are altered, affecting coordination, physical response, perception, mood, and other functions.

To some degree, we might compare this mechanism with looking through a clear water stream followed by looking through the stream after it became darkened with mud. Through the clear water, the rocks below are easily visible. The muddy stream on the other hand, either may block our vision of the rocks below altogether or may alter their appearance. They might appear smaller or deeper than they are. Because the fluid is clouded by mud, the ability of light to travel through the water is affected.

This is illustrated by the same general effects of intoxication. A heavy drinker will usually have cloudy or bloodshot sclera. The pupils will not readily be responsive to light, and thus may appear overly dilated or constricted for that environment. They may speak with lethargic or slurred speech. They may find difficulty forming words from their thoughts, or may find it difficult to control their language. They might also be easily angered or upset, as their perception may be clouded. They may misinterpret an events and or context. They may also have a lack of control over their emotions or appropriateness. Alcohol intoxication in particular will often also result in a decreased sense of balance and coordination with a heightened sense of confidence. These are all symptoms of an altered ion channel motion. The ionic—thus magnetic—imbalances within the body's fluids created by the intoxicant disrupt the normal ionic flow of minerals, nutrients and neurotransmitters through the various ion channels.

Much of the body's biochemical processes are *hydrolytic*. In other words, most of the body's biochemical metabolic reactions are water-dependent, requiring hydrolysis. The hydroelectric energy and ion transport through the cell membrane allows many of these processes—such as the ATP energy manufacturing cycle—requiring water as the essential ion buffering and transport foundation. Thus water is one of the main substrates within a vast range of metabolic biochemical processes within the body.

When the body becomes dehydrated, a number of physiological responses take place. Initially, when the cells among the least vital areas of the body become exhausted of water, various ionic channels will close to preserve fluid for vital tissues. As this happens, the movement of ions, nutrition, and fluids in and out of those cells will slow down or even shut down. Typically the body prioritizes and rations its availability of water very pragmatically and intelligently. The areas where cell membrane channels close first will be the less vital regions of joints, tendons and other less active areas—away from the vital circulatory-rich organs. Various messenger cells such as histamine, vasopressin, rennin-angiotensin, along with supportive prostaglandin and kinin activity support and communicate the body's water level adaptation processes. After the body orchestrates its prioritization routines, should enough water still be unavailable, channels of the surrounding tissues also begin to close down.

As a result, we find that a number of disorders are related to chronic dehydration. For example, many arthritic and joint issues appear be directly related to dehydration. In the case of joint issues, water is reprioritized to other parts of the body. As this effect matures, a lack of hydration can either directly cause or contribute to the deterioration of joints and their supporting structures (Batmanghelidj 1992).

Negative effects upon cognition and psychomotor performance has been observed when at least 2% of the water by body weight is lost due to dehydration according to Grandjean and Grandean (2007). This has been established through the use of various neurological testing and other neurophysiology tests.

Other pathologies appear to be related to even mild dehydration as illustrated by Manz (2007). These include cystic fibrosis, renal toxicity, urinary tract infections, constipation, hypertension, various coronary and artery disorders, and glaucoma. Evidence from the CF/Pulmonary Research and Treatment Center of the University of North Carolina (Boucher 2007) has revealed the possible link between hydration and cystic fibrosis as "low airway surface liquid volume." This is another way of saying that the mucosal membranes lining the airways require good body hydration.

We also can link a lack of water consumption with various digestive disorders such as GERD (gastroesophageal reflux disease), ulcers, and irritable bowel syndrome (Batmanghelidj 1992). In a state of dehydration, the pH chemistry of the stomach radically changes. Again, the mucous membranes of the esophagus and stomach wall become thinner and less protective. This is because water is the central component of mucous and gastrin, which in turn buffers the

HCL component of stomach secretions. Water is also a major element in the sloughing and division of the cells of the walls of the stomach and intestines. Intestinal cells are some of the shortest living cells of the body. Cells of a healthy digestive tract will divide and slough off within days, leaving the body with virtually a new stomach mucosal lining within days. Should these dividing cells become dehydrated, genetic mutation may also take place during division. This mutation may allow the cell to function with less water, but often at a price. It may also result in other adjustments, which may decrease the healthy functioning of the stomach and its lining. Once mutation occurs, the cell may assume foreign attributes. As the immune system is exposed to these foreign attributes, a condition referred to as *autoimmunity* may arise.

These are only a few of the potential effects of chronic dehydration in the human physiology. Others may include headaches, heart problems, hypertension, allergies, asthma, hiatus hernia, low back pain, diabetes, and so many other ailments—many of which have interestingly been described as "autoimmune diseases."

Nature's Laws

The processes of the natural environment are driven by living organisms. This component is illustrated by the fact that specific plants help cure specific ailments. Is this not a curious mechanism? What connects these particular botanicals to particular ailments? Why does ginger treat digestive ailments while eucalyptus treats respiratory ailments? Why does cayenne stimulate circulation while skullcap slows metabolism and nerve firing to help us relax and sleep?

The connection between the botanical species and the disease is more clearly understood from the perspective of consciousness. This issue was discussed in great detail by early twentieth century Dr. Edward Bach, a well-educated British physician. Dr. Bach described that at its very fundamental aspect, a disease is an expression of a particular deficiency or malignment between the inner self and its physical body. He taught that this deficiency created the need for learning particular lessons. In other words, particular diseases are associated with particular lessons to learn. This concept was also shared by a German physician now considered the father of homeopathy, Dr. Samuel Hahnemann a century earlier. Though Ayurvedic and Greek physicians also utilized homeopathy, Dr. Hahnemann perfected the techniques and discovered hundreds of different natural remedies. Dr. Hahnemann also introduced the concept of *miasms*. A miasm, Dr. Hahnemann proposed, was a particular deficiency of the inner being, expressed through physical tendencies and disease models.

The ability of plants to produce reflective medicinal effects yields a rather complex yet revealing discussion. As the thousands of years of traditional research have been compiled, it has become evident that while certain botanicals have particular medicinal effects, there also appears to be a connection between the medicinal effect and the physical appearance of the botanical. This link between botanicals' physical shape and medicinal benefit is illustrated in the North American Indian medical *Doctrine of Signatures*. This doctrine stated that each medicinal herb reveals its therapeutic properties through a *sign*. This sign shows a visual relationship between plants and ailments. This might be the shape of the root, the shape of the leaf, the color of the plant, or another aspect. For example, milkweed and plants with milky fluids are linked with ailments of the breasts, while roots like ginger—twisted and contorted like the digestive tract—is linked with stomach and intestinal health. It is also interesting that the root is where plant nutrient absorption takes place, while plant milky fluids are often a byproduct of their procreative activities.

The healing practice of the North American Indians, like so many indigenous medicines, also (independently) utilized the famed Hippocratic theory (and later homeopathic concept) of the *law of similars,* or *"like cures like."* Many medicinal botanicals reflect their properties by mimicking some of the same symptoms they treat. As these ancient pretexts have wound their way into modern medicine practice, there has been confirmation by research for much of these basic tenets. Today we find the same law of similars being applied in the form of vaccination, allergy treatment, and digestive issues.

As Ayurvedic medicine began to utilize thousands of years earlier, Dr. Hahnemann further documented the effective use of the law of similars with thousands of *provings*. A proving is the clinical establishment of the therapeutic effects of a natural element by observing the effects upon a healthy person. If the element created symptoms, that element was considered curative for precisely those symptoms in diluted doses. Elements used in *provings* over the last 250 years of clinical homeopathy have included botanicals, rock minerals, venoms, and animal secretions. In all, over 2000 homeopathic treatment elements have been *proved*.

Dr. Bach extended the curative nature of homeopathics beyond physical ailments, by disclosing and proving the curative effects of various flower essences for psychological and mood disorders. In addition, many centuries before, Ayurveda elaborated on the curative effects of gemstones for healing not only physical ailments but specific mood and psychological issues.

As we examine again the usefulness of botanical biochemicals for therapeutic purpose, we cannot escape connecting the living nature of these botanicals with their therapeutic properties. Just as our weight, skin complexion; even hair color and eye color our consciousness, we may consider each plant's nature a reflection of that plant's inner self. If we consider that each plant is also housing an individual inner self, just as the higher forms like animals and humans portray an individual self within. When we assume that our physical body reflects our conscious intentions, we can then cross-reference our ailments with the strengths expressed by the consciousness of certain medicinal plants. In other words, their expression perfectly juxtaposes with our expression of deficiency. This understanding was arrived at by Dr. Bach.

Because plants are stationary, they must protect themselves with their various biochemicals. This means the biochemicals they produce interact with environmental threats in the same way those biochemicals will interact with environmental threats within the human body. The consistency of nature's rhythms allows for a consistency of therapeutic biochemistry.

Flower essence biochemistry provides the ideal expression of plant consciousness as it interacts with its environment and other plants. While the constituents of plant roots and plant leaves will each have different effects when we apply them medicinally, the essence of the flower produces yet another effect. Furthermore, each type of flower produces a distinct effect. From biology we learn the flower of a plant is its expression of its sexual activity. A flower will display color and delicate beauty, just as a female human looking to attract a man might wear a colorful dress with delicate high heels. The flower appropriately expresses the plant's personality and moods on during its pollinating season. This contrasts with the photosynthetic activities of the plants' leaves, or the nutrient-absorptive root activities. As Dr. Bach illustrated and evidenced by the billions of people who have benefited from Dr. Bach's flower remedy discoveries, these expressive flower essences happen to help us with our expressive areas of emotions and moods.

Though research on flower remedies overall appears scant, a famous flower essence blend called rescue remedy has undergone a variety of controlled studies with humans and animals (Muhlack *et al.* 2006). Made from essences of the flowers of the cherry plum, clematis, impatiens, rockrose, and the star of Bethlehem, this remedy quickly treats mood-related issues of anxiety, trauma, and emergency-related stress. The efficacy of the rescue remedy has not only been used successfully by humans over the years, but on a variety of animals, including pets and horses. In both animal and human use following a traumatic experience, a few drops of rescue remedy consumed directly, or in a glass or basin of water has repeatedly been shown to bring about a state of relaxation without any side effects. For this reason, rescue remedy is a favorite among many who are feeling nervous before traumatic events such as driving tests, public speeches, or following accidents and other traumas. While Dr. Bach's research focused on thirty-seven flowers growing throughout England, further research over the years has revealed hundreds of other flower essences with a variety of effects.

This discussion illustrates how consciousness is expressed through the biochemistry of our environment. We can see this directly as we review the thousands of studies linking moods and emotions with the various neurotransmitters and hormones produced by the body. We have observed that a conscious emotion of fear will stimulate the body to produce adrenaline, acetylcholine and other 'fight or fight' biochemicals. We have observed how the conscious feeling of love or joy stimulates the production of oxytocin and dopamine. These different chemicals are produced by the body in response to the self's conscious feelings and emotions. Connecting consciousness with the production of biochemistry is not such a far-fetched concept after all.

As we ponder the fundamental differences in consciousness between the intention to respect and work with nature and the intention to manipulate nature, we can each individually examine our own attitudes regarding this discussion. What, we may ask, is the difference between harvesting a natural herb or a natural fiber from the fields and the production of synthetic chemicals for the same ultimate purpose?

The difference is our consciousness. Synthetic chemical production expresses a consciousness of *arrogance*. While we are aware of many of the nuances associated with the delicate nature of the nature's biochemistry, we ignore this delicate balance while we seek to accomplish our goals. When arrogance is combined with greed, we surge with self-confidence. This self-confidence directs us to believe we can duplicate nature's processes better with our own technologies.

Humankind's recent need to create this massive industrial chemical complex—with its infrastructure of chemical manufacturers and large-scale distribution centers around the globe—is built upon a falsehood: That falsehood is that we can do better. That falsehood assumes that something is missing from nature. That there is no design in place. That there is no meaning and reason for our existence. As a result, we assume we can do what we want without any consequences.

We can see this particular virus of arrogance deeply entrenched when we hear of many scientists' views of the future and how technology and synthetic chemicals will bring about greater luxuries and happiness. Meanwhile, there is no net increase in happiness or ease existing today as a result of our modern technologies. We are only experiencing an increase in complexities and problems. For every chemical we manufacture and release into the environment, we are faced with the problem of how to remove or neutralize that chemical to avoid our own extinction.

It is not hard to rediscover the natural biochemical options that can provide immediate balance. Over the past decade, as a society we are rediscovering natural alternatives to just about every synthetic chemical. The environment gives us natural antibiotics, natural pesticides, natural cleaning agents, natural pharmaceuticals, natural health and beauty agents and of course natural foods. Some of us have found we can clean with natural soaps, disinfect with vinegars and citrus, repel insects with various oils and soaps, and fertilize with compost, to name a few. Some of us have recently discovered that the same creativity that went into making synthetic chemicals can also be applied in working intelligently with nature's own biochemistry. These realizations are still a tiny drop in a large ocean of destructive forces at work in our pursuit of a synthetic chemical environment. A mass change will require a big dose of humility: An admission that our environment has been designed by a greater Intelligence for a purpose greater than our self-gratification. Will a mass environmental disaster be required to force this humility?

Clocks

The human body paces to an array of rhythmic cycles, each ebbing and flowing with a different frequency. A cycle charted against time is simply another waveform. The body's various cycles, encompassing just about every activity including eating, sleeping, defecation, labor and relaxation—along with every biochemical rhythm that supports them—are all cycling each day, driven by various external clockworks. These have loosely been called the body's *biowaves*. Generally, there are four types of human biowaves: *Circadian (circa*=about; *dian*=a day) cycles occur more or less in the range of one day. *Ultradian* cycles occur in less than a day. *Infradian* cycles occur in multiple days. Finally, *circannual* cycles occur annually.

Over the past century, researchers have been vigorously hunting for the source for the body's biological clockworks. In 1929, two Harvard researchers John Fulton and Percival Bailey studied disrupted sleep rhythms among patients with hypothalamus lesions. They concluded a mysterious link between the endocrine system and sleep cycles.

In 1958, Harvard's Dr. Woody Hastings and Dr. Paul Mangelsdorf illustrated how the marine species *G. polyedra* lit up the night's ocean timed to the sun's path. Exposing the tiny plant to various light pulses at different times, Dr. Hastings concluded some internal biological mechanism within the organism must respond to the sun, switching on and off its illuminating appearance. Over the next decade, various other organisms—including humans—were observed maintaining rhythmic biological responses in conjunction with light.

This research began a focused hunt to corner the body's biological connection to light. Researchers assumed that plants and animals possessed cell-switching mechanisms sensitive to light. Controversy took hold in the 1960s when researchers from Germany's Max Planck Institute published a study showing that human biological rhythms were not light-driven as had been suggested. Charles Czeisler, M.D., Ph.D., an eminent Harvard sleep researcher for several decades with over 180 research papers under his belt, questioned that research. Upon visiting the Planck facility, he found that although the subjects' outside lighting was controlled, they were still able to switch on and off indoor lights within their rooms. Apparently, even weak indoor lights could disrupt or entrain the body's clocks. In the years following, numerous light studies done elsewhere confirmed humans' biological clockworks responded to light—many led by Dr. Czeisler.

Most human light research has put subjects into caves or other light-controlled dwellings. These dwellings were removed of any cues as to time and place. Multiple studies indicated that the human circadian rhythm was about 25 hours. In 1985, Max Planck's Dr. Rutger Wever monitored temperature cycles, illustrating daily cycles of 21 and 28 hours instead of this 25-hour daily cycle. Furthermore, he found that body core temperatures quickly adjusted to the new light schedules. These studies indicated that the body's circadian cycles, which include the daily cycling of cortisol, melatonin and other hormones and neurotransmitters through the body, appear to be governed by the sun's path.

In 1972, University of Chicago researcher Dr. Robert Moore dropped radioactive label material in rats' eyes and traced its pathway from retinal neurons to two small clusters of neurons deep within the hypothalamus. This was traced to two centrally located pinhead-sized clusters of about 10,000 nerve cells called the *suprachiasmatic nuclei* (or SCN cells). The SCN cells were heralded as the biological clock researchers had been looking for over so many decades. Over the next few years, Dr. Moore, together with Lenn and Beebe, traced synaptic contacts with retinal afferent dendrites though the metabolism of young rats, eventually confirming that the SCN cells entrained their switching mechanisms to light (Lenn *et al.* 1977).

For the next two decades, Dr. Moore and other researchers, including Dr. Charles Weitz, Dr. David Welsch, and Dr. Eric Herzog, investigated these SCN cells from various aspects. Without synchronized SCN cells, an animal's body rhythms would collapse into chaotic patterns. These SCN cells were observed primarily residing within the hypothalamus. It was assumed that the body's clock was located within the hypothalamus.

These SCN cells appear to connect the hypothalamus with the activities of the pineal gland—a small conical structure lying above the posterior end of the third ventricle. The pineal gland receives impulses directly from the optic nerves. This seemed to confirm that SCN cells were the human body's switching mechanisms for light.

SCN cells are implicated in the secretion of most if not all the major hormones and neurotransmitters within the body. They appear to switch on in response to light pulses as they are received by the pineal gland. The mechanism for this appeared to be a double-neuron oscillation guided by a combination of light and genetic expression (Ilonomov *et al.* 1994, Fukada 2002).

As the research on the genetic connection to SCN cell activity unfolded, it became evident the activities of the thousands of oscillating nerve cells making up the SCN cell region are somehow expressed through a set of clock-oriented genes (Kalsbeek *et al.* 2006). Recent genetic research has identified several clockwork genes. The central CLOCK gene has been identified as 3111T/C; rs1801260 (Benedetti *et al.* 2007) and APRR9 in plants. Other clockwork genes have been identified as BMAL, PER, CRY (cryptochrome-12q23q24.1), and DEC genes (Gomez-Abellan 2007, Kato *et al.* 2006). These genes have been identified through responses to light and measured circadian biowaves.

Early suspicions were raised about the assumption that SCN cells only existed within the hypothalamus. Gradually, *in vitro* and *in vivo* testing demonstrated that other cells throughout the body also contain individual SCN cells. In 1970, Yamaoka reported finding SCN cells in the region of the thyroid gland. Over the next few years, enough dissecting had been done to demonstrate that SCN cells exist throughout the human body. Studies on light inducement have confirmed that these genetically expressed switches around the body respond to light, and exist within the testes, ovaries, kidneys, and most other organs. They have also been found in adipose cells, various nerve cells, and even cartilage cells. Each of the SCN genes is expressed through a unique disposition. The PER expression, for example, is increased by light exposure during the night, yet remains unstimulated by increased light exposure during the day (Shearman *et al.* 1997).

Further research concluded that SCN cells are not only responsive to light. They also respond to selected mRNA and prostaglandin switching molecules. It was found that every cell seems to have its own independent clockworks, but groups of cells synchronize their clocks to a common setting. The genetic structures of the SCN cells have been further investigated, indicating these clockworks have precise genetic switching mechanisms (Buijs *et al.* 2006).

The work of Dr. H. Okamura (2005) from the Kobe University School of Medicine confirmed that SCN clock cell genes are located throughout most of the body's major tissue and organ systems. Apparently, the genetic expressions of SCN cell oscillations are coupled with the independent clockwork genes in these various locations of the body. This coupling (or resonating) of genetic expressions appears to synchronize the pacing of the SCN-stimulated activities within the cell.

This tells us that the body's clockworks create an alignment between consciousness and sensory stimuli from the environment. A variance or misalignment between these two would logically lead to a diseased state. Through a combination of *in vitro* elimination and research on animals, a number of studies have confirmed that damage or mutation to these clockwork genes can result in various disease models. For example, damage to the Per1 and Per2 genes has been linked with a number of human cancer models (Chen-Goodspeed and Cheng 2007).

Clockwork genes have also been undeniably linked to the rhythmic release of hormones and neurotransmitters. Clockwork genes are now considered the key regulators (or mediators) for all metabolic processes. Mutations of human clock genes have been linked to metabolic syndrome (Gomez-Abellan *et al.* 2007), bone marrow CD34 immune cell availability (Tsinkalovsky *et al.* 2007), depression (Benedetti *et al.* 2007), and glutathione function (Igarashi *et al.* 2007). Clock genes are disrupted in mania-like behavior (Roybal *et al.* 2007). The clock genes have also been observed mediating expression of the plasminogen activator inhibitor, yielding a greater risk of heart attack (Chong *et al.* 2006). In 2005, researchers from the University of Pittsburgh's School of Medicine found that bipolar disorder was also linked to a disruption of clock genetic expression (Mansour 2005).

The clock genes correlate information from the SCN cells with various cues from around the body as well. One of the more important synchronizing mechanisms for these genes along with light is feeding schedules. There is an apparent entrainment to feeding cycles and energy metabolism connected with the SCN/CLOCK gene interaction (Mendoza 2007). Alcohol consumption also appears to substantially alter the expression patterns of a large population of clock genes. The PER genes—especially among brain cells—are significantly affected by alcohol consumption (Spanagel *et al.* 2005).

Recent research indicates that the clock genes engage in a feedback loop of genetic transcription and translation. This takes place with protein phosphorylation via kinases that reactivate alternating expression loops of the WC-1 and WC-2 proteins. These sequences become switched on and off through the induction of light to heat (Lakin-Thomas 2006). Cry1 seems to mediate CLOCK/Bmal1 complex repression, which sets up the feedback response (Sato *et al.* 2006). Further research has uncovered the potential of prostaglandin-2 as an activation-switch for resetting these genes, leading researchers to propose a connection between pain and the biological clock. These feedback loops have also been referred to as rhythmic, with a conserved control of gene transcription regulation (Hardin 2004).

It also appears that these SCN neurons are coupled to (or resonate with) other cells. Through a co-signaling process linked to glucocorticoid production, sympathetic nerve activity and other metabolic systems, activation of genetic alterations by SCN are stimulated by light and other waveforms. Organ-based SCN neurons also have their own waveform switching mechanisms, which turn on and off the various functions of that particular organ.

SCN cells participate in the production of critical neurotransmitter-hormones melatonin and serotonin. The major on and off switches for these biochemicals include light along with a biochemical switching (inhibitory) neurotransmitter messenger called GABA (Gamma-aminobutyric acid) (Perreau-Lenz *et al.* 2005). The dense network of serotonergic neurons within the central nervous system connects with networks of SCN cells. Light-driven oscillations of the SCN cells thus stimulate rhythmic serotonin release through these neurons' activity (Moore and Speh 2004).

The photoreceptor signaling process is still somewhat mysterious. It appears, however, that a protein called malanopsin is involved in a photo pigmentation process stimulating SCN cells. The signaling transduction pathway proposed with respect to the gene phosphorylation system is Glu-Ca2+-CaMKII-nNOS-GC-cGMP-cGK—>—>clock genes. This is obviously a waveform transmission and semiconductance pathway. The body's crystalline transmission and reception sequences within DNA translate these waveforms into intelligent instructional signals.

In 2005, Dr. Erik Herzog and Sara Aton discovered a peptide that lies between SCN neurons, polarizing their rhythmic oscillations. The *vasoactive intestinal polypeptide,* so named because it was found in the gut, became noteworthy because it is apparently produced within the SCN cell pathway. Dr. Herzog proposes the VIP lying between SCN neurons *"is like a rubber band between the pendulums of two grandfather clocks, helping to synchronize their timing"* (Aton *et al.* 2005).

Dr. Paolo Sassone-Corsi's 2006 studies at the University of California revealed that the CLOCK genes function in a fashion comparable to enzymes in the switching process. A year later, Dr. Sassone-Corsi's research found that a single amino acid within the BAL1 protein provides the initial switching signal that influences a single modification. This amino acid bonding modification appears to stimulate other body clock switching systems.

Other body clock signaling pathways have been discovered as the research has continued. These involve a myriad of biochemicals and gene sequences. The irony here is that scientists have been looking for a particular single biochemical or gene that is ultimately responsible for the entire body's clock mechanisms. Instead, soon after one biochemical, molecule or gene is located and thought to be the clock mechanism; another seems to emerge to replace it. The apparent weakness seems to be in the theory of one particular clock mechanism. We propose that the real weakness lies within the assumption that the clock is a single biochemical switch.

One of the mysteries illustrating a weakness in this single switch theory is that blind people have functional biological clocks. A blind body's clockworks will tune precisely to the sun's clockworks despite no obvious entry of light to the pineal gland's SCN region. It has been proposed that retinal cells contain another type of neural photoreceptor system—one receiving electromagnetic rhythms outside the visual relay system. Another theory proposes a few photoreceptor cells remain in blind people allowing them to stimulate the pineal/SCN system while not having enough activity to stimulate the LGN and visual cortex.

A larger mystery is how these various clockwork genes and cells communicate and synchronize throughout the body. In 2004, Dr. David Welsh and a team of researchers observed individual fibroblasts under various conditions. Fibroblasts are cells that will differentiate into connective tissue cells, osteoblasts and other cells. It turns out that fibroblasts also contain self-regulating circadian clockwork genes, somehow synchronizing their behavior with the rest of the rhythmic activities of the body.

The missing link is consciousness. Imagine a house full of thousands of clocks, each having different timing mechanisms and different alarms, dials, pace, and functions, all requiring occasional resetting to stay coordinated. Who oversees the process of resetting? Who governs the objectives or purpose of the resetting? Without a purpose, we would find a room of coo-coo clocks, ticking away separately without a governor.

The rhythms of all these clockworks remain harmonious through consciousness. A good example is the cycle between cortisol and melatonin. Each is driven by different cascading pathways. Cortisol—known to increase metabolism—levels tends to increase and peak as melatonin—known to decrease metabolism and induce sleep—levels recede in the morning. Then, as cortisol levels recede in the evening, melatonin levels increase correspondingly, peaking around midnight as the cortisol levels have wound down. Seemingly independent pathways are driven by seemingly independent endocrine systems. Somehow, these cycles synchronize with each other, yet do not overlap. Through some intelligent mechanism, one gradually recedes while the other increases. This single feat, repeated billions of times every second, is orchestrated. What is the orchestrating mechanism? What provides the baseline direction or controlling purpose?

DNA Information Conductance

In 1869, the Swiss Dr. Friedrich Miescher isolated an interesting conglomeration of molecules extracted from discarded surgical bandages. Believing this substance was derived from the nuclei of human cells, he called this substance *nuclein*. Two decades earlier the Swiss botanist Karl von Nageli observed this same material dividing in plant cells. They were named *chromosomes* because they so conveniently received identifying colored dyes, making them very visible (chromo) when peering through a microscope. In a series of discoveries from 1905 to 1929, Dr. Phoebus Levene demonstrated the existence of ribose and deoxyribose linked together in phosphate-sugar base units. Dr. Levene was convinced, however, that these units were isolated and did not contain any kind of coding information.

In 1944, physicist Erwin Schrödinger proposed in a book called *What is Life?* that the cell contained an information element within the chromosomes, which he surmised, scripted the activities of the cell and life in general. This consideration lay dormant until in 1948, using x-ray diffraction imaging, Dr. Linus Pauling pointed out that most proteins inside the cell were made not only of complex 20-amino acid combinations, but were often curiously helical in shape. These observations led to a deepening curiosity regarding the nucleus' protein content, and a suspicion they provided the instructional foundation for cellular growth and metabolism. Between 1950 and 1953, again utilizing x-ray diffraction, Dr. Rosalind Franklin and Dr. Maurice Wilkins independently developed scans of base pairings that demonstrated the possibility of a much larger helical molecule with numerous base pairings. Working from these unpublished results, Dr. Francis Crick and Dr. James Watson were the first to publish a presentation of a double-helixed deoxyribonucleic acid, or DNA, in a series of articles for *Nature* magazine.

Proteins are the primary biochemical structures involved in the execution of nearly every cellular process throughout biological life. Proteins are the body's soldiers: Some proteins act as enzymes and catalysts to assist in metabolic reactions. Some proteins are hormones. They stimulate cells and various organs to perform certain activities. Other proteins will assist in cell growth, energy production, or immune systems. Most other proteins are made up of a distinctive arrangement of up to twenty different amino acids. A typical protein molecule will contain hundreds of different combinations of these twenty amino acids. Many protein molecules are twisted, helical or semi-helical molecules. An example of this is the interleukin-6 molecule, a complex immune protein produced by the body's T-cells.

DNA is actually a very large protein. DNA might be aptly considered a protein library, as its sequencing and transcription with RNA predicates the formation of specific proteins. DNA is a very complex molecule. It is elegantly designed, made up of long sugar-phosphate chains linked to combinations of four possible purine or pyrimidine nucleotide pairs. The DNA molecule has two complementary strands bound between the pairs, which form its double-helix structure. The two strands are not precisely identical. They are described as complementary because they have a slightly different polarity. This polarity bends DNA into its beautiful spiral structure.

The order of nucleotides on the DNA chain and the particular amino acid each nucleotide associates with creates distinctive sequencing combinations. These are typically called the *genetic code,* or the *hapmap.* Portions of a hapmap or sequenced combinations are referred to as *alleles.* It has been estimated that one human DNA molecule can have over 3 billion base (purine or pyrimidine) pair and amino acid combinations. Together, the combination of sequences is called a *genome*.

The DNA pairs making up the sequencing are connected by weak electromagnetic hydrogen bonds. These electromagnetic bonds allow the DNA molecule to quite easily separate its framework under stress, depending upon the length of the strand. Shorter DNA strands will fall apart more easily in a heated solution or from radiation for this reason. These weak bonds are easily breakable, but their sequencing combinations provide a framework for a translation mechanism for information. Several decades of progressive genetic research has confirmed that DNA sequences match up with unique characteristics and functions within individual cells and organisms.

The reason for DNA's mysterious complexity is not its double helix shape or its intricate coding system: Its coding system is actually rather simple. The incredible complex nature of DNA lies primarily with ribonucleic acid or RNA. RNA molecules are very similar to DNA molecules, except most are single-stranded. Most RNA are still helical, however. RNA also have slightly different chemical base systems, but their sequencing is programmed via the copying—or *transcription*—of sections of the DNA's hapmap.

RNA transcription allows DNA to be replicated—or copied to make a new DNA molecule with the same coding sequences. To accomplish this, special DNA enzymes such as DNA polymerase will split apart a DNA strand. RNA strands are then somehow stimulated to wrap up against the DNA strand to extract and record the code. Once it records the coding, RNA uses this to help make another DNA set by transferring the coding on to structures that assemble proteins.

RNA is the molecule implicitly required not only for the survival of DNA, but also for the production of the millions of proteins, which in turn perform most of the body's metabolic processes. The various types of RNA will translate selected sections of the DNA's sequencing information for different purposes: Transfer RNA (tRNA) transfer amino acids to protein sequences to assemble active proteins. Messenger RNA (mRNA) are considered metabolic information carriers: They communicate specific action plans from DNA sequencing to specialized ribosomes—where many proteins are assembled. This process of making proteins in the ribosomes is also assisted by another RNA type, the ribosomal RNA (rRNA). Catalytic RNA or ribozymes are catalysts for specialized biochemical reactions. Double-stranded RNA (dsRNA) appear to be intermediaries for another active double-stranded RNA called small interfering RNA (siRNA) which apparently interfere with the expression of certain DNA sequences. This seems to create a protective function in circumstances where invasion or mutation is possible.

A number of other RNA types have been classified as non-coding RNA (ncRNA). These include micro RNA (miRNA) and germline RNA. These were proposed by Rassoulzadegan (2006) as being heritable—or able to be passed through to new generations. Non-coding forms of RNA provide the new frontier in understanding RNA function.

In essence, RNA appear to provide the mechanisms to copy and transmit the informational coding contained in the DNA. After copying the DNA master hapmaps, RNA seem to effectively pass on that information into executive form by enabling protein mechanisms to perform their particular activities. RNA enable the process of manufacturing specialized protein molecules, and even contribute particular amino acids themselves. RNA's activities also provide a storage and retrieval function for DNA's coded sequencing, thereby guaranteeing the DNA's survival as cells divide and become replaced.

Noting that RNA provide a form of information biocommunication, most researchers have assumed that all of this information is chemically transmitted through the transcription process. Recent research from Stanford Medical Center's John Rin and Dr. Howard Chang (2007) has confirmed that RNA can also communicate their instructional messages remotely. RNA can remotely silence individual genes by interfering in their expression, for example. ncRNA were observed regulating and suppressing genes on remote chromosomes at remote distances within the cell.

Over the last two decades, geneticists have focused on assembling the combined gene combinations that together would make up the genome of particular organisms. The human genome research combined with an institution-wide focus on establishing the genome of other species. The assumption in the beginning of this research project—which involved hundreds of scientists from different specialties over two decades—was that we would find within the genome the answers to all the mysteries of the body, disease, evolution, and our ultimate identity. Surprisingly, none of this was found. The evolutionary assumption, for example, was that they would find an increasingly complex assembly of genes up the evolutionary 'hierarchy' of species. This fell on its ear as the research revealed that humans only have about 25,000 gene combinations—about the same amount that a small fish or a mouse has. Plants contain more genes than humans. In other words, gene combinations were no more complex in humans than they were in many other creatures.

Furthermore, the initial assumption was that the combination of genes in humans would unfold and unlock the key to all disease pathologies. Preliminary research connected certain gene combinations or gene expressions to particular diseases. It was assumed that every disease had a particular genetic trait to match. This worked out pretty well until researchers began discovering that sometimes two or three diseases were connected to the same genetic trait or expression. For example, Angelman Syndrome and Prader-willy Syndrome both relate to the same chromosome 15 deletion. This revealed some further factor involved.

The other mystery for geneticists, which we will discuss later in more detail, was that identical twins—which have the same DNA at some point, seemingly at conception—do not develop the same diseases. Identical twins, in fact, often have very different physiological outcomes. This was apparently related to whether the genes were switched on.

This has forced a calibration of the genetic theory with the concept of *epigenetics*. In general, epigenetics is the acceptance of additional factors that affect the switching of gene expression and non-expression. It was hypothesized—and confirmed by the research—that ones DNA was not as important as how gene expressions—or *phenotypes*—were turned on or off. If the genes were expressed, particular metabolism consequences resulted. If they were not expressed, there would be other consequences.

The original concept of epigenetics was penned by geneticist Conrad Waddington in the early 1940s to explain in general how environmental circumstances could effect ones genetic instructions. The concept, however, was given increasing focus in the 1990s and early 2000s as geneticists discovered the various many holes genome assumptions contained.

The biochemical relationships between gene expressions have focused upon the action of DNA methylation or histone regulation. These biochemical messengers were observed switching alleles on or off. Experiments on mice at McGill University's Douglas Hospital Research Center (Szyf *et al.* 2008) found that phenotype switching could be turned on and off with the exchange of increased nurturing from the mother. Those baby mice receiving the nurturing from mama would switch on genes differently than those mice that received less nurturing from mama.

Biochemical mechanisms like phosphorylation, sumoylation, acetylation, methylation, and ubiquitylation appear to be mechanically responsible for phenotype expression—which connects them to the availability of nutrients like vitamin B and Co-Q-10. Even so, a critical element of the *epigenome* bridges these messaging systems with consciousness.

These illustrate the very elements that nature stimulates through the conductance of natural materials. These include our foods, our nutrients, sunlight, fresh air, water and so on. Nature's waveforms pulse through our bodies just as our man-made pollutants do. The difference is that man-made pollutants degrade our bodies while nature supports them.

Homeopathy is a homuncular element of nature. In homeopathy, these natural elements are being diluted to their most fundamental electromagnetic information.

How do we know this? Nature provides homuncular elements in every dilution process. When rain inundates the ground and becomes absorbed into the soil, it is taken up by plants and other organisms who present that water back in the form of their excrement and waste streams. These provide nutrients and nourish the soils and the plants reflectively. It all folds in together, creating arrays of ecological balance. This is illustrated by the very cyclic nature of our environment.

Dilution is part of nature, and the dissolving of substance into water and creating increasing dilution simply extends the natural processes of solvents and solutes. They mirror them.

We are thus constantly consuming nature's elements in a homeopathic manner. With every breath we take in minute quantities of trees that produced the oxygen, and the ocean waters that were evaporated to produce humidity. Thus we cannot be disconnected with the homeopathic tendency of nature. We can only get closer to it by embracing it and understanding it better.

Chapter Six

Mind and Homeopathy

The sciences of psychology and mental health have a rather obtuse history. Psychological disorders such as depression and anxiety were considered and treated in Ayurvedic medicine, ancient Chinese medicine, the Egyptian healing arts, and the medicines of the Greeks and Romans. In the middle ages, however, a religious fanaticism took hold of Europe, which led to the widespread belief that mental disease was the result of demonic possession.

There is a significant amount of knowledge and research on the mind over the thousands of years of traditional medicine amongst those cultures. Psychology and psychiatry as a science is considered today to have arose only during the late nineteenth century: A limited view to say the least. Wilhelm Wundt is thus considered the father of modern psychological research. He founded an 1879 laboratory at the University of Leipzig—where he was a professor. Two years later, he founded the first European psychology journal, and wrote a number of books on the subject. Professor Wundt's *structuralism* model of the mind proposed a dividing of the mind into various parts, with each part performing different tasks. This theory later gave way to the modern theories of *functionalism* and *behaviorism*.

The role of the unconscious part of the mind has been studied for thousands of years. The Greeks were known to use hypnosis, and they studied the undercurrent of the mind, together with the dreamscape. The art of hypnosis was somewhat lost, however, until it was revived by Franz Mesmer in the eighteenth century. Mesmer's proposal was that hypnosis was created by a force of nature called *animal magnetism,* which overwhelmed his subjects as they encountered magnets—adjusting the body's tidal influences. Interestingly, Mesmer also proposed that life moves through the body via thousands of tiny channels. The flow of life through these channels, he thought, was subject to various environmental influences, including spiritual forces and the movement of planets. One might wonder whether Mesmer studied the ancient Ayurvedic and/or Chinese systems. Nonetheless, hypnotism became controversial to say the least.

It was not until the respected Scottish surgeon James Braid announced hypnotism as genuine in the 1840s that the hypnotic trance was accepted as anything other than a form of hysteria in Europe and America. Hypnosis was largely overlooked during the years following. Its use as a form of treatment only became more prominent in the late nineteenth century and the early twentieth century. Today it is widely used.

The concept that prevailed in the nineteenth century was one describing the mind as consisting of different levels of sections. A number of theories were proposed on the nature and functions of these portions. Probably the most famous were those of Dr. Pierre Marie Félix Janet and Dr. Sigmund Freud, both prominent psychologists during the late nineteenth and early twentieth century. Janet is attributed to have arrived at the theory of the mind being divided into *conscious, unconscious* and *preconscious* parts. In the 1920s, Freud proposed the mind contained three different components: the *ego*, the *super-ego* and the *id*. Freud's theory took center stage as a possible explanation of various behavioral problems confronting physicians and psychologists since that time. Both Freud and Janet gathered a great deal of information through hypnotism. By hypnotizing people, Freud and Janet *regressed* them to re-experience the behavior or thinking that occurred prior to a current disorder. Though many insights and disease pathologies came out of this research, it was generally regarded as having fallen short of proving the existence of the three parts of the mind.

The proposal regarding mental disease stemming from the three sections of the mind was rooted in the assumption that the mind is constantly in conflict. Freud proposed that a conflict between these three parts of the mind creates mental disturbance, while a balance between them creates mental health. He proposed that the id is the unconscious source encouraging the gratification of desires, rooted in the most basic desires of survival. Meanwhile the super-ego supposedly stands in opposition with these desires, acting as the conscience. The ego supposedly mediates between the id and super-ego, presenting the conscious portion of the mind to the world. The science of psychology has accepted the assumption of a conscious and subconscious apportionment of the mind. However, various ancillary theories have been presented over the years since Janet and Freud.

Unsatisfied with the ability to change a person's behavior using hypnotism, Janet and Freud embarked on their now-famous methods of *psychoanalysis*. These methods are still used today by psychologists and psychiatrists, and are actually quite basic: The patient is simply encouraged to discuss problems and issues the patient feels is related to the dilemma at hand.

The process of hypnosis for psychological treatment is based upon the use of *autosuggestion*. The process usually begins with the hypnotist positioning before the patient and suggesting the patient is becoming sleepy and relaxed. Sometimes distractive rhythmic devices are used, the most famous of which is a small pendulum. As the trust in the hypnotist develops within the patient, the patient dozes off into a state of *suggestibility*—being open to suggestion. During this time, the patient may be clearly aware of the events transpiring—or not, depending upon the suggestions of the hypnotist. Depending upon the type of hypnosis given, the patient may also be drawn into a deeper state where the patient may not be able to recall the hypnosis episode consciously. This has often been described as an altered state of consciousness.

One discipline, which has its roots in Freud and hypnotism, is *autogenics*, introduced by Dr. Malcolm Caruthers in the 1970s. The word autogenic refers to something generated from within. The *autogenic training system* consisted of becoming aware of the body's autonomic nervous system, and being able to control both sympathetic and parasympathetic physical responses to stress. This was accomplished primarily through visualization techniques.

Another important psychological system, also deeply steeped in these concepts of the conscious and unconscious mind was behaviorism. Research into behavior modification was made famous by the work of Ivan Pavlov, who in the early twentieth century worked with both animals and humans to understand how the mind can connect pleasure and pain with particular *triggers,* which bring about a trained response. The dog-salivation experiments of Pavlov's dog experiments are quite famous, and they have given birth to a number of behavioral psychological theories and practices. One of the more notable behavioral theorists is B. F. Skinner. Professor Skinner's research into conditioning and behavior modification has become a foundation for many of the psychological theories assumed today.

A distant relative of behaviorism is functionalism. This concept was advanced by Dr. Alan Turing. In 1950 Dr. Turing laid out the fundamentals of the theory with his article *Computing Machinery and Intelligence.* Dr. Turing proposed that the mind is a learning machine of sorts, accumulating experience throughout ones lifetime.

Of course, behavior modification and conditioning—or *operant conditioning*—has been commonly used by parents, teachers and authoritarians over the duration of human existence. This system is also embedded into the natural world. It is not hard to observe that as we experience events and the consequences of our actions, we begin to learn that certain activities have better results than do others. This realization theoretically changes our behavior, leading to a gradual process of evolution. Those who do not adjust their behavior or learn the lessons, on the other hand, are destined to face a recurrence of those lessons until they are learned.

After many years of hypnotherapy, the fundamental mechanisms— along with the supposed conscious and unconscious mind themselves—are still considered mysterious by western science. Some propose suggestibility is simply a state of mind and hypnosis is simply the succumbing to suggestion. However, there is enough documented evidence of hypnotized patients retrieving historical information not accessible when conscious to consider the alternatives. This lends credence to the position of the mind held by the ancient sciences.

Neuronal Information Exchange

Over the past couple of decades, the study of the mind has been directed towards the electromagnetic properties of the brain's neurons. This trend towards a physiological interpretation of the mind through the transduction of electrical activity between neurons necessitates the assumption that the mind and brain are one and the same. The primary means for research promoting this assumption has been the use of various radiative imaging systems such as electroencephalography (EEG), magnetoencephalography (MEG), magnetic resonance (MRI), positron emission tomography (PET), and computed tomography using x-rays. These imaging systems each focus on different waveform attributes of brain neurons, as they are altered by these different forms of radiation.

This mapping of the brain was pioneered during the 1920s by Dr. Wilder Penfield, who touched various parts of subjects' brains with electrode sensors while they lay conscious on the operating table prior to or following brain surgery. Dr. Penfield began noticing commonalities between patient responses as he touched certain parts of the brain. Dr. Penfield accumulated enough data over time to develop a map of the various cortex regions and sensory regions. Dr. Penfield co-authored the landmark *Epilepsy and the Functional Anatomy of the Human Brain* (1951) with Dr. Herbert Jasper, a reference still used today.

Dr. Penfield's research focused on epileptics initially. He observed that certain parts of the brain were more active than others during certain types of thoughts, memories, and/or behaviors. Dr. Penfield found that if he stimulated a part of the brain with the electrode, he could provoke a particular type of memory. This led to Dr. Penfield and the rest of the medical community surmising that memory is retained within particular specialized brain cells within certain regions. Furthermore, he concluded that particular parts of the brain specialized in certain types of thoughts or activities. The subsequent mapping not only identified functional parts of the brain. It also identified which types of memories were theoretically stored within that particular region. These mapped locations were called *engrams*.

In the 1940s, a psychologist named Dr. Karl Lashley conducted research that contradicted this notion that memories were located in specific brain neurons. Dr. Lashley trained mice to particular tasks and then removed different parts of their brains. He then reintroduced the mice to the same circumstances, and found that despite brain cell areas associated with those memories being removed, they were still able to remember the tasks learned prior to the surgery. Furthermore, even when most of the rats' brains were removed, the rats were unexpectedly still able to remember what was taught to them prior to the surgery.

A prominent neuroscientist Dr. Karl Pribran followed this research with many years of study on memory and engrams. Dr. Pribran's initial research focused on the frontal cortex of monkeys and cats, and his research identified specific areas of the brain associated with particular cognitive functions. However, he was intrigued by repeated results—like Dr. Lashley—indicating that when specific neurons or regions were removed or severed, cognition predominantly continued. For example, he found when the optic nerve was severed, an animal could still perceive an image in detail. This led to Dr. Pribran's conclusion that perception and cognition went deeper than simply particular brain neurons and brain regions.

Years earlier, Dr. Lashley had entertained the notion of a wave interference pattern for memories. Dr. Pribran, worked closely with renowned physicists Dr. David Bohm and Dr. Dennis Gabor—the 1971 Nobel laureate in physics. Together they arrived at the notion that cognition and memory were related to the mechanics of wave transmission. Using *Fourier analysis*—in which sine wave function is calculated within the context of the action, the *holonomic brain model of cognitive function* was born. This theory was proposed along the lines of the *Gabor function,* which was put forth by Dr. Gabor to propose the natural existence of the hologram within light (Pribran 1991).

When we examine some of the expansive research done in the field of brainwaves, we see how both brain function and the mind are closely related to rhythmic wave mechanics. The electroencephalogram measures the voltage potential differences among different regions of the brain. These voltage differences result in a wave formation, which can range in wavelength, frequency and amplitude among a collection of neurons. These brainwaves are not single units in themselves. They are surges of collective interference patterns created by the billions of reflecting waves of billions of neurons, cells and the various other waveforms large and small moving through the body.

Delta waves cycle from one to three hertz, and tend to predominate during NREM (non-rapid eye movement) sleep, and some meditation. During this type of sleep, dreaming is minimal and the body is often in motion. Delta waves tend to resonate more actively in the frontal cortex. Delta waves correlate with an increase in the production and circulation of growth hormone. One of growth hormone's more important attributes within the body is its ability to advance the healing and regeneration process.

Theta waves cycle at four to seven hertz and dominate during mid-stage sleeping. Theta waves are more elusive, but seem to most active during memory retrieval and consolidation during sleep, and become more active in creative endeavors and behavior modification during waking hours. The hippocampus appears to actively accommodate and transduce these waves. Observations have noted peak hippocampus activity during predominantly theta wave periods. The hippocampus is associated with spatial recognition and short-term memory consolidation.

Alpha waves will cycle at eight to thirteen cycles per second, and are dominant during light sleep and dreaming, as well as some meditation states. Alpha waves are seen dominant during memorization tasks, especially those related to words, persons and visual impressions.

They tend to be most prominent at the back of the skull and towards the side of the body most favored by the organism. The earth's predominating waveforms cycle in the alpha range. This is called the *Schumann resonance,* discovered by Dr. Winfried Otto Schumann in 1952. The earth has several Schumann Resonance nodes, including the alpha level eight hertz (rounded), fourteen hertz, twenty hertz, twenty-six hertz, thirty-two hertz, thirty-nine hertz and forty-five hertz. The harmonic here is approximately six to eight hertz. Audio testing has concluded that listening to an eighth hertz beat will increase alpha brainwave levels. This essentially establishes a harmonic between the body's wave activity and the earth's.

Beta waves will cycle at fourteen to thirty hertz and are dominant during active, waking consciousness. These waves tend to be prominent towards the front of the brain on the side predominating during that activity. Beta waves reflect a state of focused attention and activity. A lack of beta waves during waking hours—or lower frequency beta waves—tends to occur with a lack of focus or concentration. On the other hand, as the brainwave levels increase toward the higher range of beta and into the gamma range at over thirty cycles per second, a higher level of focus and concentration occurs.

Gamma waves are higher frequency brain waves, and are often referred to as high-frequency beta waves. Gamma waves predominate during intense problem solving and focused learning. Gamma waves cycle at thirty to sixty hertz. Recent research has determined that gamma waves will be synchronized and coded by phase within the visual cortex. This phase shifting creates a coherence mechanism—a sorting process where gamma waves with the same phases are segregated and commingled. The resulting sorting process allows the gamma waves to interfere and provide associations of particular thoughts, images or impressions of sensual information.

High gamma waves cycle from sixty to two hundred hertz, and have only become obvious to researchers using more sensitive equipment. These brainwaves are seen during the most intense cognitive functions. The slower waves of theta, delta and alpha tend to resonate with distinct physical attributes. The high gamma waves tend to relate to higher states, and tend to be more diverse in their connection points and locations around the regions of the central nervous system. In one study of eight subjects, for example, high gamma brainwave activity increased during the practice of *pranayama*—a method of concentrated meditative breath control (Vialatte *et al.* 2008).

Another type of brainwaves were found using sensitive microelectrodes. These have been termed *ripples*. Ripples are high frequency oscillations that appear to be generated in the hippocampus. They have been observed oscillating with the negative portion of slower brainwaves. Ripples appear to transduce through the medial temporal lobe, notably between the hippocampus and the rhinal cortex—a region associated with the processing of explicit memory recall. Explicit memory includes active intentional recall during conscious cognition. In other words, ripples appear to function as informational waveform 'bites' used to access recent, conscious memories and instructions. It is part of our active information biocommunication system.

The discovery of ripples augments our position that EEG research has tended to oversimplify the role of brain waveforms that oscillate through the various neurons. The brain's mapping has focused on larger regions of the brain. There are still intra-neuronal networks that function on a more subtle basis. For example, a central pivoting exchange factor of the brain's networking system includes the *pyramidal neuron networks*. Pyramidal neurons lie within the cortex regions of the brain. Regions more dense with pyramidal neurons are often collectively referred to as the *neocortex*. Here their densities can be as high as 75%. Researchers have estimated the total number of pyramidal neurons in the brain to be in the neighborhood of fifteen to twenty billion. These specialized neurons crystallize and transduce waveform signals between the cortices and the rest of the central nervous system. Some of these signals have different frequency attributes. They appear to transduce through the polar gateway systems of ion channels. These are not unlike the on-off states of computer machine code, except there is typically more than one type of on-off state among each gateway, to allow for feedback loops. Another, more dimensional description of this transduction is called *signal coupling*. This is when multiple waveforms are "coupled" to create a unique pattern. We might refer to this as a *multiple wave interference model.*

Research has clocked the brain's activity has speeds of between 1/1000 and 10/1000 of a second, which would convert to 100-1000 meters/second. As these frequencies relate to the wave nature of the electrical activity of the brain, they also imply that there is a rhythmic function to the mechanics of the mind. The fact that the frequency increases as our mind becomes more active indicates that higher activity exerts a greater wave speed.

Certainly if we consider how instantaneous reactions and thoughts move around the body, we are talking not only about speed. We are dealing with a network broadcasting system allowing for nearly instantaneous communication. Not that this communication system is not linear as well; it is linear yet still global: concurrently spreading into the vast territories of organs, tissues and muscles. Allopathy compares all of this activity moving through the body to electricity. We would rather compare this biocommunication process to the network access of a website to billions of browsers connected on the internet. This certainly requires an information technology quite a bit more complicated than a home electricity circuit. This type of technology utilizes a mechanism of simultaneous information data coherence.

One example of how multiple waveform coherence works is the *potassium channels*—discovered several decades ago. Potassium channels are specialized proteins found in brain neurons, which regulate the voltage moving between neurons around the brain. As we look closer at these channels, we find they oscillate between gateway states, regulating ionic electrical pulses. These channels provide just one of the conduits for transmitting information. As we examine the instructional pathways connecting neurons together with the physical activity of the body, we can conclude these circuits crystallize and broadcast complex waveforms, disseminating conscious intention from one part of the body throughout various regions of the anatomy.

These pathways for waveform broadcasting from one part of the brain to another appear to be necessary for the mind to develop complete images. Multiple researchers have confirmed that neurons of the visual cortex do not readily pick the full spectrum of frequencies necessary to form a complete image of what we perceive. The ramification of this is significant, simply because we typically assume that what we perceive is "out there" in the physical domain. We assume that we are receiving a complete picture.

Russian scientist Dr. Nikolai Bernstein performed film studies on human perception for several decades in the mid-twentieth century, illustrating that human movement could be translated into wave patterns using Fourier calculations. This is illustrated as we watch television or a movie. When we perceive movement on the TV or movie screen, we are not actually seeing any movement. We are merely seeing a series of still pictures flashed in sequence faster than we can consciously notice. Between the flashed images is a significant dead space or dark image. Our minds fill in the blanks and create the illusion of movement.

The work of neuroscientist Dr. Russell DeValois focused on this element of visual perception over the past several of decades. His research papers documented how the mind integrates batches of visual inputs such as color and motion. His years of groundbreaking research culminated in a 1990 compendium *Spatial Vision*, co-authored with his wife Kathleen—also a professor in the subject. His memorial quoted him describing his lifetime's work in visual perception as, *"the physiological and anatomical organization underlying visual perception. In particular, how wavelength information is analyzed and encoded, the contribution of wavelength and luminance information to spatial vision, and how spatial information is analyzed and encoded in the visual nervous system."*

In one study performed by Dr. DeValois at the University of California at Berkeley, the responses of cats and monkeys were analyzed while responding to visual checkerboard patterns. Rather than responding to the patterns themselves, the animals responded to the interference patterns created by the complementary aspects of the design, consistent with Fourier-calculated interference waves.

The work of Dr. Fergus Campbell at Cambridge University has confirmed that the human cerebral cortex picks up particular frequencies and not others. The cerebral component neurons are 'tuned' to specific wavelengths and frequencies. Dr. Pribran also confirmed this in his research on cats and monkeys. During these tests, it became apparent that combinations of waves of particular frequencies were being received, processed and converted into perceived images as they were combined with internally created waveforms. These internal waveforms are drawn from memory through a hierarchical cortical mapping sorting process.

In the 1970s, Dr. Benjamin Libet began researching decision-making and brain electrical response at the University of California at San Francisco. His goal was to explore a concept first introduced by Luder Deeke and Hans Kurnhuber called *bereitschafts-potential*—which translates to *readiness potential*. In Dr. Libet's studies, human volunteers hooked up to an electroencephalograph were told to perform activities such as button pressing or finger flicking. Dr. Libet's research compared three points in time: When the subject consciously made the decision to press the button; when the button was pressed; and when brainwaves indicated an instruction from the motor cortex was made using the EEG. As expected, the conscious decision preceded the button pushing by an average of about 200 milliseconds (or 150 milliseconds considering a 50 msec margin of error). Surprisingly, however, the brainwaves associated with the instruction to press the bottom actually preceded the subject's conscious decision to take the action. Stunned by these results, Dr. Libet and others spent several years confirming the results. Several scientific articles documented the findings (Libet *et al.* 1983; Libet 1985). These results indicated that the action somehow was not originating from the conscious mind, but must be coming from a deeper source. Still, as Dr. Libet wrote in 2003, the gap between the conscious mind and the physical act gives the conscious mind an ability to *"block or veto the process, resulting in no motor act."* This, Dr. Libet said, is confirmed by the common experience of consciously blocking urges incompatible with social acceptability.

In 2004—more than two decades after his groundbreaking discovery—Dr. Libet proposed a theory based on his and others' research in this area. He called this the *conscious mental field* theory. This theory proposed the mind is a sphere of activity bridging the various rhythmic pulsing of physical nerve cells with the subjective conscious experience. He described this subjective experience as an outgrowth of the various pulses, a sort of gathering or convergence of various inputs.

A neuron is made up of a cell body with a nucleus, and two types of nerve fibers that extend outward from the cell body. The fibers include *dendrites,* which conduct informational waveforms into the neural cell body. *Axons,* on the other hand, project waveforms outward, away from the cell body. Most neurons have multiple dendrites that spider outward making several connections. Sensory nerves typically have only one dendrite, however. Sensory nerves are also typically longer—sometimes measuring up to a meter in length. Dendrites act as receptors. They are tuned into the pulsed waveform messages that pass from neuron to neuron. They carry this rhythmic information into the neuron cell body where it may be translated or even transmuted before being conducted or broadcasted. In some cases, the neuron may simply conduct and amplify the waveform.

In addition to specialized sensory neurons referred to as *afferent nerves,* there are also motor neurons, which are usually referred to as *efferent neurons.* The efferent or motor neurons are designed to carry instructional waveforms outward through the central nervous system to specific skeletal or organ cells. In these locations, these cells respond as instructed by the information provided by these waveform interference patterns. We note this because a single waveform does not necessarily contain enough information to drive a complex motor process. It takes a waveform combination to affect these specialized cells. Some are stimulated into metabolism responses, secretions, or contractions. Because they are stimulated by the efferent neurons, these cells are called *effectors.*

The intentional self ultimately stimulates the effector neurons through the facilities offered by the neural network. The neural network generally has three basic types of processes: The first is to receive and translate afferent sensory waveforms from the senses and environment. The second is to project instructional waveform combinations outward through the appropriate neural tracts. The third process of the neural net is to prioritize, sort and catalog memories and various autonomic programs.

The brain grows and develops in the body from a tubular canal called the *neural tube*. The entire brain is made up of billions of neurons. These are networked into bundles of groupings, which include *nerve tracts, gyri, fissures, sulci* and *cerebrum lobes*. These groupings of specialized neurons work conjunctively to accomplish specialized tasks, while transmitting information back and forth through neural superhighways. The locations of these nerve groupings will be common. Most nerve functions thus have location *plasticity*. Plasticity is the ability of the organism to move or reorganize the location or processes involved in accomplishing particular tasks. In other words, should one location not be able to function, the organism will relocate the function to another region of the brain.

The self primarily utilizes the brain's functions through the frontal cortex. Here the various waveforms provided by the senses and the body's feedback are observed by the self. The self utilizes a command center called the prefrontal cortex to respond to these images. This is located towards the front of the brain, behind and on top of the forehead, almost the precise position described by *Ayurveda* as the region between the sixth and seventh *chakra* regions—the *soma chakra*. Indeed this region provides a gateway for the self to not only observe the condition of the body and the environment, but also submit executive orders in response. For these reasons, researchers have determined that the frontal lobes are stimulated during the processing of decisions related to right and wrong, the prioritization of consequences, and logical thinking. Through the prefrontal region, the self expresses personality and submits executive orders.

The *motor cortex* lies just behind the frontal cortex as we comb back over the head. It normally resides within a band of neural grey matter (neuron cells) that wrap around the top of the head onto the two sides. Here physical instructions from the frontal cortex begin their transduction towards execution. Within the motor cortex reside specialized networks of neurons, each network coordinated with specific types of motor activity. The *premotor* region contains billions of specialized *mirroring* neurons, which mirror and sort the executive decisions transmitted from the frontal cortex. Behind the premotor cortex is the *primary motor cortex*. This region contains specialized neurons that are able to broadcast specific neural waveforms out through the neural network for specific parts of the body. One section will govern the toes, while another will govern the feet, and so on. This organized vertical arrangement of specialized motor neurons is also referred to as the *homunculus motor* region, because each location is connected to specific body locations.

Behind the region of the motor cortex neurons is another set of regions grouped into what is called the *sensory cortex*. This region has several individual cortices, and spreads from the top of the head (*parietal lobe*) through the back of the head (*occipital lobe*) and along the sides (*temporal lobe*). Among these lobes lie the *visual cortex*, the *auditory cortex*, the *olfactory cortex*, the *postcentral gyrus*, and the *gustatory cortex*. In these respective regions, the various incoming sensory waveforms are translated and processed. The first three cortices—the visual, auditory and olfactory—are self-explanatory, being the centers that process waveforms of seeing, hearing and smelling, respectively. The postcentral gyrus processes the sensory waveforms of touch and balance, while the gustatory cortex processes taste waveforms from the tongue. Into each sensory cortex, specialized neural tracts conduct in and blend waveforms from the sense organs. The interference patterns of these waveforms blend together to provide an image screen of sorts for the self to observe.

The critical limbic system is positioned inside these cortex regions, towards the center of the brain. The limbic system is made up of the thalamus, the hypothalamus, the hippocampus, the cingulates, the fomix and the amygdala. Each of these has a slightly different function, but together they translate waveform data from the body in to be processed for memory and observance by the self. The limbic system's role is to prioritize and sort information according to crystallized neural programming. The hypothalamus and thalamus are the central translation system for waveforms traveling between the brain and the rest of the body. They also stimulate endocrine release of hormones and neurotransmitters, and translate incoming communications from around the body. The cingulates are programmed to govern the autonomic systems such as the heartbeat, breathing, hunger, and so on. The amygdala on the other hand, provides a gateway to the lower *chakra* centers, channeling the self's focus upon survival into fear and anger into the information processing. The hippocampus sorts and prioritizes all this information for memory storage. The fomix channels the waveform information from the hippocampus through a circuitry of memory processing (called the *Papex circuit)*, which we will examine in detail. Together the limbic system provides a translation and staging service for waveform information. We might compare the limbic system to a computer's operating system. The software might be stored in a particular location within the computer. Nevertheless, its programming instructions govern information translation, assembly, prioritization, storage, and transmission out to processing among peripheral devices and specialized programs.

The brain receives several types of input. The first is called *exteroception*, which means information gathered by the five basic senses of hearing, taste, smell, vision and touch. *Interoception* is the reception of signals received by the internal neurons, such as pain and other internal responses. The third reception type is *proprioception*, which is the internal feedback mechanism gauging coordinated movements, balance and motor efficiency—often referred to as *kinesthesia*. Meanwhile *equilibrioception* is the feedback of motor balance information, which is coordinated with waveforms passing through the vestibular system. *Nociception* is the reception of pain signals that accompany a threat of damage to tissues or cells. Finally, *thermoception* is the sensing of heat or coldness within the body. Other interoceptions include the sense of time, the esophageal senses and others. A few other sensations have been proposed, though most could also be considered a subset of interoception.

Each of these types of signals is associated with a particular region of the brain—though most interact in one respect or another within the limbic system and its components. For example, proprioception appears to resonate at the cerebellum. Thermoception resonates with thermoceptor cells in the hypothalamus. Nociception is thought to biocommunicate through the *anterior cingulated gyrus* (part of the cingulates).

As waveforms are stepped up through neural tracts toward the brain, the waveforms are boosted or converted by neural gateways into waveform configurations that can be managed by the limbic system. It is through the limbic system that various cortex regions are fed interoception from around the body. Programming sequences drive autonomic responses from the cortices primarily via the limbic system as well. As waveforms travel through the limbic system, the amygdale—channeling survival concerns of the self—is able to interact and alter these waveforms on their route to the particular cortex. This emotional interference system also works in reverse. Even if a particular decision is being channeled from the motor cortex to initiate a particular response in the body, the amygdale can alter or influence that instructional waveform as it moves back through the limbic system on its way out to stimulate particular motor nerve centers and endocrine responses (initiated primarily through the hypothalamus-pituitary pathway). In this way, motor responses may be exaggerated or muted through fear responses or other emotional responses.

Research has demonstrated an ionic channel based electrochemical *beta-adrenergic modulation* (Strange and Dolan 2006) facility within the amygdale. This modulation process requires a sophisticated level of waveform collaboration between the sensual inputs coming from the cortices and those arising from the mind web. As mentioned, the amygdale sorts images or impressions with an emotional or fearful perspective, which provides a sorting and priority criteria to the information. Research has concluded that by pegging information with emotional criteria, greater memory recall is established as compared to images without emotional tags (Dolcos *et al.* 2006).

This blending and transduction system could be compared to the internet or worldwide web. The internet or 'web' accomplishes a peer-accepted platform for the convergence of a variety of information gateways—or website portals. The convergence of all these website portals through the internet platform allows a particular user with a computer to choose to view any of the information portals. On the internet, the computer operator can choose to view a sorted compilation of websites through a search engine. The search terms are of course decided by the computer operator. In the case of the mind's web, the viewer is the self, and the gateways are the various types of pathways for waveform information being received and retained by the billions of brain cells. The limbic system offers to the self a platform where these information waves can be sorted and compiled. The self uses the sorting facility of the mind to program the search terms and the priorities for search compilation. In acquisition mode, once a search string is established, the limbic system coordinates a search through the standing waves of the various neuron gateways to locate information with similar waveform specifications.

The hippocampus is a central locator and search center to the mind's web. We might compare it to the placement of information throughout a hard disk, or even the assembly of information by search engine spiders. Located on each side of the brain in the temporal lobe, information from the senses and the body are converted by the hippocampus through a complex staging process. As was first published in a 1957 report by Scoville and Milner and later confirmed by Squire *et al.* (1991) along with other researchers, when the hippocampus becomes damaged, the first symptom is typically disorientation, memory acquisition loss, and recall deficiency. This is also evidenced in cases of encephalitis, where the hippocampus does not receive enough oxygen. When the hippocampus is damaged, new memories cannot be retained or recalled.

Within the hippocampus is an intricate pathway called the *Papex circuit* for electromagnetic rhythms, which can be likened to the cochlear passageway that stages and converts air pressure waves into electromagnetic nerve pulses. In the hippocampal pathway, waveforms from the cortical field (*entohinal cortex, perihinal cortex, cerebral cortex,* and so on), the subcortical field (*amygdale, broca, claustrum, substantia innominata,* and so on) mix with pulses from the thalamus and hypothalamus. These pulses are channeled through the *perforant path* consisting of three regions of the *dentate gyrus.* The signals pass through the CA3 and CA1 regions and on to the *subiculum* and *parahippocampal gyrus.* Here, between the subiculum and the parahippocampal gyrus, information in the form of interference waveform patterns is processed and translated to higher frequency waveforms—and broadcast into the neural net for storage or processing. In all, this circuit vets, tags and prioritizes information, preparing it to be cataloged. The various regions of the brain are also identified during this circuitry, which also identifies potential storage locations for information. In this way, the various neural networks of the different regions of the brain are mapped for waveform information storage and further processing.

In the pathway for visual impressions, for example, waveform combinations of different frequencies strike the retina and pass through the LGM to the visual cortex. Here in the cortex, waveforms drawn from memory through the amygdale are combined with internal stimuli waveforms and the LGM waveform data to create impression waveform interference patterns. These interference patterns create the specific information images for the self to see. We might compare this with creating an image by blending light rays of different colors and shapes onto a dark screen. Alone each light ray does not create much of an image, but together the different rays and colors can create a more complete image on the screen.

The images the self observes within the cortex are thus altered by context and history. The waveforms from the amygdale and memory alter the interference patterns. This accounts for the expression that we 'see what we want to see.' The interference patterns from these different sources eventually deliver convincing impressions to the hippocampus. Because the cortex combines all these waveforms together, the waveform information is forever altered. This creates the reality that each of us actually perceives a slightly different world around us.

In order to attempt to 'standardize' our perception, the self will seek confirmation from others. Information is thus gathered from others and the different forms of media. This creates a feedback loop between the amygdale, the hippocampus, and the cortices to constantly adjust our perception of reality towards the apparent perception of others. This is an intentional process because the self is constantly seeking affirmation from others in our never-ending quest for love and fulfillment.

Mapped brain regions also sort and translate incoming waveforms from the hippocampus. These are ultimately governed and coordinated by the prefrontal cortex. The intentions of the self stimulate a form of waveform programming mechanism that modulates neuron channels for particular waveform biocommunications. This creates a sorting system among those programmed neurons. The ion channel gateway states, neurotransmitter fluid content, and even genetic structures within the neuron may be manipulated by the executive initiatives programmed by the mind—under the intentions of the self. Many pre-programmed responses are crystallized within our static DNA. Still, neurons accommodate the executive authority of the inner self, expressed and translated through the prefrontal cortex and communicated via messenger pathways.

Chakras have been described in esoteric terms in much of the literature. However, we should realize that the *chakras* are inseparable from the waveform translating gateways existing within key networking regions of the brain and central nervous system. This is why the first five elemental *chakras* are described as regions aligned along the spine, and the last two within the brain. While not all neural tracts are *chakras*, all *chakras* utilize neural tracts to translate and transmit waveform conversions. These neural gateways of the *chakras* each accommodate a different medium and type of waveform, as we have described. Each also utilizes other pathways outside the neural system.

The limbic system is a part of the sixth *chakra* energy center, for example. Here waveforms from all over the body are converged and translated together with remodeled waves from the sensory cortices and the various feedback centers throughout the body. After translation, the limbic system coordinates instructions out to the body, together with a reflective broadcasting of waveform signals to the frontal cortex for executive review. Should the self respond to these inputs, executive waves are fed back to the body through the limbic system and the motor cortex. Here again the limbic system is acting as a transfer station, stimulating the release of various hormones through the hypothalamus and pituitary gland, which cascade through the various glands of the endocrine system. This provides the feedback pathway of executive instruction that Dr. Libet's research illustrated, allowing conscious decisions to take place after (programmed) responsive nerve impulses are detected.

Ultimately, it is the inner self—utilizing the various equipment of the brain—who initiates executive action. Once converted through the prefrontal and frontal cortices, this is accomplished directly through executive stimulation of the motor cortex and limbic system. This is like a car driver who sets up the proper cruise control speed, then removes his foot from the gas pedal. The cruise control will maintain the speed of the car by accelerating up hills and decelerating down hills automatically. However, should the driver decide to change speeds, avert running into the car ahead, or even stop the car, the driver can immediately take over the gas pedal and control the car's speed directly. In the same way, the self is driving the vehicle of the body, through both autonomic programming and executive control. Most autonomic functions can be manipulated directly should the self consciously intend to change them. In some cases, this takes practice, as biofeedback research illustrates. This conscious insertion of executive command can be initiated even during an autonomic response, just as the car driver can hit the gas pedal at any time to change the car's speed while it is running on cruise control.

As waveform messages from sensory nerves combine with physiology feedback and enter the brain's mapping network through the limbic system, they can be observed by the self on the interference 'screens' of a particular cortex or a combination of cortices. (The self can also manipulate, prioritize and distort these incoming physiological waveforms through the amygdale, however.) As they blend in the cortex, the self is able to review the waveforms and if need be, respond with intention. By this time, however, the programming already in place to process the particular situation is also ready to respond. Should a conscious 'executive' decision be made by the self, instructional waveforms are initiated through the prefrontal cortex. These are channeled through the motor cortex, which formats the waveforms for the hypothalamus. The hypothalamus in turn transduces these waveforms into physical response through the endocrine system and central nervous system. These instructional messengers may also contain a stop order to override whatever other instructions may already be in place.

Autonomic responses are established through initialized intentions and a subsequent programming of key web hubs by the mind. Most of these intentions are related to the survival of the body, translated from the self's fear of dying. This fear becomes translated into various scenarios that stimulate the programming features of mind. The programming waveforms stimulated by the mind are stored in neurons just as memories are, in the form of standing waves, crystallized by ionic molecular polarity and bonding sequences. Some autonomic programs are more permanently 'wired' into the standing waveforms that make up DNA bonds. These 'hard-wired' programs ultimately are passed on to the body's successors through the DNA.

These 'coded' standing waveforms with neurons are activated by certain types of waveforms incoming through sensory nerves and from interoception translated through the hypothalamus and thalamus. As information moves through this network, the neural programming indirectly relays the self's ultimate intentions of keeping the body alive with specific autonomic responses. The information will also be stepped up to the mind's web for viewing through the cortices. When we burn our finger, our autonomic programming will immediately respond by pulling the hand away. The self will also be able to view the incoming information separately, and initiate a separate, conscious response, such as tending to the injury or turning off the flame.

The self's recognition of information within the frontal cortex (or *mind screen*) is called *cognition*. In humans and primates, the central interface or bridge between the incoming impulse pathways of the nervous system and executive control is located in the *dorsolateral prefrontal cortex* (Otani 2002). It is here waveforms are examined, responded to and their responses relayed onto the motor cortex. Simultaneously, goal-directed intentions from the self stimulate the broadcast of waveform messages back into the neural net through the frontal cortex. Instructive waveforms are simultaneously pulsed through the hypothalamus, the specific regions of the motor cortex, and then the lower *chakras*. These instructive waveforms together stimulate the various elemental channels to respond. In other words, the body is not shocked or jerked into motion solely from pulses moving out from the brain. There are several pathways of activity initiated during a full-body response. The body's endocrine systems are stimulated. The body's heat-producing centers are stimulated. The body's insulin and energy releasing centers are stimulated. The body's pacemaker, vasomotor, perfusive and respiratory functions all are simultaneously stimulated into immediate response. How else could the body react so instantaneously and thoroughly from head to toe following an intentional decision? We certainly have to characterize the chemical binding process as too cumbersome to exclusively provide these broadcasting mechanisms.

The connection between the cognitive functions of higher decision-making and the mind screen web are illustrated by the size of the frontal lobe cortex areas of the brain in more evolved organisms. Behavioral studies with animals and humans have also confirmed that complex executive functions with goal-directed behavior, language and higher cognition in general is associated with a larger, more developed prefrontal cortex (Fuster 2002). The developed frontal lobe cortex enables the self to command a greater volume of switchboard control and the ability to specify intention through a complex mental capacity. We also note that all highly evolved organisms also have advanced backbones and high-energy entry-points to carry out full-body *chakra* responses. As for less evolved organisms, we still find key neural points that transduce that self's intentions, albeit less complexly.

Neurotransmitter Transmission

As we examine the incoming waveforms received by the neural cell body through the neuron dendrites, we note the dendrites do not actually touch. They are not connected in the physical sense. Rather, between them exists a space called the *synapse*. The synapse contains a special chemistry called the *neurotransmitter fluid*. The neurotransmitter chemistry provides the medium for the waveform pulses traveling between neurons. Through this chemistry, waves of various frequencies are transmitted, moving information from one neuron to another, and as described above, enabling a broadcasting of the information through various other channels around the body.

This tiny sea of neurotransmitter fluid contains various biochemical components, most of which are ionic in nature. These ions combine with the protein neurotransmitters to create a system that drives an electromagnetic *synaptic potential*. Each CNS neuron can range in synapse count. Some might have several thousand while others have significantly less. Through these synapses, each neuron may be firing up to 100,000 electromagnetic pulse inputs into this fluid at one time. Depending upon its particular makeup at the time, the fluid will provide a combination of *excitatory potential* and *inhibitory potential.* This balance serves to escort or conduct waveform information from one nerve to another, while at the same time dampening or filtering these waveforms to prevent overload and over-stimulation. This process might well be compared to the process of transistors and resisters we see in integrated circuits. Neurotransmitters are tremendous semiconductors. Their delicate ionic balance precisely buffer and conduct waveform biocommunications within neurotransmitter fluids.

Two examples of neurotransmitters are acetylcholine and adrenaline (or epinephrine). These two messenger substances conduct and/or magnify specific wave rhythms, which reflect either programmed (autonomic) intention or conscious intention. Acetylcholine will modulate an instruction to muscle fibers to contract, while adrenaline will modulate instructions that perpetuate the 'fight or flight' response: Causing a quickening of heart rate and blood flow, immediate motor muscle response, visual acuity, and so on. Each of these biochemicals conducts particular types of waveforms. They will affect the neurotransmitter fluid, but they also interact with waveforms outside the confines of the fluid. For example, acetylcholine also stimulates skeletal muscle cells directly. This means the intentional response and programming to protect the body in specific ways is being conducted through these messenger molecules—and they are effectively translating that information into physical response.

Neurotransmitters and their cousins the hormones are secreted by various glands of the body. Epinephrine, for example, is secreted by the adrenal gland. Sex hormones are secreted by the gonads and ovaries. Metabolic hormones are secreted by the thyroid. Most secretions of the body follow a chain of command, however. Their secretions are stimulated by other secreted messengers produced by the pituitary gland. The pituitary gland is the master gland stimulating most of the various neurochemical messengers. This master gland not only responds to the stimulation of the hypothalamus and cortices, but also resonates with the higher frequencies of the *chakra* programming.

The pituitary gland is about the size of a cherry. It is located behind the eyes in a depression of the sphenoid bone, just behind where the optic nerves cross. It is also lying within the region of the sixth *chakra*. The pituitary produces hormone messengers that directly stimulate the body, such as growth hormone (GH), vasopressin, oxytocin and others. The pituitary gland connects to the hypothalamus by the *infudibulum,* a stalk of portal veins and nerves tracts. It is through this stalk the pituitary gland's activities are regulated by the hypothalamus. The hypothalamus sends *releasing hormones* to the pituitary. This regulatory process might be considered a balancing or filtering mechanism, compiling various waveforms into a balanced set of instructions.

Neurotransmitter chemistry acts as a conductor for these informational waveforms. There are many types of neurotransmitters. Some neurotransmitters such as epinephrine and glutamate increase transmission, while others such as dopamine subdue transmission. Other neurotransmitters—such as acetylcholine—facilitate muscle stimulation response, while others—such as serotonin—facilitate biocommunication of emotion and mood responses between nerves. The specific neurotransmitter chemistry provides a medium for particular types of wave transmissions, allowing the endocrine system (where most neurotransmitters are produced) to exert some feedback control into the process of conducting information around the body.

The biochemistry is intricate in this biocommunication process. We must be careful not to confuse chemicals with waves, however. Waves are informational, and conduct through chemicals. Their interference patterns can be stored within biochemicals in the form of standing waves between atoms. This is why biomolecules have unique properties. Biochemicals serve primarily as echo chambers, reflecting the informational waveforms being transmitted around the body. We might compare this to hearing a radio playing a song broadcast from a distant station. The radio does not contain the song, nor is it the source of the radiowaves that are being broadcast to millions of radios from the same radio station. The radio does not contain the singer either. Rather, the radio is simply a conducting vehicle, which temporary crystallizes and transforms the radiowaves into the speaker sounds that we can hear. In the same way, biochemicals reacting throughout the body during metabolism are merely vehicles of wave conduction. Waves and their informational interference patterns are being broadcast in multiple bandwidths through biomolecular processes.

Neurotransmitter conduction also might be compared to opening our eyes under water. Were we to dive into a river during a rain storm and attempt to open our eyes and look through its murky, muddy waters, we would not see much. We would be lucky to see our hand in front of our face underneath the muddy brown waters. That same river during a warm summer day might be so clear that we could see the bottom ten feet down. The difference between seeing within the two rivers is due to the muddy river mud being stirred up by the rain and stormy weather. It is not that our vision has gotten worse.

In the same way, an imbalanced chemistry in the neurotransmitter fluid will alter the waveforms passing from neuron to neuron. Some chemicals will interfere in the transmission of waves through the fluid. Certain chemicals affect neurotransmitter fluids in such a way that can subdue or distort the biocommunications as they are conducted across the neurotransmitter chemistry.

Case in point: When we drink alcohol, the alcohol will affect the chemistry of the synaptic junction—the neurotransmitter fluid—in such a way that distorts the electrical signals that travel from one neuron to another. This creates a situation where the brain cells controlling motor functions receive slow or even inaccurate signals. As these are stepped up into the neural net, the distorted signals create an unrealistic impression of the circumstances. This distorts perception, leading to coordination impairment, irrational behavior and mood swings: A potentially disastrous combination.

The key role of the neurotransmitter is to create an electrical potential for the waveform. This creates a bridge of sorts for the wave to transverse. The type of neurotransmitter also dictates which type of channel gateway will be opened on the post-synaptic nerve—the receiving nerve. The type of ion channel will typically dictate what kind of information will be transduced through the linkage of neurons.

One of the more interesting players in neurotransmitter biochemistry is GABA, which stands for *gamma-aminobutyric acid.* GABA is considered an inhibitory neurotransmitter in that it slightly slows down the wave conduction. This actually has a positive effect upon the synaptic transmissions, allowing nerve signals to pass through without as much distortion. GABA appears to be manufactured in the brain. GABA is known for its calming, regulating, and clear-thinking effects upon the brain and nervous system. Research has indicated that various mood disorders like depression, anxiety and even insomnia are related to the body having lower GABA levels within the neurotransmitter fluid. Epileptics typically have insufficient amounts of this neurotransmitter as well. Many of the popular anti-depressant pharmaceuticals increase the levels of GABA. It should be noted, however, that these drugs also produce various side effects as well.

Healthy amounts of GABA in the neurotransmitter fluid have been shown to accompany a state of physical relaxation with greater alertness. This state naturally also facilitates the conductance of alpha brainwaves. GABA research has confirmed that this molecule will induce increases in alpha brainwaves. In one study, L-theanine (a GABA precursor) was given to thirteen subjects. Electroencephalography examinations were conducted, and each recipient was observed having heightened alpha waves and reduced beta waves (beta waves are associated with nervousness and anxiety while alpha waves accompany increased concentration) (Abdou 2006).

Abdou's research also demonstrated the effect chemical neurotransmitters have upon the biocommunication of fear around the body. Two groups of eight volunteers were divided into a non-GABA (placebo) group and a GABA group. Both groups were monitored for IgA immunoglobulin levels following the crossing of a suspension bridge. Because IgA levels tend to shut down during anxious or fearful moments as the adrenal gland prepares for 'fight or flight,' this test illustrated GABA's effects upon fear-based immune response. The GABA group had normal IgA levels while the non-GABA group experienced significantly lower IgA levels. It was thus concluded that GABA levels are associated with reducing inappropriate fear responses as well as facilitating alpha waves.

As we assess this last trial, we can conclude that GABA created a calming or clearing effect upon the neurotransmitter fluid, which allowed the subjects to realistically assess the dangers involved. Using the senses to realistically assess the strength of the bridge and the likelihood of the bridge actually collapsing would be considered a clear-headed response. On the other hand, a heightened fear of falling simply by looking down (acrophobia) would not be considered a realistic assessment of the situation simply because the bridge could be easily crossed and was obviously strong enough to handle all of the walkers.

GABA provides a neurotransmitter environment at the synapse allowing a clearer and less distorted broadcasting of waveform information through the neural pathways. This allows the information to flow more clearly between the mind, the neural network and the sense organs. We might wonder how a seemingly simple biochemical molecule has such a drastic affect upon perception.

Microtubular Spirals

During the 1970s, Dr. Stewart Hamerhoff from the University of Arizona, and Dr. Kunio Yasue and Dr. Mari Jibu from the Okayama University began researching the pathway of conscious activity between neural cells. One of the mysteries they probed in independent research was how anesthesia agents such as chloroform and nitrous oxide could disable the consciousness of a patient. Through their respective research, they independently discovered that conscious activity within the body had to do with a curious matrix of twisted spiral filaments they called *tubulins*. These tubulins are arranged into networked pathways that wind through the neural cells in three-dimensional protein spirals called *microtubules*. These microtubules appear to be conducting tracts for waveform activity. The research illustrated that the microtubules make up a previously unseen network for subtle waveform biocommunication through the neural net (Hameroff 1974; Hameroff 1982; Hameroff *et al.* 1984; Hameroff 1987; Hameroff and Penrose 1996).

As the larger waveforms of the physical realm are processed and transmitted through dendrites, they conduct through the neurotransmitters between the synapses. As they are conducted through this medium, the waveforms meet with other waveforms traveling within the neural network. This convergence creates coherent interference patterns. The resonating results of these interference patterns are then transmitted through the subtle network of the microtubules. In this state, these subtle waveforms are 'stepped up' to a higher frequency format. These subtle high frequency waveforms in turn create holographic wave patterns, which are ultimately reflected (or mirrored) onto the 'screens' of the cortices. Once on the screens, these holograms interact with others to create a 'picture' of the body and the world around us. The self interacts with these cortices through the primary screening device of the frontal cortex to view this holographic 'picture.'

Within these microtubules also travel the various subtle waveforms that conduct the intentions of the self through the body. The discovery of these microtubule pathways confirms much of the ancient wisdom of the *nadis* and *meridians*. These channels were also described as being pathways for living energy flow. We might consider nerve tracts as pathways of lower-frequency reflexive waveforms, while the microtubules broadcast higher-frequency, complex information waves.

We might compare the microtubular process of projecting wave interference patterns onto the mind to the recording of a musical composition in a modern studio. The studio producer will record the guitar onto one track, the piano onto another track, the drums onto another and the voice onto another track. The producer may even overlay background singers' voices onto other tracks. Then using these various individual sounds, the producer will assemble all the tracks together at particular sound levels to form the entire piece of music. This is often referred to as a *composition*. Each track makes up a piece of the total song. To listen to each track alone without the other tracks will sound weird. In much the same way, the mind captures the various waveform frequencies coming through the microtubular network, neural net and biochemical messengers—combining them to form unified holographic images of the outside world.

One of the basic principles of holography is that each part mirrors the entire image. This is accomplished through a splitting of waves as they interfere, creating a multitude of waves, each containing all the information via the composition of waveforms. Using waveform interference, the mind orchestrates holographic assembly in both directions. The mind reflects its images semiconducted through particular neurons. The mind also stimulates effector neurons to act reflectively in response to the intentions of the self. The mind projects the whole image using the various cortex images, each assembling waveforms from different locations. This collection of images is broadcast through crystallized neuron pathways. Each neuron is constructed with the appropriate crystal DNA structure, ion channel system and microtubules, giving it the ability to join with others to relay multiple waveform interference patterns simultaneously.

Electromagnetic Memory

Modern neuroscience divides memory into short-term and long-term processes. Long-term memory is further divided into three types: *Episodic*—when memories are unique to the time and place; *semantic*—when memories involve concepts or learning; and *procedural*—when memories revolve around skills. Episodic memories relate to events that happened in the past, or people we knew from the past. Semantic memories relate more to concept understanding. Procedural memories relate to remembering how to ride a bike, write or use a telephone.

Interestingly, memory loss of one type will not typically accompany the loss of another type. Thus in many amnesia cases, long-term memory may appear erased while short-term memory is retained. The person may forget older events yet continue to remember what just happened.

Furthermore, all too frequently one type of long-term memory may be lost while another type may be retained. For example, a person may suffer the loss of their episodic memory—forgetting their name, family, school history, phone number, birth date and other personal details or events of the past. At the same time they may remember how to write, drive, talk on the phone and even retain concepts such as how economic markets work.

Often a particular trauma or event may cause the forgetfulness of either what happened just before the event, or what happened just after the event. The former case is referred to as *retrograde amnesia*— a loss of memory just prior to a trauma. The latter is referred to as *anterograde amnesia*—a loss of memory just after a trauma. Both may also occur. The causes of these types of forgetfulness are considered quite mysterious. This is because memory has been miscalculated.

There are other types of memory loss. Many are unconnected to any particular event, while others follow injury to particular brain regions or involve trauma. Trauma-associated amnesia may or may not involve physical injury. It may follow a head injury or automobile accident. Traumatic amnesia may also follow a witnessing of a traumatic event, or may involve abuse. Rape is an example of traumatic amnesia involving abuse. *Psychogenic* or *dissociative fugue* is another type of memory loss, which also may occur following a trauma, and may result in a person re-identifying him- or herself as someone else, and even taking an unexpected trip to a place previously unknown. Other events that can cause memory loss include alcohol and drug related blackouts, and *Wernicke-Korsakoff's,* which is thought to be caused by thiamin deficiency.

A more common type of amnesia involves the loss of memory of a particular event. This may be the forgetting of certain childhood events, for example. Forgetting certain events may also be referred to as traumatic memory loss. Many of us forget events in the distant past that were not necessarily traumatic as well. It is not unusual for us to forget our younger childhood events. We also may recall something without remembering how we knew it—called *source amnesia.*

One illness overwhelming modern medicine and capturing research attention is *Alzheimer's disease.* The first documented case of AD was discovered by a Bavarian psychiatrist named Dr. Alois Alzheimer. Dr. Alzheimer treated a 51-year old patient who suffered from memory loss and hallucinations. The patient, "Auguste D" was frequently delirious and had extreme short-term memory deficit. She complained of having "lost myself." She was committed to the Frankfurt asylum in 1901 and died five years later. Autopsy revealed a sticky plaque among brain cells and nerve tissue entanglement. The disease was named after the diagnosis given by Dr. Alzheimer, and this variant of dementia became associated with physical damage to the brain apparently relating to a build-up of beta amyloid plaque among certain regions of the brain. The definite cause of AD has not been determined, although there appear to be a number of potential contributing factors, including stress, heavy metal toxicity, and certain diets. Recent research seems to point at a lack of phosphatidylserine among brain cell membranes as well.

This sort of research contributes to our notion that memory is chemical-based. The frontal and medial temporal lobe is the prevailing theory for long-term memory storage location—based on EGG and magnetic resonance scans. Still, researchers have observed numerous instances where memories are retained when specific regions of the brain thought to control a particular type of memory are removed or incapacitated. This occurred in hemicortication surgeries—a frequent treatment of childhood epilepsy for many years. Episodic memories were retained even through the brain regions thought to be involved were removed. We must therefore question the assumption that memories are specific to particular neurons. Yet we still need to address the fact that many memory losses occur following brain damage to particular locations. What is going on here?

The first clue is that most of these cases are specific to short-term memory loss. Long-term memories remain a mystery. In one study (Piolino *et al.* 2006), thirteen patients with early stage dementia, ten patients with semantic dementia and fifteen patients with frontotemporal dementia were compared to assess the connection between memory loss and damage to the medial temporal lobe. One of the central areas of focus in this study was the *autobiographical amnesia of episodic memories,* or the lack of ability to acquire or remember events of ones past. The results of this study concluded no consistency between memory loss and frontal lobe impairment. In some cases, short-term memories were difficult to acquire as a whole, and in other cases, the memory acquisition depended upon the details and importance of the event. In many cases, long-term "remote" memories were retained and preserved while short-term details and events were not. This led the study authors to support a newer theory called the *multiple trace theory,* which says that memory acquisition occurs through more than one physical mechanism, and can be stored in multiple locations.

In a similar study (Matuszewski *et al.* 2006) on autobiographical episodic memory loss among frontotemporal dementia patients, near learning abilities with semantic memories revealed a shifting executive function with multiple processes. As for other possible models of memory acquisition, several studies have indicated that the hippocampus complex was significantly involved in the storage and recall of recent memories, but not for older memories. Other research has offered evidence that the hippocampal complex is responsible for autobiographical episodic memory and special memory, but the storage of other types of memory was shifted to other locations (Nadel and Moscovitch 1997).

In a 2002 report (Nester *et al.*) published in *Neuropsychologia* on autobiographical memories among semantic dementia patients, the preservation of recent memories and the loss of remote memories supported the trace theory of memory retention and acquisition. This report confirms, as so many animal studies have, that memories are not chemically retained within specific neurons. We can logically compare memories to data stored on a computer's hard drive. However, modern science has yet to locate the program, the language nor the methods used to categorize, place and retain memories.

This is because modern science does not understand the most basic understandings of living biology. Again, we first must know who the driver of the vehicle of the body is. From there we must understand the means for the operation of the vehicle. Just as a car's driver uses the wheel, the clutch and the gas pedal to move the car, the driver of the body also utilizes particular equipment to drive the body. The reality is, the mind is the software of the brain, and the brain assembles information as programmed by the mind. The self dictates the functioning of the mind through conscious intention: desire.

This was clearly exposed in a study of memory-challenged patients with different brain disorders (Thomas-Anterion 2000). Twelve Alzheimer's disease patients and twelve frontotemporal dementia patients with functionally similar semantic memory, logical memory and retrograde memory test scores were studied for antegrade verbal memory and frontal lobe activity. Despite similar memory acquisition scores and types of memory loss, physiological brain function occurred in different locations among the subjects. This illustrated flexibility in brain region utilization, quite similar to practical daily living: Should we be unable to pick up something with one hand, we will quickly adjust and pick up the item with the other hand. In the same way, the self, using the utility of the mind, can often accomplish the same purpose using different neurons, cortices and/ or limbic components.

Should the intent to remember exist, memory can be retained using a variety of external physical mechanisms as well. Humans have indeed resorted to various tools to replace or augment memory function for thousands of years. For example, a person may retain memories within a diary to assist in the recall of particular thoughts, emotions and events. Projects or objectives may be recorded onto daily planners, or onto digital voice recorders for later recall. Most students and businesspeople carry notebooks to every class and meeting to assist with the retention and recall of lectures and discussions. These external memory devices replace or augment limited memorization abilities. They also illustrate an intention to remember.

The memory experiments by Dr. Wilder Penfield at the Montreal Neurological Institute in the 1970s clearly illustrated that memories typically accompanied emotions and intentions. When Dr. Penfield's weak electrical currents excited locations within the brain, the subject would recall historical facts associated with past experiences. Their recollections included songs connected to feelings from the past, aromas connected to experiences, people connected to personal relationships, and events connected to other emotional events. Dry information such as what score a person received twenty years ago on a test or sporting event might seem like raw data, but even this data are connected to personal intentions to win or receive a good score. Without an emotional, intentional attachment, the ability to recall that event subsides as the self's intention to remember it weakens.

The sensual information we absorb with our senses is transmitted via waveform mechanics. Our senses convert waveforms from one medium into waveforms that can travel within the medium of the neural biology. As these waveform pulses are stepped into higher frequency waveforms, they are transmitted through the various neural pathways, including the microtubules, as we have discussed. These waveforms come together within our cortices to create coherent interference patterns, which tie together with the brainwaves arising from our limbic system. Together these interference patterns create networks of standing waveform patterns that bond molecule and ion sequences within our neurons. They accumulate to create a web of networked waveforms.

This might be compared to looking at a pond after many stones have been tossed into it. The confluence of intersecting and interfering ripples contain the data that reveal the original event to an intelligent observer. The interference patterns reveal whether a single stone or multiple stones were thrown in. They may reveal how large the stones were, how long ago they were thrown in and how far apart the stones were thrown in. Even one of the stones' waves, ripped up by interference patterns, can be followed back to the original stone throws, because they have each become interconnected through the medium of the pond. In this way, the ripples and waves of the stone throws are all interconnected into a web of waveforms.

In the case of the mental web, we are speaking of a convergence of millions of sensory, neural and brain waveforms all interacting within the system. This wave interaction keeps each memory associated with various other events and memories. This interactive pattern might also be compared to that of a spider's web—weaved and linked with silk strands interlaced into a sturdy net.

One strand alone will not hold much. Networked together, they are strong. In the same way, our holographic memory retention is based upon a linking of emotions with sensory images, all wrapped together by the intention to succeed and enjoy the physical body. As some strands become older or less important, they gradually become pushed further away from the priority strands that are tied to the current events now central to our current goals. These older memories might still available in the grand web of interlocking waveforms. However, they become increasingly difficult for us to recall, as they fade from our intentional priorities.

The reason tumors in the hippocampus have been known to cause amnesia is because the hippocampus is a conversion tool used by the mind to transmute event waveform combinations from one type to another. The ability of the limbic system to translate impulses into the memory web map and also access that map—translating the webbed memories back into physical recall—has been damaged. In the same way, if we got cancer of the vocal cords, we would not be able to convert our thoughts into words.

Losing the conversion tool does not bode well for that activity. The bridge between the physical waveforms of the neural net and the subtle mapping of those rhythms has been broken. As research has indicated, should another part of the limbic system be available for web building and should the intent remain, the self may still be able to shift that function elsewhere, though it will be difficult. It is easier to shift cortex functions because there are several cortex regions situated around the brain, each having similarly structured neurons.

We can compare the mapping technology of the memory web or net to the tracking location system of a computer hard drive memory disk. The computer hardware is compared to the limbic system, which coordinates the mapping and retrieval of particular memory waveforms. The hippocampus, hypothalamus and amygdale work together with the rest of the limbic system to coordinate the storage and retrieval of particular informational waveforms. These are of course fed in from the senses along with feedback from the body, converted, and then escorted through the particular neurotransmitter messenger relays.

Together this sorted information is both sent to memory and projected in the frontal cortex for the self to view. Together these waveforms create a harmonic coherence, because the events are strung together by our emotional intent. Our intentions are thus inserted into the sorting process of the limbic system. The waveform synchronization is finally projected upon the mind screen web for the self's direct interaction. The self's feedback from this viewing becomes tied together historically using the formatting and storage mechanisms of the hippocampus and prefrontal cortex. This reformatting sorts specific types of waveform patterns to resonate with other historical information, tying them together within the particular region of the brain that resonates with that wave format.

Each memory waveform or set of interference waveforms is held in resonance and crystallized within a region of neural cell molecules. Protein crystal semiconductors provide the platform for these waveform combinations to be retained in standing waves. Though this statement might deceive us into thinking the memories are contained in the neuron chemistry, this is immediately refutable. Research has illustrated that when we sleep, the mind quietly shuffles and reprioritizes the memory banks, aligning them with the self's current objectives. Less important memories are shuffled out, while memories considered more critical to the self are retained. The rejected memories are discarded, yet those neurons remain, albeit with newly crystallized waveform interference patterns.

Succussing and Placebos

The inability of the "verifiers" to duplicate Dr. Benveniste's laboratory results appears to be as easily explainable as how the mixture was treated prior to and after dilution. In an interview shortly before his death in 2004, Dr. Benveniste explained his and the other labs' process of dilution and memory-testing. He described agitating the diluted solution for twenty seconds with a spinning motion, creating a spiral or funnel shape inside the beaker. He called this motion a *vortex*. Dr. Benveniste explained, *"Only then do you get the transmission of the information."*

Succussing has been standard practice of homeopathy since the father of modern homeopathy Dr. Samuel Hahnemann began his clinical provings. (*Ayurvedic* doctors practiced a form of homeopathy for many centuries before Hahnemann.) The process of homeopathic dilution as described by Dr. Hahnemann also required this process of *sucussion,* which was a swirling and knocking of the substance upon the heel of the hand in order to mix the memory components. This practice of sucussion is still widely practiced amongst homeopathic manufacturers and physicians conducting clinical dilutions for patients. This succussion process is quite consistent with the process of vortex shaking documented in Dr. Benveniste's research.

As we convert this process to waveform language, we would explain that succession is stimulating coherent interference between the substance's molecular waveforms and the water's molecular waveforms. This type of interference would logically imbed a sustained impact upon the waveforms and magnetic fields of the remaining water molecules.

As we will explore further later, water clustering illustrates one of water's many interesting attributes. Over the past four decades, chemists and physicists have been observing very organized yet weak-hydrogen-bond clusters forming and breaking up within water, seemingly on a spontaneous basis. Initially it was supposed that these structures were simply randomly forming these complex structures. However, upon further observation it became evident that once a cluster broke apart another cluster would form in its place. Many of the new clusters often replicated the shape of the previous clusters. It was also noticed that most of these clusters took on symmetrical shapes, such as icosahedrons. Is this not an indication of some sort of molecular memory among water molecules?

Controlled laboratory research has concluded that catalytic enzyme activity will vary greatly, depending upon the nature of the organic solvents in the solution (Zaks and Klibanox 1988; Lee and Dordick 2002). From this, we can determine that different solutes affect catalysts differently. The exact mechanisms for the catalytic activity are mysterious in many instances. As we consider the quantum nature of these types of molecules, we can appreciate that reactions do not simply take place between molecules or particles. Reactions take place through an interactive process between the electromagnetic bonding forces inherent within the reactive species. Still the surrounding environment is involved. The environment will either facilitate or buffer a particular reaction.

In a downgrading *allosteric regulation* for example, a molecule is bound with an effector atomic structure at the molecule's active bonding site—controlling its ability to continue that particular reaction. The mechanics of reactions such as these are not exclusive of water—water is surely a conductor and sometimes buffer of reactivity with its ever-changing, short-lived hydrogen-bond ion structures. Thus, water logically should have at least the same electromagnetic impact any other reactive substrates might have. As we will discuss later, water actually has an extraordinary capacity in this respect.

Consider the ability of an iron-oxide tape to memorize data or sounds through electromagnetic field manipulation. Our ability to tape-record a song or speech onto a magnetizing substance like iron oxide occurs simply by impinging a magnetic influence upon the surface with a magnetized head. Is this not the same occurrence as water's ability to memorize? Are we not manipulating iron oxide's polarity to memorize a particular electromagnetic contact? Not only can we read the magnetically charged iron oxide tape later, but the playback of the recording will be quite precise. We can then store magnetically recorded information for extended periods, erasing it to make way for new information.

When we press a bar magnet upon another magnetic metal we change the polarity of a majority of the molecules making up the metal. The polarity is changed through a restructuring of the electron wave orbital orientation, rendering an electron-heavy side and a proton-heavy side. This polarization causes an effective means for memorization. After removing the magnet, some molecules will revert to their original polarity. Others will remain in the same direction. In either case, there is a recollection of positioning and orientation long after the bar magnet encounter.

When a solution is diluted many times and the theoretical amount of molecules left in the solution is seemingly too small for probability equations, there are certainly still innumerable hydrogen ions left in the water that were once part of the original solute. If we envision these ions not as "particles" but as rhythmic waveforms, we can incorporate the dilution into an ongoing information wave technology: Coherent waveform interference patterns create the basis for memory.

As researchers have come to understand the placebo effect over the past century, double-blind studies have become the norm to isolate the treatment's success from various biases, notably expectations affecting the results. Following the results of thousands of trials, it has been commonly accepted that the placebo effect may skew results by as much as 33%. In other words, up to 33% of the test subjects will improve simply because they expected improvement from the therapy, or their doctors expected improvement. When we consider this is one-third of the population being tested, a placebo-range result has quite an influence on healing. What causes the placebo-result and why are results in the placebo range so frowned upon?

Placebo effects have gotten a bad rap. A study's results will be considered insignificant if the trends are under 33% of the study's population even if the study was double-blinded. This is because of the effect expectations have upon results.

Expectations are no more than conscious intentions for a particular result. These intentions can affect research results in either a positive or negative way. In medical research, it would be considered positive if the placebo effect increased the efficacy of the treatment. Perhaps the treatment required some personal interaction between the researcher or clinician and the patient. Perhaps this created a placebo effect and increased the effects of the therapy. Should we then say that clinicians should not have personal interaction with patients so we do not create any additional opportunities for healing? Certainly not.

The viability of the *non-local effects* and *local effects* of personal consciousness, clinician consciousness and group consciousness has significant implications toward healing. Certainly the placebo effect illustrates the non-local effect conscious expectations have upon healing. If consciousness can have up to a 33% positive effect upon treatment and the health of the body, then we must accept the notion that consciousness can somehow be retained, memorized, and transmitted within the waveforms exchanged during these studies (Leder 2005).

Whether or not we relate the clinical results of homeopathy to the effects of water retaining memory, we can illustrate through the placebo effect that intention and expectation can influence physical results. Therefore, should a substance be diluted down to the infinitesimal solute state by a therapist who intends for a particular therapeutic effect, there is some likelihood that the resulting solution will contain some molecular waveform memory of the substance. This will be accompanied by the effects of the conscious intentions of the healer. We could see the combination of these two effects taking place in homeopathy just as it takes place in pharmaceutical research.

We see this effect everyday: When we give a gift to someone, they might look upon and remember the gift decades later. As they look upon the gift, there will be a retrieval of the conscious intent of its giver. Does the gift itself physically contain that consciousness? Possibly not, but certainly the physical gift connects to the memory of the intention of its purchase. Certainly, the gift is a vehicle for the transmission of the consciousness of the giver. How did it arrive at that point? A connection between the giver's intent and the gift had to take place at some point—perhaps when the giver picked out the gift. Therefore, we would say that the gift *reflects* the consciousness of the giver. As soon as the giver interacted with the gift by taking possession of it, the gift has taken on a new character: It is now irrevocably tied to the consciousness of the giver. Does the gift physically contain the consciousness of the giver? By perception it certainly does. Perhaps it simply serves as a reminder or a trigger for the memory. In either case, the perceived effect is the same. The gift triggers the memory of the original conscious intent.

Chapter Seven

In Conclusion: The Challenges of Homeopathy

The question before us is whether homeopathy has a scientific foundation. Hopefully this book has established without a doubt that it does.

Yet this does not necessarily answer the question of whether homeopathy necessarily works, and works consistently.

While we cannot prove that homeopathy works in all cases, we have scientifically established that homeopathy has the ability to work. It has the potential to influence our physiology, behavior, mind and nervous systems by conducting part of a substance's electromagnetic information potential through the body's various channels of conductance.

This might be like asking whether an electric wire has the potential to electrocute us. It certainly does, because the wire is a conductor, and should the wire be electromagnetically hot, and should we touch the wire and thus become a current to that wire's electromagnetic current, we may certainly become electrocuted.

But perhaps the wire is not currently 'hot'—and not conducting electricity. Or perhaps the wire itself is rusted and not a good conductor. Or maybe we are using an insulated tool that blocks the electricity from getting to our body. Or maybe we are grounded somehow and the electricity safely passes through us.

In other words, if any of the requirements of conductance are not met, our touching the wire will not electrocute us at all.

We have the same issue with homeopathy. In order for a diluted substance to retain and conduct the biomolecular electromagnetic information through our bodies, all of the elements for conductance must be in place.

These would include, first, the proper extraction of the initial substance. If it is Rhus tox, the essential oils of the poison oak or ivy plant must be extracted intact. If the extract is overheated or otherwise not treated well, it may lose its potency. This same issue takes place with many herbal extracts that have been extracted or stored incorrectly, losing their potential ability to provide their therapeutic benefits. Garlic, for example, will lose most of its antibacterial qualities if it has been overheated during extraction.

Secondly, the dilution must provide the right conducting elements. For some remedies, this may mean the calcium, magnesium or other ions in the water that allow the remedy's electromagnetic properties to transfer and be retained in the solution as it is diluted.

This may also occur with the Van der Waals forces between the container and the substance's molecules—creating adhesion. When adhesion is accomplished, the electromagnetic bonding information of the material will be retained on the surface of the container, and carried through to the final dilution, no matter how small the dilution.

This conductance may also be achieved through the water or milk or other solvent used for the dilution. But again, this depends highly upon the particular solute (homeopathic) substance, the solvent and the resulting solution obtained after dissolving.

In other words, one substance may carry its electromagnetic information through the calcium ions of the water, while another may utilize the $H+$ ions resident in the water itself. Another may be carried through the Van der Waals forces of the glass container's walls.

The research indicates that the ability of the initial remedy to pass on its electromagnetic information is increased when succussing is used. This 'swirling' of the solution during the dilution process creates a greater opportunity for the electromagnetic information of the solute to bond or disperse among the solvent and its resident participants.

While this has been observed in more than 275 years of homeopathy, it was also observed by French INSERM scientists such as Dr. Benveniste as we discussed. As for the *Nature* publication 'myth-buster' team that went in to the laboratory to repeat Dr. Benveniste yet refused to accept the succussing process as part of its protocol, an open-minded and extended do-over is called for.

We have discussed the technology of nature in this text, showing how information becomes conducted through waveforms and spirals. The spiraling vortex is a common feature among these occurrences in nature, and this is precisely what classical homeopaths have utilized in their traditional treatments.

With all of this said, there is a great potential—given any number of variables just as the *Nature* team found—for homeopathy not to work.

In other words, on the flip side of everything we present here, electromagnetic information can quite be blocked or inhibited during dilution. This may occur because there is no conductance through the solvent or its accompanying elements. Or the substance may not provide enough Van der Waals forces to carry through to the dilution.

Or perhaps a particular solvent does not provide the mineral properties utilized in other dilutions of that particular homeopathic remedy. This renders a case for production standardization for homeopathic remedy production—which there is currently little due to the proprietary methodologies utilized by leading producers.

Or perhaps the container used to make the dilution did not allow for adherence. Many classical homeopaths will insist, for example, that plastic or metal containers cannot be used for dilution of homeopathy, while others utilize plastic or metal containers.

For that matter, there are many other rules that classical homeopaths insist upon in order to produce the effects of a homeopathic remedy. Most of these are the result of clinical observations over the years. These include dosing on an empty stomach, having no food in the mouth, not drinking coffee near dosing and other rules. Many also insist upon a calm mind at the time of dosing. As to the reasoning, classical homeopaths suggest these things can interfere with the remedy's ability to affect the body.

The larger point here is that there are many many variables at play in homeopathy. Providing a clear pathway of conductance from tangible substance to a diluted homeopathic remedy and its eventual effects within the body might be compared to trying to escape from a prison by burrowing under the ground. You never know what barriers may be found—pipes, sewers, concrete and so on. Any one of these barriers may block the escape.

In the same way, from a scientific perspective, the homeopathic pathway is wrought with uncertainty. Will the electromagnetic bonding information resonate with the solvent, the solvent's other solutes or with the container material? Or will there be elements of interference which block the conductance of the information through the dilution process?

There are more than 2,000 homeopathic remedies, and each has distinct properties and effects. Each also comes from a unique substance before dilution, and each has the potential to produce a unique homeopathic remedy following dilution.

This also means there are also many different electromagnetic characteristics among these substances. Suggesting a 'one size fits all' methodology for diluting all homeopathics, therefore, would not make much sense.

Added to this uncertainty for patient and physician, there are numerous manufacturers of homeopathic remedies. Many of these utilize proprietary methods—distinct from each other—to produce their homeopathic end products. Are they sharing their bench testing? Some have. There is still a lot of secrecy involved among manufacturers, however.

Added to this mix of uncertainty is the application of the remedy. As any classical homeopath will tell you, finding the right remedy for a particular person and his/her condition can seem more like an art than a science. There are many things that are considered, including the person's range of symptoms, stage of illness, mental condition, dreams and behavior. The homeopath also tends to incorporate intuition into his interpretation of the relationship between the symptoms and the patient's underlying issues. And how does the power of suggestion play a role in the homeopath-patient relationship?

These notions make western medical scientists shudder, because diagnosis and prescription in conventional medicine has become very hard-edged and mechanical. There is little leeway for intuition and behavioral investigation. The conventional doctor's clock runs out in about ten minutes: He or she must produce the diagnosis and prescription immediately. The method is thus computer-like: Symptoms in, diagnosis out. Diagnosis in, prescription out. This is not to suggest that homeopathy should align with western medicine: But this is the medical environment we deal with and homeopaths must be able to navigate this environment.

On top of the uncertainty related to matching the right remedy to the condition is the actual dosage and consumption of the remedy. According to classical homeopathy, higher dilutions can have stronger and more internal effects, yet these stronger effects can also be easily inhibited by the wrong environment or method of consumption of the remedy.

For example, many classical homeopaths will insist that the person should be in relative quiet and peaceful surroundings to bring the full effects of the remedy to bear. This is in addition to the other rules mentioned.

This naturally adds to the incredible variability of a homeopathic remedy's success when this is added to the other variables. Is there any wonder why so many doubt the ability of homeopathy to therapeutically treat a condition?

It also means that homeopathy requires a new vision and approach in order for it to be accepted as a genuine medicine.

This vision relates to a new realm of research and development that provides a solid foundation to each substance's dilution process. It requires that the electromagnetic 'fingerprint' of the substance is no longer the subject of trial and error and a mix of seemingly disconnected rules and regulations relating to dilution methods, dosage, storage and consumption.

While the current methods may well still be required to provide therapeutic remedies, the mechanisms of those methods need to be sorted out. We now have the capability and the knowledge to do this that we simply did not have 250 years ago. Or even 50 years ago.

This is why the Benveniste research is so important, and it is important to continue this research in earnest, utilizing modern laboratories and advanced research capabilities.

For example, if a particular remedy's electromagnetic information is carried through Van der Waals forces, then we can measure that conducting process through dilution and provide a tangible measurement through dilution. This provides a clear pathway towards a mechanism of action.

No longer can we afford as a society to spend billions of dollars on homeopathic remedies without spending more on substantiating and quantifying the electromagnetic information being transferred.

This is precisely what Benveniste did, and must continue if we expect homeopathy to carry on into the future.

The challenge is important. The fate of our future existence and the existence of humanity also lies in the balance. Why? Because the continued pursuit of chemical solutions to our illnesses is destroying immune systems and the environment at the same time. Pharmaceutical chemicals are now polluting our waterways and producing disastrous effects among our fellow creatures.

If we do not establish the mechanisms of action related to the healing by herbal treatment and homeopathic treatment—natural treatments that harmonize with nature instead of destroy it—herbal and homeopathic treatment will be relegated to being unscientific myth.

The evidence increasingly shows that herbal therapy is everything but myth. Herbal remedies are therapeutic, and this reality is becoming increasingly found in modern research. But it is only through understanding their mechanisms of action that modern medical science has allowed herbal treatment to become increasingly used and accepted.

Homeopathy has been accepted by modern conventional medicine as generally safe—because of its dilution methods. But proving its therapeutic mechanisms is a more difficult challenge.

Yet this must be done if we expect homeopaths to be ushered into generally-accepted medical treatment going forward.

Hopefully we have provided with this book the basic elements involved in the mechanisms of action in homeopathy. What is needed from this point is focused research to establish the specific mechanisms involved from dilution to dosing for each homeopathic remedy. We can start with the most successful of the homeopathics, and work back through additional remedies until at least we have established some waypoints to navigate with clarity from there with.

For example, if we find that a particular active constituent of Rhus tox—say the catechols within the urushiol—bond with the calcium ions of water as the dilution process takes place. Should these produce a distinct electromagnetic waveform reading using liquid chromatography, mass spectrometry or both combined (HPLC-MS)—or perhaps using Dr. Benveniste's laboratory audio waveform analyzing equipment—that translates through homeopathic dilutions with succussing, then this understanding of electromagnetic conductance can be extended to other remedies that contain catechols as active constituents.

Until this type of meticulous and homeopathic-remedy intensive research can be accomplished and published, classical homeopaths are encouraged to cloak themselves in the science and connect the dots between what we know as scientific fact and the effectiveness of our remedies. Vague discussions of "vibrations" and the like should be replaced by grounded scientific discussions of electromagnetic and electrostatic waveform bonding between substances, solvents and solutes. These discussions can include the evidence of provings, and how those effects are precisely conducted through to dilution, but these are unconvincing without an acceptable mechanism of action.

In other words, the science of homeopathy must emerge from the eighteenth century. Dr. Hahnemann was certainly a medical genius of his day, but we should be taking what he discovered to the next level. This is what Dr. Benveniste's work was beginning to do. We simply need to continue that research with more intensity and clarity of purpose.

There will be no losers in such an effort. Open-minded yet focused scientific investigation can only guide us to a better understanding of the incredible nature swirling around us.

References and Bibliography

Abdou AM, Higashiguchi S, Horie K, Kim M, Hatta H, Yokogoshi H. Relaxation and immunity enhancement effects of gamma-aminobutyric acid GABA). *Biofactors.* 2006;26(3):201-8.

Abou-Seif MA. Blood antioxidant status and urine sulfate and thiocyanate levels in smokers. *J Biochem Toxicol.* 1996;11(3):133-138.

Ackerman D. *A Natural History of the Senses.* New York: Vintage, 1991.

Ackermann RT, Mulrow CD, Ramirez G, Gardner CD, Morbidoni L, Lawrence VA. Garlic shows promise for improving some cardiovascular risk factors. Arch Intern Med. 2001 Mar 26;161(6):813-24.

Airola P. *How to Get Well.* Phoenix, AZ: Health Plus, 1974.

Aissa J, Harran H, Rabeau M, Boucherie S, Brouilhet H, Benveniste J. Tissue levels of histamine, PAF-acether and lysopaf-acether in carrageenan-induced granuloma in rats. *Int Arch Allergy Immunol.* 1996 Jun;110(2):182-6.

Aissa J, Jurgens P, Litime M, Béhar I, Benveniste J. Electronic transmission of the cholinergic signal. *FASEB Jnl.* 1995;9: A683.

Aissa J, Litime M, Attias E, Allal A, Benveniste J. Transfer of molecular signals via electronic circuitry. *FASEB Jnl.* 1993;7: A602.

Aissa J, Litime MH, Attis E., Benveniste J. Molecular signalling at high dilution or by means of electronic circuitry. *J Immunol.* 1993;150:A146.

Aissa J, Nathan N, Arnoux B, Benveniste J. Biochemical and cellular effects of heparin-protamine injection in rabbits are partially inhibited by a PAF-acether receptor antagonist. *Eur J Pharmacol.* 1996 Apr 29;302(1-3):123-8.

Albrechtsen O. The influence of small atmospheric ions on human well-being and mental performance. *Intern. J. of Biometeorology.* 1978;22(4): 249-262.

INDEX

Alexandre P, Darmanyan D, Yushen G, Jenks W, Burel L, Eloy D, Jardon P. Quenching of Singlet Oxygen by Oxygen- and Sulfur-Centered Radicals: Evidence for Energy Transfer to Peroxyl Radicals in Solution. *J. Am. Chem. Soc.,* 120 (2), 396 -403, 1998.

Allais G, Bussone G, De Lorenzo C, Castagnoli Gabellari I, Zonca M, Mana O, Borgogno P, Acuto G, Benedetto C. Naproxen sodium in short-term prophylaxis of pure menstrual migraine: pathophysiological and clinical considerations. *Neurol Sci.* 2007 May;28 Suppl 2:S225-8.

Allen SJ, Okoko B, Martinez E, Gregorio G, Dans LF. Probiotics for treating infectious diarrhea. The Cochrane Library. 2004;3. Chichester, UK: John Wiley & Sons, Ltd.

Amassian VE, Cracco RQ, Maccabee PJ. A sense of movement elicited in paralyzed distal arm by focal magnetic coil stimulation of human motor cortex. *Brain Res.* 1989 Feb 13;479(2):355-60.

American Dietetic Association; Dietitians of Canada. Position of the American Dietetic Association and Dietitians of Canada: vegetarian diets. *Can J Diet Pract Res.* 2003 Summer;64(2):62-81.

Ammor MS, Michaelidis C, Nychas GJ. Insights into the role of quorum sensing in food spoilage. *J Food Prot.* 2008 Jul;71(7):1510-25.

Anderson GC, Moore E, Hepworth J, Bergman N. Early skin-to-skin contact for mothers and their healthy newborn infants. *Cochrane Database Syst Rev.* 2003;(2):CD003519.

Anderson RC, Anderson JH. Acute toxic effects of fragrance products. *Arch Environ Health.* 1998 Mar-Apr;53(2):138-46.

Anderson RC, Anderson JH. Respiratory toxicity of fabric softener emissions. *J Toxicol Environ Health.* 2000 May 26;60(2):121-36.

Anderson RC, Anderson JH. Toxic effects of air freshener emissions. *Arch Environ Health.* 1997 Nov-Dec;52(6):433-41.

Anim-Nyame N, Sooranna SR, Johnson MR, Gamble J, Steer PJ. Garlic supplementation increases peripheral blood flow: a role for interleukin-6? J Nutr Biochem. 2004 Jan;15(1):30-6.

Anonymous. Cimetidine inhibits the hepatic hydroxylation of vitamin D. *Nutr Rev.* 1985;43:184-5.

Aoki T, Usuda Y, Miyakoshi H, Tamura K, Herberman RB. Low natural killer syndrome: clinical and immunologic features. *Nat Immun Cell Growth Regul.* 1987;6(3):116-28.

Appleman P ed. *Darwin: A Norton Critical Edition.* New York: Norton, 1970.

Armstrong BK. Absorption of vitamin B12 from the human colon. *Am J Clin Nutr.* 1968;21:298-9.

Aronne LJ, Thornton-Jones ZD. New targets for obesity pharmacotherapy. *Clin Pharmacol Ther.* 2007 May;81(5):748-52.

Asimov I. *The Chemicals of Life.* New York: Signet, 1954.

Askeland D. *The Science and Engineering of Materials.* Boston: PWS, 1994.

Aspect A, Grangier P, Roger G. Experimental Realization of Einstein-Podolsky-Rosen-Bohm Gedankenexperiment: A New Violation of Bell's Inequalities. *Physical Review Letters.* 1982;49(2): 91-94.

Aton SJ, Colwell CS, Harmar AJ, Waschek J, Herzog ED. Vasoactive intestinal polypeptide mediates circadian rhythmicity and synchrony in mammalian clock neurons. *Nat Neurosci.* 2005 Apr;8(4):476-83.

Atsumi T, Tonosaki K. Smelling lavender and rosemary increases free radical scavenging activity and decreases cortisol level in saliva. *Psychiatry Res.* 2007 Feb 28;150(1):89-96.

Avanzini G, Lopez L, Koelsch S, Majno M. The Neurosciences and Music II: From Perception to Performance. *Annals of the New York Academy of Sciences.* 2006 Mar;1060.

Aymard JP, Aymard B, Netter P, Bannwarth B, Trechot P, Streiff F. Haematological adverse effects of histamine H2-receptor antagonists. *Med Toxicol Adverse Drug Exp.* 1988 Nov-Dec;3(6):430-48.

Bach E. *Bach Flower Remedies*. New Canaan, CN: Keats, 1997.

Bach E. *Heal Thyself*. Saffron Walden: CW Daniel, 1931-2003.

Bache C. *Lifecycles: Reincarnation and the Web of Life*. New York: Paragon House, 1994.

Bachmann KA, Sullivan TJ, Jauregui L, Reese J, Miller K, Levine L. Drug interactions of H2-receptor antagonists. *Scand J Gastroenterol Suppl*. 1994;206:14-9.

Backster C. Primary *Perception: Biocommunication with Plants, Living Foods, and Human Cells*. Anza, CA: White Rose Millennium Press, 2003.

Bader J. The relative power of SNPs and haplotype as genetic markers for association tests. *Pharmacogenomics*. 2001;2:11-24.

Bai H, Yu P, Yu M. Effect of electroacununcture on sex hormone levels in patients with Sjogren's syndrome. *Zhen Ci Yan Jiu*. 2007;32(3):203-6.

Baker DW. An introduction to the theory and practice of German electroacupuncture and accompanying medications. *Am J Acupunct*. 1984;12:327-332.

Baker SM. *Detoxification and Healing*. Chicago: Contemporary Books, 2004.

Balch P, Balch J. *Prescription for Nutritional Healing*. New York: Avery, 2000.

Ballentine R. *Diet & Nutrition: A holistic approach*. Honesdale, PA: Himalayan Int., 1978.

Ballentine RM. *Radical Healing*. New York: Harmony Books, 1999.

Bannerjee H. *Americans Who Have Been Reincarnated*. New York: Macmillan, 1980.

Banyo T. The role of electrical neuromodulation in the therapy of chronic lower urinary tract dysfunction. *Ideggyogy Sz*. 2003 Jan 20;56(1-2):68-71.

Baranauskas G, Nistri A. Sensitization of pain pathways in the spinal cord: cellular mechanisms. *Prog Neurobiol*. 1998 Feb;54(3):349-65.

Barber CF. The use of music and colour theory as a behaviour modifier. *Br J Nurs*. 1999 Apr 8-21;8(7):443-8.

Barker A. *Scientific Method in Ptolemy's Harmonics*. Cambridge: Cambridge University Press, 2000.

Barron M. Light exposure, melatonin secretion, and menstrual cycle parameters: an integrative review. *Biol Res Nurs*. 2007 Jul;9(1):49-69.

Bastide M, Doucet-Jaboeuf M, Daurat V. Activity and chronopharmacology of very low doses of physiological immune inducers. *Immun Today*. 1985;6: 234-235.

Bastide M. Immunological examples on ultra high dilution research. In: Endler P, Schulte J (eds.): *Ultra High Dilution. Physiology and Physics*. Dordrech: Kluwer Academic Publishers, 1994:27-34.

Bates DW, Cullen DJ, Laird N, Petersen LA, Small SD, Servi D, Laffel G, Sweitzer BJ, Shea BF, Hallisey R, *et al*. Incidence of adverse drug events and potential adverse drug events. Implications for prevention. ADE Prevention Study Group. *JAMA*. 1995 Jul 5;274(1):29-34.

Batmangheilidj F. Neurotransmitter histamine: an alternative view point, *Science in Medicine Simplified*. Falls Church, VA: Foundation for the Simple in Medicine, 1990.

Batmanghelidj F. *Your Body's Many Cries for Water*. 2nd Ed. Vienna, VA: Global Health, 1992-1997.

Beauvais F, Bidet B, Descours B, Hieblot C, Burtin C, Benveniste J. Regulation of human basophil activation. I. Dissociation of cationic dye binding from histamine release in activated human basophils. *J Allergy Clin Immunol*. 1991 May;87(5):1020-8.

Beauvais F, Burtin C, Benveniste J. Voltage-dependent ion channels on human basophils: do they exist? *Immunol Lett.* 1995 May;46(1-2):81-3.

Beauvais F, Echasserieau K, Burtin C, Benveniste J. Regulation of human basophil activation; the role of Na+ and Ca2+ in IL-3-induced potentiation of IgE-mediated histamine release from human basophils. *Clin Exp Immunol.* 1994 Jan;95(1):191-4.

Beauvais F, Shimahara T, Inoue I, Hieblot C, Burtin C, Benveniste J. Regulation of human basophil activation. II. Histamine release is potentiated by K+ efflux and inhibited by Na+ influx.. *J Immunol.* 1992 Jan 1;148(1):149-54.

Becker R. *Cross Currents.* Los Angeles: Jeremy P. Tarcher, 1990.

Becker R. *The Body Electric.* New York: William Morrow, 1985.

Beckerman H, Becher J, Lankhorst GJ. The effectiveness of vibratory stimulation in anejaculatory men with spinal cord injury. *Paraplegia.* 1993 Nov;31(11):689-99.

Beeson, C. The moon and plant growth. *Nature.* 1946;158:572–3.

Bell B, Defouw R. Concerning a lunar modulation of geomagnetic activity. *J Geophys Res.* 1964;69:3169-3174.

Bell IR, Baldwin CM, Schwartz GE, Illness from low levels of environmental chemicals: relevance to chronic fatigue syndrome and fibromyalgia. *Am J Med.* 1998;105 (suppl 3A).:74-82. S.

Beloff J. Parapsychology and radical dualism. *J Rel & Psych Res.* 1985;8, 3-10.

Benatuil L, Apitz-Castro R, Romano E. Ajoene inhibits the activation of human endothelial cells induced by porcine cells: implications for xenotransplantation. *Xenotransplantation.* 2003 Jul;10(4):368-73.

Benedetti F, Radaelli D, Bernasconi A, Dallaspezia S, Falini A, Scotti G, Lorenzi C, Colombo C, Smeraldi E. Clock genes beyond the clock: CLOCK genotype biases neural correlates of moral valence decision in depressed patients. *Genes Brain Behav.* 2007 Mar 26.

Bengmark S. Curcumin, an atoxic antioxidant and natural NFkappaB, cyclooxygenase-2, lipooxygenase, and inducible nitric oxide synthase inhibitor: a shield against acute and chronic diseases. *JPEN J Parenter Enteral Nutr.* 2006 Jan-Feb;30(1):45-51.

Bennett GJ, Update on the neurophysiology of pain transmission and modulation: focus on the NMDA-receptor. *J Pain Symptom Manage.* 2000;19 (suppl 1):S.:2-6.

Benor D. Healing Research. Volume 1. Munich, Germany: Helix Verlag, 1992.

Bensky D, Gable A, Kaptchuk T (transl.). *Chinese Herbal Medicine Materia Medica.* Seattle: Eastland Press, 1986.

Bentley E. *Awareness: Biorhythms, Sleep and Dreaming.* London: Routledge, 2000

Benveniste J, Aïssa J, Guillonnet D. A simple and fast method for in vivo demonstration of electromagnetic molecular signaling (EMS) via high dilution or computer recording. *FASEB Jnl.* 1999;13: A163.

Benveniste J, Aïssa J, Guillonnet D. Digital Biology : Specificity of the digitized molecular signal. *FASEB Jnl.* 1998;12: A412.

Benveniste J, Aïssa J, Guillonnet D. The molecular signal is not functional in the absence of "informed" water. *FASEB Jnl.* 1999;13: A163.

Benveniste J, Aïssa J, Litime M, Tsangaris G, Thomas Y. Transfer of the molecular signal by electronic amplification. *FASEB J.* 1994;8:A398.

Benveniste J, Arnoux B, Hadji L. Highly dilute antigen increases coronary flow of isolated heart from immunized guinea-pigs. *FASEB J.* 1992;6:A1610.

Benveniste J, Davenas E, Ducot B, Spira A. Basophil achromasia by dilute ligand: a reappraisal. *FASEB Jnl.* 1991;5: A1008.

Benveniste J, Ducot B, Spira A. Memory of water revisited. *Nature.* 1994 Aug 4;370(6488):322.

Benveniste J, Guillonnet D. QED and digital biology. *Riv Biol.* 2004 Jan-Apr;97(1):169-72.

Benveniste J, Jurgens P, Aïssa J. Digital recording/transmission of the cholinergic signal. *FASEB Jnl.* 1996;10: A1479.

Benveniste J, Jurgens P, Hsueh W, Aïssa J. Transatlantic transfer of digitized antigen signal by telephone link. *Jnl Aller Clin Immun.* 1997;99: S175.

Benveniste J, Kahhak L, Guillonnet D. Specific remote detection of bacteria using an electromagnetic / digital procedure. *FASEB Jnl.* 1999;13: A852.

Benveniste J. Benveniste on Nature investigation. *Science.* 1988 Aug 26;241(4869):1028.

Benveniste J. Benveniste on the Benveniste affair. *Nature.* 1988 Oct 27;335(6193):759.

Benveniste J. Diagnosis of allergic diseases by basophil count and in vitro degranulation using manual and automated tests. *Nouv Presse Med.* 1981 Jan 24;10(3):165-9.

Benveniste J. Meta-analysis of homoeopathy trials. *Lancet.* 1998 Jan 31;351(9099):367.

Berg A, Konig D, Deibert P, Grathwohl D, Berg A, Baumstark MW, Franz IW. Effect of an oat bran enriched diet on the atherogenic lipid profile in patients with an increased coronary heart disease risk. A controlled randomized lifestyle intervention study. *Ann Nutr Metab.* 2003;47(6):306-11.

Bergner P. *The Healing Power of Garlic.* Prima Publishing, Rocklin CA 1996.

Berk M, Dodd S, Henry M. Do ambient electromagnetic fields affect behaviour? A demonstration of the relationship between geomagnetic storm activity and suicide. *Bioelectromagnetics.* 2006 Feb;27(2):151-5.

Berman S, Fein G, Jewett D, Ashford F. Luminance-controlled pupil size affects Landolt C task performance. *J Illumin Engng Soc.* 1993;22:150-165.

Berman S, Jewett D, Fein G, Saika G, Ashford F. Photopic luminance does not always predict perceived room brightness. *Light Resch and Techn.* 1990;22:37-41.

Bernardi D, Dini FL, Azzarelli A, Giaconi A, Volterrani C, Lunardi M. Sudden cardiac death rate in an area characterized by high incidence of coronary artery disease and low hardness of drinking water. *Angiology.* 1995;46:145-149.

Bertin G. *Spiral Structure in Galaxies: A Density Wave Theory.* Cambridge: MIT Press, 1996.

Bhandari U, Sharma JN, Zafar R. The protective action of ethanolic ginger (Zingiber officinale) extract in cholesterol fed rabbits. *J Ethnopharmacol.* 1998 Jun;61(2):167-71.

Bharani A, Ganguli A, Mathur LK, Jamra Y, Raman PG. Efficacy of Terminalia arjuna in chronic stable angina: a double-blind, placebo-controlled, crossover study comparing Terminalia arjuna with isosorbide mononitrate. *Indian Heart J.* 2002 Mar-Apr; 54(2):170-5.

Bharani A, Ganguly A, Bhargava KD. Salutary effect of Terminalia Arjuna in patients with severe refractory heart failure. *Int J Cardiol.* 1995 May;49(3):191-9.

Bhattacharjee C, Bradley P, Smith M, Scally A, Wilson B. Do animals bite more during a full moon? *BMJ.* 2000 December 23; 321(7276): 1559-1561.

Bishop B. Pain: its physiology and rationale for management. Part III. Consequences of current concepts of pain mechanisms related to pain management. *Phys Ther.* 1980 Jan;60(1):24-37.

Bishop, C. Moon influence in lettuce growth. *Astrol J.* 1977;10(1):13-15.

INDEX

Bitbol M, Luisi PL. Autopoiesis with or without cognition: defining life at its edge. *J R Soc Interface.* 2004 Nov 22;1(1):99-107.

Blackmore SJ. Near-death experiences. J R Soc Med. 1996 Feb;89(2):73-6.

Bockemühl, J. *Towards a Phenomenology of the Etheric World.* New York: Anthroposophical Press, 1985.

Bodnar L, Simhan H. The prevalence of preterm birth varies by season of last menstrual period. *Am J Obst and Gyn.* 2003:195(6);S211-S211.

Boivin DB, Czeisler CA. Resetting of circadian melatonin and cortisol rhythms in humans by ordinary room light. *Neuroreport.* 1998 Mar 30;9(5):779-82.

Boivin DB, Duffy JF, Kronauer RE, Czeisler CA. Dose-response relationships for resetting of human circadian clock by light. *Nature.* 1996 Feb 8;379(6565):540-2.

Borchers AT, Hackman RM, Keen CL, Stern JS, Gershwin ME. Complementary medicine: a review of immunomodulatory effects of Chinese herbal medicines. *Am J Clin Nutr.* 1997 Dec;66(6):1303-12.

Borets VM, Lis MA, Pyrochkin VM, Kishkovich VP, Butkevich ND. Therapeutic efficacy of pantothenic acid preparations in ischemic heart disease patients. *Vopr Pitan.* 1987 Mar-Apr;(2):15-7.

Bose J. *Response in the Living and Non-Living.* New York: Longmans, Green & Co., 1902.

Bottorff JL. The use and meaning of touch in caring for patients with cancer. *Oncol Nurs Forum.* 1993 Nov-Dec;20(10):1531-8.

Bourgine P, Stewart J. Autopoiesis and cognition. *Artif Life.* 2004 Summer;10(3):327-45.

Bowler PJ. *The Eclipse of Darwinism: Antievolutionary Theories in the Decades Around 1900.* Baltimore: Johns Hopkins, 1983.

Brasseur JG, Nicosia MA, Pal A, Miller LS. Function of longitudinal vs circular muscle fibers in esophageal peristalsis, deduced with mathematical modeling. *World J Gastroenterol.* 2007 Mar 7;13(9):1335-46.

Braude S. *First Person Plural: Multiple Personality and the Philosophy of Mind.* Landham, MD: Rowman & Littlefield, 1995.

Braunstein G, Labat C, Brunelleschi S, Benveniste J, Marsac J, Brink C. Evidence that the histamine sensitivity and responsiveness of guinea-pig isolated trachea are modulated by epithelial prostaglandin E2 production. *Br J Pharmacol.* 1988 Sep;95(1):300-8.

Brighenti F, Valtueña S, Pellegrini N, Ardigò D, Del Rio D, Salvatore S, Piatti P, Serafini M, Zavaroni I. Total Antioxidant Capacity of the Diet Is Inversely and Independently Related to Plasma Concentration of High-Sensitivity C-Reactive Protein in Adult Italian Subjects. *Br J Nutr.* 2005;93(5):619-25.

Brinkhaus B, Witt CM, Jena S, Linde K, Streng A, Hummelsberger J, Irnich D, Hammes M, Pach D, Melchart D, Willich SN. Physician and treatment characteristics in a randomised multicentre trial of acupuncture in patients with osteoarthritis of the knee. *Complement Ther Med.* 2007 Sep;15(3):180-9.

Britt R. Hole Drilled to Bottom of Earth's Crust, Breakthrough to Mantle Looms. *LiveScience.* 2005. 07 Apr. http://www.livescience.com/ technology/050407_earth_drill.html. Acc. 2006 Nov.

Britton WB, Bootzin RR. Near-death experiences and the temporal lobe. Psychol Sci. 2004 Apr;15(4):254-8.

Brodeur P. Currents of Death. New York: Simon and Schuster, 1989.

Brody J. *Jane Brody's Nutrition Book.* New York: WW Norton, 1981.

Brosseau LU, Pelland LU, Casimiro LY, Robinson VI, Tugwell PE, Wells GE. Electrical stimulation for the treatment of rheumatoid arthritis. *Cochrane Database Syst Rev.* 2002;(2):CD003687.

Brown V. *The Amateur Naturalists Handbook.* Englewood Cliffs, NJ: Prentice-Hall, 1980.

Brown, F. & Chow, C.S. Lunar-correlated variations in water uptake by bean seeds. *Biolog Bull.* 1973;145:265-278.

Brown, F. The rhythmic nature of animals and plants. *Cycles.* 1960 Apr:81-92.

Brown, J. Stimulation-produced analgesia: acupuncture, TENS and alternative techniques. *Anaesthesia &intensive care medicine.* 2005 Feb;6(2):45-47.

Browne J. Developmental Care - Considerations for Touch and Massage in the Neonatal Intensive Care Unit. *Neonatatal Network.* 2000 Feb;19(1).

Brownstein D. *Salt: Your Way to Health.* West Bloomfield, MI: Medical Alternatives, 2006.

Brummer RJ, Geerling BJ, Stockbrugger RW. Initial and chronic gastric acid inhibition by lansoprazole and omeprazole in relation to meal administration. *Dig Dis Sci.* 1997;42:2132-7.

Buck L, Axel R. A novel multigene family may encode odorant receptors: A molecule basis for odor recognition. *Cell.* 1991;65(April 5):175-187.

Buckley NA, Whyte IM, Dawson AH. There are days ... and moons. Self-poisoning is not lunacy. *Med J Aust.* 1993 Dec 6-20;159(11-12):786-9.

Buijs RM, Scheer FA, Kreier F, Yi C, Bos N, Goncharuk VD, Kalsbeek A. Organization of circadian functions: interaction with the body. *Prog Brain Res.* 2006;153:341-60.

Bulsing PJ, Smeets MA, van den Hout MA. Positive Implicit Attitudes toward Odor Words. *Chem Senses.* 2007 May 7.

Burgess JF. Causative Factors in Eczema. *Can Med Assoc J.* 1930 Feb; 22(2): 207-211.

Burnham K, Andersson D. *Model Selection and Inference. A Practical Information-Theoretic Approach.* New York: Springer, 1998

Burr H, Hovland C. Bio-Electric Potential Gradients in the Chick. *Yale Journal of Biology & Medicine.* 1937;9:247-258

Burr H, Lane C, Nims L. A Vacuum Tube Microvoltmeter for the Measurement of Bioelectric Phenomena. *Yale Journal of Biology & Medicine.* 1936;10:65-76.

Burr H, Smith G, Strong L. Bio-electric Properties of Cancer-Resistant and Cancer-Susceptible Mice. *American Journal of Cancer.* 1938;32:240-248

Burr H. *The Fields of Life.* New York: Ballantine, 1972.

Buzsaki G. Theta rhythm of navigation: link between path integration and landmark navigation, episodic and semantic memory. *Hippocampus.* 2005;15(7):827-40.

Cajochen C, Jewett ME, Dijk DJ. Human circadian melatonin rhythm phase delay during a fixed sleep-wake schedule interspersed with nights of sleep deprivation. *J Pineal Res.* 2003 Oct;35(3):149-57.

Cajochen C, Zeitzer JM, Czeisler CA, Dijk DJ. Dose-response relationship for light intensity and ocular and electroencephalographic correlates of human alertness. *Behav Brain Res.* 2000 Oct;115(1):75-83.

Callender ST, Spray GH. Latent pernicious anemia. *Br J Haematol* 1962;8:230-240.

Calvin W. *The Handbook of Brain Theory and Neural Networks.* Boston: MIT Press, 1995.

Campbell A. The role of aluminum and copper on neuroinflammation and Alzheimer's disease. *J Alzheimers Dis.* 2006 Nov;10(2-3):165-72.

Capitani D, Yethiraj A, Burnell EE. Memory effects across surfactant mesophases. *Langmuir.* 2007 Mar 13;23(6):3036-48.

INDEX

Carlsen E, Olsson C, Petersen JH, Andersson AM, Skakkebaek NE. Diurnal rhythm in serum levels of inhibin B in normal men: relation to testicular steroids and gonadotropins. *J Clin Endocrinol Metab.* 1999 May;84(5):1664-9.

Carlson DL, Hites RA. Polychlorinated biphenyls in salmon and salmon feed: global differences and bioaccumulation. *Environ Sci Technol.* 2005 Oct 1;39(19):7389-95.

Carroll D. *The Complete Book of Natural Medicines.* New York: Summit, 1980.

Cassileth B, Trevisan C, Gubili J. Complementary therapies for cancer pain. *Curr Pain Headache Rep.* 2007 Aug;11(4):265-9.

Cavalli-Sforza L, Feldman M. *Cultural Transmission and Evolution: A quantitative approach.* Princeton: Princeton UP, 1981.

Celec P, Ostatníková D, Hodosy J, Skoknová M, Putz Z, Kúdela M. Infradian rhythmic variations of salivary estradioland progesterone in healthy men. *Biol Res.* 2006;37(1): 37-44.

Celec P, Ostatníková D, Putz Z, Hodosy J, Burský P, Stárka L, Hampl R, Kúdela M. Circatrigintan Cycle of Salivary Testosterone in Human Male. *Biol Rhythm Res.* 2003;34(3): 305-315.

Celec P. Analysis of rhythmic variance - ANORVA. A new simple method for detecting rhythms in biological time series. *Biol Res.* 2004;37:777-782.

Cengel YA, *Heat Transfer: A Practical Approach.* Boston: McGraw-Hill, 1998.

Cesarone MR, Belcaro G, Nicolaides AN, Ricci A, Geroulakos G, Ippolito E, Brandolini R, Vinciguerra G, Dugall M, Griffin M, Ruffini I, Acerbi G, Corsi M, Riordan NH, Stuard S, Bavera P, Di Renzo A, Kenyon J, Errichi BM. Prevention of venous thrombosis in long-haul flights with Flite Tabs: the LONFLIT-FLITE randomized, controlled trial. *Angiology.* 2003 Sep-Oct;54(5):531-9.

Chaitow L, Trenev N. *ProBiotics.* New York: Thorsons, 1990.

Chaitow L. *Conquer Pain the Natural Way.* San Francisco: Chronicle Books, 2002.

Cham, B. Solasodine glycosides as anti-cancer agents: Pre-clinical and Clinical studies. *Asia Pac J Pharmac.* 1994;9: 113-118

Chaney M, Ross M. *Nutrition.* New York: Houghton Mifflin, 1971.

Chao A, Thun MJ, Connell CJ, McCullough ML, Jacobs EJ, Flanders WD, Rodriguez C, Sinha R, Calle EE. Meat Consumption and Risk of Colorectal Cancer. *JAMA.* 2005 January 12: 172-182.

Chapat L, Chemin K, Dubois B, Bourdet-Sicard R, Kaiserlian D. Lactobacillus casei reduces CD8+ T cell-mediated skin inflammation. Eur J Immunol. 2004 Sep;34(9):2520-8.

Chapidze G, Kapanadze S, Dolidze N, Bachutashvili Z, Latsabidze N. Prevention of coronary atherosclerosis by the use of combination therapy with antioxidant coenzyme q10 and statins. Georgian Med News. 2005 Jan;(1):20-5.

Characterization and quantitation of Antioxidant Constituents of Sweet Pepper (*Capsicum annuum* - Cayenne). *J Agric Food Chem.* 2004 Jun 16;52(12):3861-9.

Chen HY, Shi Y, Ng CS, Chan SM, Yung KK, Zhang QL. Auricular acupuncture treatment for insomnia: a systematic review. *J Altern Complement Med.* 2007 Jul-Aug;13(6):669-76.

Chen-Goodspeed M, Cheng Chi Lee. Tumor suppression and circadian function. *J Biol Rhythms.* 2007 Aug;22(4):291-8.

Chilton F, Tucker L. *Win the War Within.* New York: Rodale, 2006.

Chirkova E. Mathematical methods of detection of biological and heliogeophysical rhythms in the light of developments in modern heliobiology: A platform for discussion. *Cybernet Sys.* 2000;31(6):903-918.

Chirkova EN, Suslov LS, Avramenko MM, Krivoruchko GE. Monthly and daily biorhythms of amylase in the blood of healthy men and their relation with the rhythms in the external environment. *Lab Delo.* 1990;(4):40-4.

Choi DW. Glutamate neurotoxicity and diseases of the nervous system. *Neuron.* 1988;1:623-34.

Chong AS, Boussy IA, Jiang XL, Lamas M, Graf LH Jr. CD54/ICAM-1 is acostimulator of NK cell-mediated cytotoxicity. *Cell Immunol.* 1994 Aug;157(1):92-105.

Chong NW, Codd V, Chan D, Samani NJ. Circadian clock genes cause activation of the human PAI-1 gene promoter with 4G/5G allelic preference. *FEBS Lett.* 2006 Aug 7;580(18):4469-72.

Christopher J. *School of Natural Healing.* Springville UT: Christopher Publ, 1976.

Christophersen, A. G., Jun, H., Jørgensen, K., and Skibsted, L. H. Photobleaching of astaxanthin and canthaxanthin: quantum-yields dependence of solvent, temperature, and wavelength of irradiation in relation to packageing and storage of carotenoid pigmented salmonoids. *Z. Lebensm. Unters. Forsch.,* 1991;192:433-439.

Chu Q, Wang L, Liu GZ. Clinical observation on acupuncture for treatment of diabetic nephropathy. *Zhongguo Zhen Jiu.* 2007 Jul;27(7):488-90.

Churchill G, Doerge R. Empirical threshold values for quantitative trait mapping. *Genetics* 1994;138:963-971.

Chwirot B, Kowalska M, Plóciennik N, Piwinski M, Michniewicz Z, Chwirot S. Variability of spectra of laser-induced fluorescence of colonic mucosa: Its significance for fluorescence detection of colonic neoplasia. *Indian J Exp. Biol.* 2003;41(5):500-510.

Chwirot WB, Popp F. White-light-induced luminescence and mitotic activity of yeast cells. *Folia Histochemica et Cytobiologica.* 1991;29(4):155.

Citro M, Endler PC, Pongratz W, Vinattieri C, Smith CW, Schulte J. Hormone effects by electronic transmission. *FASEB J.* 1995:Abstract 12161.

Citro M, Smith CW, Scott-Morley A, Pongratz W, Endler PC. Transfer of information from molecules by means of electronic amplification, in P.C. Endler, J. Schulte (eds.): *Ultra High Dilution. Physiology and Physics.* Dordrecht: Kluwer Academic Publishers. 1994;209-214.

Clark D. The use of electrical current in the treatment of nonunions. Vet Clin North Am Small Anim Pract. 1987 Jul;17(4):793-8.

Cocilovo A. Colored light therapy: overview of its history, theory, recent developments and clinical applications combined with acupuncture. *Am J Acupunct.* 1999;27(1-2):71-83.

Cohen S, Popp F. Biophoton emission of the human body. *J Photochem & Photobio.* 1997;B 40:187-189.

Cohen S, Popp F. Low-level luminescence of the human skin. *Skin Res Tech.* 1997;3:177-180.

Coles JA, Yamane S. Effects of adapting lights on the time course of the receptor potential of the anuran retinal rod. *J Physiol.* 1975 May;247(1):189-207.

Coll AP, Farooqi IS, O'Rahilly S. The hormonal control of food intake. *Cell.* 2007 Apr 20;129(2):251-62.

Conely J. Music and the Military. *Air University Review.* 1972 Mar-Ap.

Conquer JA, Holub BJ. Dietary docosahexaenoic acid as a source of eicosapentaenoic acid in vegetarians and omnivores. Lipids. 1997 Mar;32(3):341-5.

Contreras D, Steriade M. Cellular basis of EEG slow rhythms: a study of dynamic corticothalamic relationships. *J Neurosci.* 1995 Jan;15(1 Pt 2):604-22.

Cook J, The Therapeutic Use of Music. *Nursing Forum.* 1981;20:3: 253-66.

INDEX

Cooper K. *The Aerobics Program for Total Well-Being.* New York: Evans, 1980.

Corkin S, Amaral DG, González RG, et al: H. M.'s medial temporal lobe lesion: findings from magnetic resonance imaging. *J Neurosci.* 1997;17:3964-3979.

Cox CB. Emory-led Study Links Metals to Alzheimer's and Other Neurodegenerative Diseases. *Emory Univ Mag.* 2007 Aug 10.

Craciunescu CN, Wu R, Zeisel SH. Diethanolamine alters neurogenesis and induces apoptosis in fetal mouse hippocampus. *FASEB J.* 2006 Aug;20(10):1635-40.

Crawley J. *The Biorhythm Book.* Boston: Journey Editions, 1996.

Creinin MD, Keverline S, Meyn LA. How regular is regular? An analysis of menstrual cycle regularity. *Contraception.* 2004 Oct;70(4):289-92.

Crick F. *Life Itself: Its Origin and Nature.* New York: Simon and Schuster, 1981.

Crofford LJ. Neuroendocrine abnormalities in fibromyalgia and related disorders. *Am J Med Sci.* 1998;315:359-66.

Cross ML. Immune-signalling by orally-delivered probiotic bacteria: effects on common mucosal immunoresponses and protection at distal mucosal sites. Int J Immunopathol Pharmacol. 2004 May-Aug;17(2):127-134.

Cruccu G, Aziz TZ, Garcia-Larrea L, Hansson P, Jensen TS, Lefaucheur JP, Simpson BA, Taylor RS. EFNS guidelines on neurostimulation therapy for neuropathic pain. *Eur J Neurol.* 2007 Sep;14(9):952-70.

Cummings DE, Overduin J. Gastrointestinal regulation of food intake. *J Clin Invest.* 2007 Jan;117(1):13-23.

Cummings M. *Human Heredity: Principles and Issues.* St. Paul, MN: West, 1988.

Curtis LH, Østbye T, Sendersky V, Hutchison S, Dans PE, Wright A, Woosley RL, Schulman KA. Inappropriate prescribing for elderly Americans in a large outpatient population. *Arch Intern Med.* 2004 Aug 9-23;164(15):1621-5.

Cuthbert SC, Goodheart GJ Jr. On the reliability and validity of manual muscle testing: a literature review. *Chiropr Osteopat.* 2007 Mar 6;15:4.

Dalmose A, Bjarkam C, Vuckovic A, Sorensen JC, Hansen J. Electrostimulation: a future treatment option for patients with neurogenic urodynamic disorders? *APMIS Suppl.* 2003;(109):45-51.

Darrow K. *The Renaissance of Physics.* New York: Macmillan, 1936.

Das UN. A defect in the activity of Delta6 and Delta5 desaturases may be a factor predisposing to the development of insulin resistance syndrome. *Prostagl Leukot Essent Fatty Acids.* 2005; May;72(5):343-50.

Davenas E, Beauvais F, Amara J, Oberbaum M, Robinzon B, Miadonna B, Tedeschi A, Pomeranz B, Fortner P, Belon P, Sainte-Laudy J, Poitevin B, Benveniste J. Human basophil degranulation triggered by very dilute antiserum against IgE. *Nature.* 1988;333: 816-818.

Davenas E, Poitevin B, Benveniste J. Effect on mouse peritoneal macrophages of orally administered very high dilutions of silica. *European Journal of Pharmacology.* 1987;135: 313-319.

Davidson T. *Rhinology: The Collected Writings of Maurice H. Cottle, M.D.* San Diego, CA: American Rhinologic Society, 1987.

DaVinci L. (Dickens E. ed.) *The Da Vinci Notebooks.* London: Profile, 2005.

Davis GE Jr, Lowell WE. Chaotic solar cycles modulate the incidence and severity of mental illness. *Med Hypotheses.* 2004;62(2):207-14.

Davis GE Jr, Lowell WE. Solar cycles and their relationship to human disease and adaptability. *Med

Hypotheses. 2006;67(3):447-61.

Davis GE Jr, Lowell WE. The Sun determines human longevity: teratogenic effects of chaotic solar radiation. *Med Hypotheses.* 2004;63(4):574-81.

Dawkins R. *Climbing Mount Improbable.* New York: Viking Press, 1996.

Dawkins R. *River out of Eden.* London: Weidenfeld and Nicholson, 1995.

Dawkins R. *The Blind Watchmaker.* Essex: Longman Scientific and Technical, 1986.

Dawkins R. *The Selfish Gene.* Oxford: Oxford UP, 1977 (1989 edition).

De Lucca AJ, Bland JM, Vigo CB, Cushion M, Selitrennikoff CP, Peter J, Walsh TJ. CAY-I, a fungicidal saponin from Capsicum sp. fruit. Med Mycol. 2002 Apr;40(2):131-7.

Dean C. *Death by Modern Medicine.* Belleville, ON: Matrix Verite-Media, 2005.

Dean E, Mihalasky J, Ostrander S, Schroeder L. *Executive ESP.* Englewood Cliffs, NJ: Prentice-Hall, 1974.

Dean E. Infrared measurements of healer-treated water. In: Roll W, Beloff J, White R (Eds.): *Research in parapsychology 1982.* Metuchen, NJ: Scarecrow Press, 1983:100-101.

Defrin R, Ohry A, Blumen N, Urca G. Sensory determinants of thermal pain. *Brain.* 2002 Mar;125(Pt 3):501-10.

Deitel M. Applications of electrical pacing in the body. *Obes Surg.* 2004 Sep;14 Suppl 1:S3-8.

Del Giudice E, Preparata G, Vitiello G. Water as a free electric dipole laser. *Phys Rev Lett.* 1988;61:1085-1088.

Del Giudice E. Is the 'memory of water' a physical impossibility?, in P.C. Endler, J. Schulte (eds.): *Ultra High Dilution. Physiology and Physics.* Dordrecht: Kluwer Academic Publishers, 1994:117-120.

Delcomyn F. *Foundations of Neurobiology.* New York: W.H. Freeman and Co., 1998.

Dement W, Vaughan C. *The Promise of Sleep.* New York: Dell, 1999.

Dennett D. *Brainstorms: Philosophical Essays on Mind & Psychology.* Cambridge: MIT Press., 1980.

Dennett D. *Consciousness Explained.* London: Little, Brown and Co., 1991.

Depue BE, Banich MT, Curran T. Suppression of emotional and nonemotional content in memory: effects of repetition on cognitive control. *Psychol Sci.* 2006 May;17(5):441-7.

Dere E, Kart-Teke E, Huston JP, De Souza Silva MA. The case for episodic memory in animals. *Neurosci Biobehav Rev.* 2006;30(8):1206-24.

Devaraj TL. *Speaking of Ayurvedic Remedies for Common Diseases.* New Delhi: Sterling, 1985.

Devulder J, Crombez E, Mortier E. Central pain: an overview. *Acta Neurol Belg.* 2002 Sep;102(3):97-103.

Dhond RP, Kettner N, Napadow V. Neuroimaging acupuncture effects in the human brain. *J Altern Complement Med.* 2007 Jul-Aug;13(6):603-16.

Dimitriadis GD, Raptis SA. Thyroid hormone excess and glucose intolerance. *Exp Clin Endocrinol Diabetes.* 2001;109 Suppl 2:S225-39.

Dobrowolski J, Ezzahir A, Knapik M. Possibilities of chemiluminescence application in comparative studies of animal and cancer cells with special attention to leucemic blood cells. In: Jezowska-Trzebiatowska, B., *et al.* (eds.). *Photon Emission from Biological Systems.* Singapore: World Scientific Publ, 1987:170-183.

Dolcos F, LaBar KS, Cabeza R. Interaction between the amygdala and the medial temporal lobe memory system predicts better memory for emotional events. *Neuron.* 2004 Jun 10;42(5):855-63.

Domonkos AN, Arnold HL, Odom RB. *Andrews' Diseases of the Skin: Clinical Dermatology.* 7th ed. Philadelphia, PA

Dong MH, Kaunitz JD. Gastroduodenal mucosal defense. *Curr Opin Gastroenterol.* 2006 Nov;22(6):599-606.

D'Orazio N, Ficoneri C, Riccioni G, Conti P, Theoharides TC, Bollea MR. Conjugated linoleic acid: a functional food? Int J Immunopathol Pharmacol. 2003 Sep-Dec;16(3):215-20.

Dotolo Institute. *The Study of Colon Hydrotherapy.* Pinellas Park, FL: Dotolo, 2003.

Drubaix I, Robert L, Maraval M, Robert AM. Synthesis of glycoconjugates by human diseased veins: modulation by procyanidolic oligomers. Int J Exp Pathol. 1997 Apr;78(2):117-21.

Dubrov, A. *Human Biorhythms and the Moon.* New York: Nova Science Publ., 1996.

Duke J. *The Green Pharmacy.* New York: St. Martins, 1997.

Duke M. *Acupuncture.* New York: Pyramid, 1973.

Dunlop KA, Carson DJ, Shields MD. Hypoglycemia due to adrenal suppression secondary to high-dose nebulized corticosteroid. *Pediatr Pulmonol.* 2002 Jul;34(1):85-6.

Dunne B, Jahn R, Nelson R. Precognitive Remote Perception. Princeton Engineering Anomalies *Res Lab Rep.* Princeton. 1983 Aug.

Dunstan JA, Roper J, Mitoulas L, Hartmann PE, Simmer K, Prescott SL. The effect of supplementation with fish oil during pregnancy on breast milk immunoglobulin A, soluble CD14, cytokine levels and fatty acid composition. *Clin Exp Allergy.* 2004 Aug;34(8):1237-42.

Durlach J, Bara M, Guiet-Bara A. Magnesium level in drinking water: its importance in cardiovascular risk. In: Itokawa Y, Durlach J: *Magnesium in Health and Disease.* London: J.Libbey, 1989:173-182.

Dwivedi S, Agarwal MP. Antianginal and cardioprotective effects of Terminalia arjuna, an indigenous drug, in coronary artery disease. *J Assoc Physicians India.* 1994 Apr;42(4):287-9.

Dwivedi S, Jauhari R. Beneficial effects of Terminalia arjuna in coronary artery disease. *Indian Heart J.* 1997 Sep-Oct;49(5):507-10.

Ebbesen F, Agati G, Pratesi R. Phototherapy with turquoise versus blue light. *Arch Dis Child Fetal Neonatal Ed.* 2003 Sep;88(5):F430-1.

Eden D, Feinstein D. *Energy Medicine.* New York: Penguin Putnam, 1998.

Edris AE. Pharmaceutical and therapeutic potentials of essential oils and their individual volatile constituents: a review. *Phytother Res.* 2007 Apr;21(4):308-23.

Edwards B. *Drawing on the Right Side of the Brain.* Los Angeles, CA: Tarcher, 1979.

Edwards R, Ibison M, Jessel-Kenyon J, Taylor R. Light emission from the human body. *Comple Med Res.* 1989;3(2): 16-19.

Edwards R, Ibison M, Jessel-Kenyon J, Taylor R. Measurements of human bioluminescence. *Acup Elect Res, Intl Jnl,* 1990;15: 85-94.

Edwards, L. *The Vortex of Life, Nature's Patterns in Space and Time.* Floris Press, 1993.

Egon G, Chartier-Kastler E, Denys P, Ruffion A. Spinal cord injury patient and Brindley neurostimulation. *Prog Urol.* 2007 May;17(3):535-9.

Electromagnetic fields: the biological evidence. *Science.* 1990;249: 1378-1381.

Electronic Evidence of Auras, Chakras in UCLA Study. *Brain/Mind Bulletin.* 1978;3:9 Mar 20.

Elias S, van Noord P, Peeters P, den Tonkelaar I, Kaaks R, Grobbee D. Menstruation during and after caloric restriction: The 1944-1945 Dutch famine. *Fertil Steril.* 2007 Jun 1.

Elwood PC. Epidemiology and trace elements. *Clin Endocrinol Metab.* 1985 Aug;14(3):617-28.

Endler PC, Pongratz W, Smith CW, Schulte J. Non-molecular information transfer from thyroxine to frogs with regard to 'homoeopathic' toxicology, *J Vet Hum Tox.* 1995:37:259-260.

Endler PC, Pongratz W, Van Wijk R, Kastberger G, Haidvogl M. Effects of highly diluted sucussed thyroxine on metamorphosis of highland frogs, *Berlin J Res Hom.* 1991;1:151-160.

Endler PC, Pongratz W, Van Wijk R, Waltl K, Hilgers H, Brandmaier R. Transmission of hormone information by non-molecular means, *FASEB J.* 1994;8:A400.

Endler PC, Pongratz W, Van Wijk R, Wiegant F, Waltl K, Gehrer M, Hilgers H. A zoological example on ultra high dilution research. In: Endler PC, Schulte J (eds.): *Ultra High Dilution. Physiology and Physics.* Dordrecht: Kluwer Academic Publishers. 1994:39-68.

Endler PC, Schulte, J. *Ultra High Dilution. Physiology and Physics.* Dordrecht: Kluwer Academic Publ, 1994.

Environmental Working Group. *Human Toxome Project.* 2007. http://www.ewg.org/sites/humantoxome/. Acc. 2007 Sep.

Erdelyi R. MHD waves and oscillations in the solar plasma. Introduction. *Philos Transact A Math Phys Eng Sci.* 2006 Feb 15;364(1839):289-96.

Ernst E. Herbal remedies for anxiety - a systematic review of controlled clinical trials. *Phytomedicine.* 2006 Feb;13(3):205-8.

Esch T, Stefano GB. The Neurobiology of Love. *Neuro Endocrinol Lett.* 2005 Jun;26(3):175-92.

Eschenhagen T, Zimmermann WH. Engineering myocardial tissue. *Circ Res.* 2005 Dec 9;97(12):1220-31.

Evans P, Forte D, Jacobs C, Fredhoi C, Aitchison E, Hucklebridge F, Clow A. Cortisol secretory activity in older people in relation to positive and negative well-being. *Psychoneuroendocrinology.* 2007 Aug 7

Exley C. Aluminium and iron, but neither copper nor zinc, are key to the precipitation of beta-sheets of Abeta in senile plaque cores in Alzheimer's disease. *J Alzheimers Dis.* 2006 Nov;10(2-3):173-7.

Ezzo JM, Richardson MA, Vickers A, Allen C, Dibble SL, Issell BF, Lao L, Pearl M, Ramirez G, Roscoe J, Shen J, Shivnan JC, Streitberger K, Treish I, Zhang G. Acupuncture-point stimulation for chemotherapy-induced nausea or vomiting. *Cochrane Database Syst Rev.* 2006 Apr 19;(2):CD002285.

Falcon CT. *Happiness and Personal Problems.* Lafayette, LA: Sensible Psychology, 1992.

Fallen EL, Kamath MV, Tougas G, Upton A. Afferent vagal modulation. Clinical studies of visceral sensory input. *Auton Neurosci.* 2001 Jul 20;90(1-2):35-40.

Fan X, Zhang D, Zheng J, Gu N, Ding A, Jia X, Qing H, Jin L, Wan M, Li Q. Preparation and characterization of magnetic nano-particles with radiofrequency-induced hyperthermia for cancer treatment. *Sheng Wu Yi Xue Gong Cheng Xue Za Zhi.* 2006 Aug;23(4):809-13.

FAO/WHO Expert Committee. Fats and Oils in Human Nutrition. Food and Nutrition Paper. 1994;(57).

Fecher LA, Cummings SD, Keefe MJ, Alani RM. Toward a molecular classification of melanoma. *J Clin Oncol.* 2007 Apr 20;25(12):1606-20.

Fehring RJ, Schneider M, Raviele K. Variability in the phases of the menstrual cycle. J Obstet Gynecol Neonatal Nurs. 2006 May-Jun;35(3):376-84.

INDEX

Feleszko W, Jaworska J, Rha RD, Steinhausen S, Avagyan A, Jaudszus A, Ahrens B, Groneberg DA, Wahn U, Hamelmann E. Probiotic-induced suppression of allergic sensitization and airway inflammation is associated with an increase of T regulatory-dependent mechanisms in a murine model of asthma. *Clin Exp Allergy.* 2007 Apr;37(4):498-505.

Felton GE. Fibrinolytic and antithrombotic action of bromelain may eliminate thrombosis in heart patients. *Med Hypotheses.* 1980 Nov;6(11):1123-33.

Ferrari R, Merli E, Cicchitelli G, Mele D, Fucili A, Ceconi C. Therapeutic effects of L-carnitine and propionyl-L-carnitine on cardiovascular diseases: a review. Ann N Y Acad Sci. 2004 Nov;1033:79-91.

Feskanich D, Willett W, Colditz G. Calcium, vitamin D, milk consumption, and hip fractures: a prospective study among postmenopausal women. *Am J Clin Nutr.* 2003 Feb;77(2): 504-511.

Fischer JL, Mihelc EM, Pollok KE, Smith ML. Chemotherapeutic selectivity conferred by selenium: a role for p53-dependent DNA repair. *Mol Cancer Ther.* 2007 Jan;6(1):355-61.

Flandrin, J, Montanari M(eds.). *Food: A Culinary History from Antiquity to the Present.* New York: Penguin Books, 1999.

Forget-Dubois N, Boivin M, Dionne G, Pierce T, Tremblay RE, Perusse D. A longitudinal twin study of the genetic and environmental etiology of maternal hostile-reactive behavior during infancy and toddlerhood. *Infant Behav Dev.* 2007 Aug;30(3):453-65.

Fox RD, *Algoculture.* Doctorate Disseration, 1983 Jul.

Fraga CG. Relevance, essentiality and toxicity of trace elements in human health. Mol Aspects Med. 2005 Aug-Oct;26(4-5):235-44.

Frawley D, Lad V. *The Yoga of Herbs.* Sante Fe: Lotus Press, 1986.

Freeman W. *The Physiology of Perception. Sci. Am.* 1991 Feb.

Frey A. Electromagnetic field interactions with biological systems. *FASEB Jnl.* 1993;7: 272-28.

Fu XH. Observation on therapeutic effect of acupuncture on early peripheral facial paralysis. *Zhongguo Zhen Jiu.* 2007 Jul;27(7):494-6.

Fuhrman B, Rosenblat M, Hayek T, Coleman R, Aviram M. Ginger extract consumption reduces plasma cholesterol, inhibits LDL oxidation and attenuates development of atherosclerosis in atherosclerotic, apolipoprotein E-deficient mice. J Nutr. 2000 May;130(5):1124-31.

Fukada Y, Okano T. Circadian clock system in the pineal gland. *Mol Neurobiol.* 2002 Feb;25(1):19-30.

Fuster JM. Prefrontal neurons in networks of executive memory. *Brain Res Bull.* 2000 Jul 15;52(5):331-6.

Gabriel S, Schaffner S, Nguyen H, Moore J, Roy J. The structure of haplotype blocks in the human genome. *Science.* 2002;296:2225-2229.

Galaev, YM. The Measuring of Ether-Drift Velocity and Kinematic Ether Viscosity within Optical Wave Bands. *Spacetime & Substance.* 2002;3(5): 207-224.

Gambini JP, Velluti RA, Pedemonte M. Hippocampal theta rhythm synchronizes visual neurons in sleep and waking. *Brain Res.* 2002 Feb 1;926(1-2):137-41.

Gandhi T, Weingart S, Borus J, Seger A, Peterson J, Burdick E, Seger D, Shu K, Federico F, Leape L, Bates D. Adverse drug events in ambulatory care. *N Engl J Med.* 2003 Apr 17;348(16):1556-64.

Garcia Gomez LJ, Sanchez-Muniz FJ. Review: cardiovascular effect of garlic (Allium sativum). Arch Latinoam Nutr. 2000 Sep;50(3):219-29.

Garcia-Lazaro JA, Ahmed B, Schnupp JW. Tuning to natural stimulus dynamics in primary auditory cortex. *Curr Biol.* 2006 Feb 7;16(3):264-71.

Gardner CD, Fortmann SP, Krauss RM. Association of small low-density lipoprotein particles with the incidence of coronary artery disease in men and women. JAMA. 1996 Sep 18;276(11):875-81.

Gau SS, Soong WT, Merikangas KR. Correlates of sleep-wake patterns among children and young adolescents in Taiwan. Sleep. 2004 May 1;27(3):512-9.

Gehr P, Im Hof V, Geiser M, Schurch S. The mucociliary system of the lung—role of surfactants. *Schweiz Med Wochenschr.* 2000 May 13;130(19):691-8.

Gerber R. *Vibrational Healing.* Sante Fe: Bear, 1988.

Ghayur MN, Gilani AH. Ginger lowers blood pressure through blockade of voltage-dependent calcium Channels acting as a cardiotonic pump activator in mice, rabbit and dogs. J Cardiovasc Pharmacol. 2005 Jan;45(1):74-80.

Gibbons E. *Stalking the Healthful Herbs.* New York: David McKay, 1966.

Gibson RA. Docosa-hexaenoic acid (DHA) accumulation is regulated by the polyunsaturated fat content of the diet: Is it synthesis or is it incorporation? Asia Pac J Clin Nutr. 2004;13(Suppl):S78.

Gionchetti P, Rizzello F, Helwig U, Venturi A, Lammers KM, Brigidi P, Vitali B, Poggioli G, Miglioli M, Campieri M. Prophylaxis of pouchitis onset with probiotic therapy: a double-blind, placebo-controlled trial. Gastroenterology. 2003 May;124:1202-9.

Gisler GC, Diaz J, Duran N. Observations on Blood Plasma Chemiluminescence in Normal Subjects and Cancer Patients. *Arq Biol Tecnol.* 1983;26(3):345-352.

Gittleman AL. *Guess What Came to Dinner.* New York: Avery, 2001.

Glover J. *The Philosophy of Mind.* Oxford University Press, 1976.

Glück U, Gebbers J. Ingested probiotics reduce nasal colonization with pathogenic bacteria (Staphylococcus aureus, Streptococcus pneumoniae, and b-hemolytic streptococci. *Am J. Clin. Nutr.* 2003;77:517-520.

Goff DC Jr, D'Agostino RB Jr, Haffner SM, Otvos JD. Insulin resistance and adiposity influence lipoprotein size and subclass concentrations. Results from the Insulin Resistance Atherosclerosis Study. *Metabolism.* 2005 Feb;54(2):264-70.

Gohil K, Packer L. Bioflavonoid-Rich Botanical Extracts Show Antioxidant and Gene Regulatory Activity. *Ann N Y Acad Sci.* 2002:957:70-7.

Goldberg B. *Past Lives, Future Lives.* New York: Ballantine, 1982.

Golub E. *The Limits of Medicine.* New York: Times Books, 1994.

Gomes A, Fernandes E, Lima JL. Fluorescence probes used for detection of reactive oxygen species. *J Biochem Biophys Methods.* 2005 Dec 31;65(2-3):45-80.

Gomez-Abellan P, Hernandez-Morante JJ, Lujan JA, Madrid JA, Garaulet M. Clock genes are implicated in the human metabolic syndrome. *Int J Obes.* 2007 Jul 24.

González ME, Alarcón B, Carrasco L. Polysaccharides as antiviral agents: antiviral activity of carrageenan. *Antimicrob Agents Chemother.* 1987 Sep;31(9):1388-93.

Gould SJ. *Eight Little Piggies.* New York: Norton, 1993.

Gould SJ. *Wonderful Life: The Burgess Shale and the nature of history.* New York: Penguin Books, 1989.

Govindarajan VS, Sathyanarayana MN. Capsicum-production, technology, chemistry, and quality. Part V. Impact on physiology, pharmacology, nutrition, and metabolism; structure, pungency, pain, and desensitization sequences. Crit Rev Food Sci Nutr. 1991;29(6):435-74.

Govindarajan VS, Sathyanarayana MN. Capsicum-production, technology, chemistry, and quality. Part V. Impact on physiology, pharmacology, nutrition, and metabolism; structure, pungency, pain, and desensitization sequences. Crit Rev Food Sci Nutr. 1991;29(6):435-74.

Grad B, Dean E. Independent confirmation of infrared healer effects. In: White R, Broughton R (Eds.): *Research in parapsychology 1983*. Metuchen, NJ: Scarecrow Press, 1984:81-83.

Grad B. A Telekinetic Effect on Plant Growth. *Intl Jnl Parapsy*. 1964;6: 473.

Grad B. The 'Laying on of Hands': Implications for Psychotherapy, Gentling, and the Placebo Effect. *Jnl Amer Soc for Psych Res*. 1967 Oct;61(4): 286-305.

Grad, B. A telekinetic effect on plant growth: II. Experiments involving treatment of saline in stoppered bottles. *Internl J Parapsychol*. 1964;6:473-478, 484-488.

Grady D, Herrington D, Bittner V, Blumenthal R, Davidson M, Hlatky M, Hsia J, Hulley S, Herd A, Khan S, Newby LK, Waters D, Vittinghoff E, Wenger N. Cardiovascular disease outcomes during 6.8 years of hormone therapy: Heart and Estrogen/progestin Replacement Study follow-up (HERS II). *JAMA*. 2002 Jul 3;288(1):49-57.

Grasmuller S, Irnich D. Acupuncture in pain therapy. *MMW Fortschr Med*. 2007 Jun 21;149(25-26):37-9.

Grasso F, Grillo C, Musumeci F, Triglia A, Rodolico G, Cammisuli F, Rinzivillo C, Fragati G, Santuccio A, Rodolico M. Photon emission from normal and tumour human tissues. *Experientia*. 1992;48:10-13.

Grasso F, Musumeci F, Triglia A, Rodolico G, Cammisuli F, Rinzivillo C, Fragati G, Santuccio A, Rodolico M. In Stanley P, Kricka L (ed). *Ultraweak Luminescence from Cancer Tissues. In Bioluminescence and Chemiluminescence - Current Status*. New York: J Wiley & Sons. 1991:277-280.

Grasso F, Musumeci F, Triglia A. Yanbastiev M. Borisova, S. Self-irradiation effect on yeast cells. *Photochemistry and Photobiology*. 1991;54(1):147-149.

Gray-Davison F. *Ayurvedic Healing*. New York: Keats, 2002.

Greger M. Bird Flu: Virus of Our Own Hatching. *Mother Earth*. 2007 Dec-Jan:103-109.

Grissom C. Magnetic field effects in biology: A survey of possible mechanisms with emphasis on radical pair recombination. *Chem. Rev*. 1995;95: 3-24.

Grobstein P. Directed movement in the frog: motor choice, spatial representation, free will? *Neurobiology of motor programme selection*. Pergamon Press, 1992.

Groneberg DA, Wahn U, Hamelmann E. Probiotic-induced suppression of allergic sensitization and airway inflammation is associated with an increase of T regulatory-dependent mechanisms in a murine model of asthma. *Clin Exp Allergy*. 2007 Apr;37(4):498-505.

Gronfier C, Wright KP Jr, Kronauer RE, Czeisler CA. Entrainment of the human circadian pacemaker to longer-than-24-h days. *Proc Natl Acad Sci USA*. 2007 May 22;104(21):9081-6.

Grzanna R, Lindmark L, Frondoza CG. Ginger—an herbal medicinal product with broad anti-inflammatory actions. *J Med Food*. 2005 Summer;8(2):125-32.

Guo J. Chronic fatigue syndrome treated by acupuncture and moxibustion in combination with psychological approaches in 310 cases. *J Tradit Chin Med*. 2007 Jun;27(2):92-5.

Gupta A, Rash GS, Somia NN, Wachowiak MP, Jones J, Desoky A. The motion path of the digits. J Hand *Surg*. 1998; 23A:1038-1042.

Gupta R, Singhal S, Goyle A, Sharma VN. Antioxidant and hypocholesterolaemic effects of Terminalia arjuna tree-bark powder: a randomised placebo-controlled trial. J Assoc Physicians India. 2001 Feb;49:231-5.

Gupta YK, Gupta M, Kohli K. Neuroprotective role of melatonin in oxidative stress vulnerable brain. *Indian J Physiol Pharmacol*. 2003 Oct;47(4):373-86.

Gutmanis J. *Hawaiian Herbal Medicine.* Waipahu, HI: Island Heritage, 2001.

Haas M, Cooperstein R, Peterson D. Disentangling manual muscle testing and Applied Kinesiology: critique and reinterpretation of a literature review. Chiropr Osteopat. 2007 Aug 23;15:11.

Hadji L, Arnoux B, Benveniste J. Effect of dilute histamine on coronary flow of guinea-pig isolated heart. Inhibition by a magnetic field. *FASEB Jnl.* 1991;5: A1583.

Hagins WA, Penn RD, Yoshikami S. Dark current and photocurrent in retinal rods. *Biophys J.* 1970 May;10(5):380-412.

Hagins WA, Robinson WE, Yoshikami S. Ionic aspects of excitation in rod outer segments. *Ciba Found Symp.* 1975;(31):169-89.

Hagins WA, Yoshikami S. Ionic mechanisms in excitation of photoreceptors. *Ann N Y Acad Sci.* 1975 Dec 30;264:314-25.

Hagins WA, Yoshikami S. Proceedings: A role for Ca2+ in excitation of retinal rods and cones. *Exp Eye Res.* 1974 Mar;18(3):299-305.

Hagins WA. The visual process: Excitatory mechanisms in the primary receptor cells. *Annu Rev Biophys Bioeng.* 1972;1:131-58.

Halliday GM, Agar NS, Barnetson RS, Ananthaswamy HN, Jones AM. UV-A fingerprint mutations in human skin cancer. *Photochem Photobiol.* 2005 Jan-Feb;81(1):3-8.

Halpern G, Miller A. *Medicinal Mushrooms.* New York: M. Evans, 2002.

Halpern S. *Tuning the Human Instrument.* Palo Alto, CA: Spectrum Research Institute, 1978.

Hamel P. *Through Music to the Self: How to Appreciate and Experience Music.* Boulder: Shambala, 1979.

Hameroff SR, Penrose R. Conscious events as orchestrated spacetime selections. *J Consc Studies.* 1996;3(1):36-53.

Hameroff SR, Penrose R. Orchestrated reduction of quantum coherence in brain microtubules: A model for consciousness. In: Hameroff SN, Kaszniak A, Scott AC (eds.): *Toward a Science of Consciousness - The First Tucson Discussions and Debates.* Cambridge: MIT Press, 1996.

Hameroff SR, Smith, S, Watt.R. Nonlinear electrodynamics in cytoskeletal protein lattices. In: Adey W, Lawrence A (eds.), *Nonlinear Electrodynamics in Biological Systems.* 1984:567-583.

Hameroff SR, Watt, R. Information processing in microtubules. *J Theor Biology.* 1982;98:549-561.

Hameroff SR. Coherence in the cytoskeleton: Implications for biological information processing. In: Fröhlich H. (ed.): *Biological Coherence and Response to External Stimuli.* Springer, Berlin-New York 1988, pp.242-264.

Hameroff SR. Light is heavy: Wave mechanics in proteins - A microtubule hologram model of consciousness. *Proceedings 2nd. International Congress on Psychotronic Research.* Monte Carlo, 1975:168-169.

Hameroff SR. *Ultimate Biocomputing - Biomolecular Consciousness and Nanotechnology.* Amsterdam: Elsevier, 1987.

Hameroff, SR. Ch'i: A neural hologram? Microtubules, bioholography and acupuncture. *Am J Chin Med.* 1974;2(2):163-170.

Hamilton-Miller JM. Probiotics and prebiotics in the elderly. London: Department of Medical Microbiology, Royal Free and University College Medical School, 2004.

Hammond BG, Mayhew DA, Kier LD, Mast RW, Sander WJ. Safety assessment of DHA-rich microalgae from *Schizochytrium* sp. *Regul Toxicol Pharmacol.* 2002;35(2 Pt 1):255-65.

Handwerk B. Lobsters Navigate by Magnetism, Study Says. *Natl Geogr News.* 2003 Jan 6.

INDEX

Hannoun AB, Nassar AH, Usta IM, Zreik TG, Abu Musa AA. Effect of war on the menstrual cycle. *Obstet Gynecol.* 2007 Apr;109(4):929-32.

Hans J. *The Structure and Dynamics of Waves and Vibrations.* New York:.Schocken and Co., 1975.

Hantusch B, Knittelfelder R, Wallmann J, Krieger S, Szalai K, Untersmayr E, Vogel M, Stadler BM, Scheiner O, Boltz-Nitulescu G, Jensen-Jarolim E. Internal images: human anti-idiotypic Fab antibodies mimic the IgE epitopes of grass pollen allergen Phl p 5a. *Mol Immunol.* 2006 Jul;43(14):2180-7.

Hardin P. Transcription regulation within the circadian clock: the E-box and beyond. *J Biol Rhythms.* 2004 Oct;19(5):348-60.

Harlow HF, Dodsworth RO, Harlow MK. Total social isolation in monkeys. *Proc Natl Acad Sci U S A.* 1965.

Harlow HF. Development of affection in primates. In Bliss E (ed): *Roots of Behavior.* New York: Harper, 1962: 157-166.

Harlow HF. Early social deprivation and later behavior in the monkey. In: Abrams A, Gurner H, Tomal J (eds): *Unfinished tasks in the behavioral sciences.* Baltimore: Williams & Wilkins. 1964: 154-173.

Hauschild M, Theintz G. Severe chronic anemia and endocrine disorders in children. *Rev Med Suisse.* 2007 Apr 18;3(107):988-91.

Haye-Legrand I, Norel X, Labat C, Benveniste J, Brink C. Antigenic contraction of guinea pig tracheal preparations passively sensitized with monoclonal IgE: pharmacological modulation. *Int Arch Allergy Appl Immunol.* 1988;87(4):342-8.

Heart Disease. New York State Department of Health. Oct. 2004.

Heckman JD, Ingram AJ, Loyd RD, Luck JV Jr, Mayer PW. Nonunion treatment with pulsed electromagnetic fields. *Clin Orthop Relat Res.* 1981 Nov-Dec;(161):58-66.

Hectorne KJ, Fransway AF. Diazolidinyl urea: incidence of sensitivity, patterns of cross-reactivity and clinical relevance. *Contact Dermatitis.* 1994 Jan;30(1):16-9.

Heinrich H. Assessment of non-sinusoidal, pulsed, or intermittent exposure to low frequency electric and magnetic fields. *Health Phys.* 2007 Jun;92(6):541-6.

Helms JA, Farnham PJ, Segal E, Chang HY. Functional demarcation of active and silent chromatin domains in human HOX loci by noncoding RNAs. *Cell.* 2007 Jun 29;129(7):1311-23.

Hendel B, Ferreira P. *Water & Salt: The Essence of Life.* Gaithersburg: Natural Resources, 2003.

Herbert V. Vitamin B12: Plant sources, requirements, and assay. *Am J Clin Nutr.* 1988;48:852-858.

Hernandez Avila M, Walker AM, Jick H. Use of replacement estrogens and the risk of myocardial infarction. *Epidemiology.* 1990 Mar;1(2):128-33.

Heyers D, Manns M, Luksch H, Gu"ntu"rku"n O, Mouritsen H. A Visual Pathway Links Brain Structures Active during Magnetic Compass Orientation in Migratory Birds. *PLoS One.* 2007;2(9): e937. 2007.

Hillecke T, Nickel A, Bolay HV. Scientific perspectives on music therapy. *Ann N Y Acad Sci.* 2005 Dec;1060:271-82.

Ho MW. Assessing Food Quality by Its After-Glow. *Inst. Sci in Society.* Press release. 2004 May 1.

Ho SE, Ide N, Lau BH. S-allyl cysteine reduces oxidant load in cells involved in the atherogenic process. *Phytomedicine.* 2001 Jan;8(1):39-46.

Hobbs C. *Medicinal Mushrooms.* Summertown, TN: Botanica Press, 1986.

Hobbs C. *Stress & Natural Healing.* Loveland, CO: Interweave Press, 1997.

Hoffmann D. *Holistic Herbal.* London: Thorsons, 1983-2002.

Hollfoth K. Effect of color therapy on health and wellbeing: colors are more than just physics. *Pflege Z.* 2000 Feb;53(2):111-2.

Hollwich F, Dieckhues B. Effect of light on the eye on metabolism and hormones. *Klinische Monatsblatter fur Augenheilkunde.* 1989;195(5):284-90.

Hollwich F. Hartmann C. Influence of light through the eyes on metabolism and hormones. Ophtalmologie. 1990;4(4):385-9.

Hollwich F. *The influence of ocular light perception on metabolism in man and in animal.* New York: Springer-Verlag, 1979.

Holmquist G. Susumo Ohno left us January 13, 2000, at the age of 71. *Cytogenet and Cell Genet.* 2000;88:171-172.

Hope M. *The Psychology of Healing.* Longmead UK: Element Books, 1989.

Hoskin M.(ed.). *The Cambridge Illustrated History of Astronomy.* Cambridge: Cambridge Press, 1997.

Hoyle F. *Evolution from Space.* Londong: JM Dent, 1981.

Hu FB, Willett WC. Optimal diets for prevention of coronary heart disease. *JAMA.* 2002 Nov 27;288(20):2569-78.

Hu X, Wu B, Wang P. Displaying of meridian courses travelling over human body surface under natural conditions. *Zhen Ci Yan Jiu.* 1993;18(2):83-9.

Huang D, Ou B, Prior RL. The chemistry behind antioxidant capacity assays. *J Agric Food Chem.* 2005 Mar 23;53(6):1841-56.

Huffman C. Archytas of Tarentum: *Pythagorean, philosopher and Mathematician King.* Cambridge: Cambridge University Press, 2005.

Hull D. *Science as a Process: An evolutionary account of the social and conceptual development of science.* Chicago: Univ Chicago Press, 1988.

Hunt V. *Infinite Mind: Science of the Human Vibrations of Consciousness.* Malibu: Malibu Publ. 2000.

Hur YM, Rushton JP. Genetic and environmental contributions to prosocial behaviour in 2- to 9-year-old South Korean twins. *Biol Lett.* 2007 Aug 28.

Ide N, Lau BH. Garlic compounds minimize intracellular oxidative stress and inhibit nuclear factor-kappa b activation. *J Nutr.* 2001 Mar;131(3s):1020S-6S.

Igarashi T, Izumi H, Uchiumi T, Nishio K, Arao T, Tanabe M, Uramoto H, Sugio K, Yasumoto K, Sasaguri Y, Wang KY, Otsuji Y, Kohno K. Clock and ATF4 transcription system regulates drug resistance in human cancer cell lines. *Oncogene.* 2007 Jul 19;26(33):4749-60.

Iizuka C. at al. Extract of Basidomycetes especially Lentinus edodes, for treatmet of human immunodeficiency virus (HIV). *Patent Application by Shokin Kogyo Co.* 1990: EP 370,673.

Ikonomov OC, Stoynev AG. Gene expression in suprachiasmatic nucleus and circadian rhythms. *Neurosci Biobehav Rev.* 1994 Fall;18(3):305-12.

Inaba H. INABA Biophoton. Exploratory Research for Advanced Technology. *Japan Science and Technology Agency.* 1991. http://www.jst.go.jp/erato/project/isf_P/isf_P.html. Acc. 2006 Nov.

Innis SM, Hansen JW. Plasma fatty acid responses, metabolic effects, and safety of microalgal and fungal oils rich in arachidonic and docosahexaenoic acids in adults. Am J Clin Nutr. 1996 Aug;64(2):159-67.

International HapMap Consortium. The international HapMap project. *Nature.* 2003;426:789-794.

INDEX

Itokawa Y. Magnesium intake and cardiovascular disease. *Clin Calcium.* 2005 Feb;15(2):154-9.

Ivanovic-Zuvic F, de la Vega R, Ivanovic-Zuvic N, Renteria P. Affective disorders and solar activity. *Actas Esp Psiquiatr.* 2005 Jan-Feb;33(1):7-12.

Iwase T, Kajimura N, Uchiyama M, Ebisawa T, Yoshimura K, Kamei Y, Shibui K, Kim K, Kudo Y, Katoh M, Watanabe T, Nakajima T, Ozeki Y, Sugishita M, Hori T, Ikeda M, Toyoshima R, Inoue Y, Yamada N, Mishima K, Nomura M, Ozaki N, Okawa M, Takahashi K, Yamauchi T. Mutation screening of the human Clock gene in circadian rhythm sleep disorders. *Psychiatry Res.* 2002 Mar 15;109(2):121-8.

Jagetia G, Aggarwal B. "Spicing up" of the immune system by curcumin. *J Clin Immunol.* 2007 Jan;27(1):19-35.

Jagetia GC, Aggarwal BB. "Spicing up" of the immune system by curcumin. *J Clin Immunol.* 2007 Jan;27(1):19-35.

Jahn R, Dunne, B. *Margins of Reality: the Role of Consciousness in the Physical World.* New York: Harcourt Brace Jovanovich, 1987.

Janelle KC, Barr SI. Nutrient intakes and eating behavior scores of vegetarian and nonvegetarian women. *J Am Diet Assoc.* 1995 Feb;95(2):180-6, 189, quiz 187-8.

Janssens D, Delaive E, Houbion A, Eliaers F, Remacle J, Michiels C. Effect of venotropic drugs on the respiratory activity of isolated mitochondria and in endothelial cells. *Br J Pharmacol.* 2000 Aug;130(7):1513-24.

Jarvis DC. *Folk Medicine.* Greenwich, CN: Fawcett, 1958.

Jensen B. *Foods that Heal.* Garden City Park, NY: Avery Publ, 1988, 1993.

Jensen B. *Nature Has a Remedy.* Los Angeles: Keats, 2001.

Jensen HK. The molecular genetic basis and diagnosis of familial hypercholesterolemia in Denmark. *Dan Med Bull.* 2002 Nov;49(4):318-45.

Jensen R, Lammi-Keefe C, Henderson R, Bush V, Ferris A.M. Effect of dietary intake of n-6 and n-3 fatty acids on the fatty acid composition of human milk in North America. J Pediatr. 1992;120:S87-92.

Jhon MS. *The Water Puzzle and the Hexagonal Key.* Uplifting, 2004.

Ji Y, Liu YB, Zheng LY, Zhang XQ. Survey of studies on tissue structures and biological characteristics of channel lines. *Zhongguo Zhen Jiu.* 2007 Jun;27(6):427-32.

Jin CN, Zhang TS, Ji LX, Tian YF. Survey of studies on mechanisms of acupuncture and moxibustion in decreasing blood pressure. *Zhongguo Zhen Jiu.* 2007 Jun;27(6):467-70.

Johari H. *Ayurvedic Massage: Traditional Indian Techniques for Balancing Body and Mind.* Rochester, VT: Healing Arts, 1996.

Johari H. *Chakras.* Rochester, VT: Destiny, 1987.

Johnston A. A spatial property of the retino-cortical mapping. *Spatial Vision.* 1986;1(4):319-331.

Johnston RE. Pheromones, the vomeronasal system, and communication. From hormonal responses to individual recognition. *Ann N Y Acad Sci.* 1998 Nov 30;855:333-48.

Jovanovic-Ignjatic Z, Rakovic D. A review of current research in microwave resonance therapy: novel opportunities in medical treatment. *Acupunct Electrother Res.* 1999; 24:105-125.

Jovanovic-Ignjatic Z. Microwave Resonant Therapy: Novel Opportunities in Medical Treatment. *Acup. & Electro-Therap. Res., The Int. J.* 1999;24(2):105-125.

Kahhak L, Roche A, Dubray C, Arnoux C, Benveniste J. Decrease of ciliary beat frequency by platelet activating factor: protective effect of ketotifen. *Inflamm Res.* 1996 May;45(5):234-8.

Kalmijn S, Launer LJ, Ott A, Witteman JC, Hofman A, Breteler MM. Dietary fat intake and the risk of incident dementia in the Rotterdam Study. *Ann of Neurol.* 1997;42(5):776-782.

Kalsbeek A, Perreau-Lenz S, Buijs RM. A network of (autonomic) clock outputs. *Chronobiol Int.* 2006;23(1-2):201-15.

Kamide Y. We reside in the sun's atmosphere. *Biomed Pharmacother.* 2005 Oct;59 Suppl 1:S1-4.

Kandel E, Siegelbaum S, Schwartz J. *Synaptic transmission. Principles of Neural Science.* New York: Elsevier, 1991.

Kang Y, Li M, Yan W, Li X, Kang J, Zhang Y. Electroacupuncture alters the expression of genes associated with lipid metabolism and immune reaction in liver of hypercholesterolemia mice. *Biotechnol Lett.* 2007 Aug 18.

Kaptchuk TJ. The placebo effect in alternative medicine: can the performance of a healing ritual have clinical significance? *Ann Intern Med.* 2002 Jun 4;136(11):817-25.

Karis TE, Jhon MS. Flow-induced anisotropy in the susceptibility of a particle suspension. *Proc Natl Acad Sci USA.* 1986 Jul;83(14):4973-4977.

Karnstedt J. Ions and Consciousness. *Whole Self.* 1991 Spring.

Kataoka M, Tsumura H, Kaku N, Torisu T. Toxic effects of povidone-iodine on synovial cell and articular cartilage. *Clin Rheumatol.* 2006 Sep;25(5):632-8.

Kato Y, Kawamoto T, Honda KK. Circadian rhythms in cartilage. *Clin Calcium.* 2006 May;16(5):838-45.

Keil J, Stevenson I. Do cases of the reincarnation type show similar features over many years? A study of Turkish cases. *J. Sci. Exploration.* 1999;13(2) 189-198.

Keil J. New cases in Burma, Thailand, and Turkey: A limited field study replication of some aspects of Ian Stevenson's work. *J. Sci. Exploration.* 1991;5(1):27-59.

Kelder P. *Ancient Secret of the Fountain of Youth: Book 1.* New York: Doubleday, 1998.

Kelley GA, Kelley KS, Tran ZV. Aerobic exercise and lipids and lipoproteins in women: a meta-analysis of randomized controlled trials. *J Womens Health.* 2004 Dec;13(10):1148-64.

Kennedy KL, Steidle CP, Letizia TM. Urinary incontinence: the basics. *Ostomy Wound Manage.* 1995 Aug;41(7):16-8, 20, 22 passim; quiz 33-4.

Keogh JB, Grieger JA, Noakes M, Clifton PM. Flow-Mediated Dilatation Is Impaired by a High-Saturated Fat Diet but Not by a High-Carbohydrate Diet. *Arterioscler Thromb Vasc Biol.* 2005 Mar 17

Kerckhoffs DA, Brouns F, Hornstra G, Mensink RP. Effects on the human serum lipoprotein profile of beta-glucan, soy protein and isoflavones, plant sterols and stanols, garlic and tocotrienols. *J Nutr.* 2002 Sep;132(9):2494-505.

Kerr CC, Rennie CJ, Robinson PA. Physiology-based modeling of cortical auditory evoked potentials. *Biol Cybern.* 2008 Feb;98(2):171-84.

Keville K, Green M. *Aromatherapy: A Complete Guide to the Healing Art.* Freedom, CA: Crossing Press, 1995.

Key T, Appleby P, Davey G, Allen N, Spencer E, Travis R. Mortality in British vegetarians: review and preliminary results from EPIC-Oxford. *Amer. Jour. Clin. Nutr. Suppl.* 2003;78(3): 533S-538S.

Kiecolt-Glaser JK, Graham JE, Malarkey WB, Porter K, Lemeshow S, Glaser R. Olfactory influences on mood and autonomic, endocrine, and immune function. *Psychoneuroendocrinology.* 2008 Apr;33(3):328-39.

Kim JT, Ren CJ, Fielding GA, Pitti A, Kasumi T, Wajda M, Lebovits A, Bekker A. Treatment with lavender aromatherapy in the post-anesthesia care unit reduces opioid requirements of morbidly obese patients undergoing laparoscopic adjustable gastric banding. *Obes Surg.* 2007 Jul;17(7):920-5.

Kinoshameg SA, Persinger MA. Suppression of experimental allergic encephalomyelitis in rats by 50-nT, 7-Hz amplitude-modulated nocturnal magnetic fields depends on when after inoculation the fields are applied. *J Neulet.*.2004;08:18.

Kirlian SD, Kirlian V, Photography and Visual Observation by Means of High-Frequency Currents. *J Sci Appl Photog.* 1963;6(6).

Klatz RM, Goldman RM, Cebula C. *Infection Protection.* New York: HarperResource, 2002.

Klaus M. Mother and infant: early emotional ties. *Pediatrics.* 1998 Nov;102(5 Suppl E):1244-6.

Klein E, Smith D, Laxminarayan R. Trends in Hospitalizations and Deaths in the United States Associated with Infections Caused by *Staphylococcus aureus* and MRSA, 1999-2004. *Emerging Infectious Diseases.* University of Florida Press Release. 2007 Dec 3.

Klein R, Landau MG. *Healing: The Body Betrayed.* Minneapolis: DCI:Chronimed, 1992.

Klima H, Haas O, Roschger P. Photon emission from blood cells and its possible role in immune system regulation. In: Jezowska-Trzebiatowska B., *et al.* (eds.): *Photon Emission from Biological Systems.* Singapore: World Scientific, 1987:153-169.

Kloss J. *Back to Eden.* Twin Oaks, WI: Lotus Press, 1939-1999.

Kniazeva TA, Kuznetsova LN, Otto MP, Nikiforova TI. Efficacy of chromotherapy in patients with hypertension. *Vopr Kurortol Fizioter Lech Fiz Kult.* 2006 Jan-Feb;(1):11-3.

Kobayashi M, Shoji N, Ohizumi Y. Gingerol, a novel cardiotonic agent, activates the Ca2+-pumping ATPase in skeletal and cardiac sarcoplasmic reticulum. *Biochim Biophys Acta.* 1987 Sep 18;903(1):96-102.

Koch C. Debunking the Digital Brain. *Sci. Am.* 1997 Feb.

Kollerstrom N, Staudenmaier G. Evidence for Lunar-Sidereal Rhythms in Crop Yield: A Review. *Biolog Agri & Hort.* 2001;19:247–259

Kollerstrom N, Steffert B. Sex difference in response to stress by lunar month: a pilot study of four years' crisis-call frequency. *BMC Psychiatry.* 2003 Dec 10;3:20.

Koo KL, Ammit AJ, Tran VH, Duke CC, Roufogalis BD. Gingerols and related analogues inhibit arachidonic acid-induced human platelet serotonin release and aggregation. *Thromb Res.* 2001 Sep 1;103(5):387-97.

Koop H, Bachem MG. Serum iron, ferritin, and vitamin B12 during prolonged omeprazole therapy. *J Clin Gastroenterol.* 1992;14:288-92.

Koszowski B, Goniewicz M, Czogala J. Alternative methods of nicotine dependence treatment. *Przegl Lek.* 2005;62(10):1176-9.

Kotani S, Sakaguchi E, Warashina S, Matsukawa N, Ishikura Y, Kiso Y, Sakakibara M, Yoshimoto T, Guo J, Yamashima T. Dietary supplementation of arachidonic and docosahexaenoic acids improves cognitive dysfunction. *Neurosci Res.* 2006 Oct;56(2):159-64.

Krause R, Buhring M, Hopfenmuller W, Holick MF, Sharma AM. Ultraviolet B and blood pressure. *Lancet.* 1998 Aug 29;352(9129):709-10.

Kräutler B. Colorless Tetrapyrrolic Chlorophyll Catabolites in Ripening Fruit Are Effective Antioxidants. *Angewandte Chemie International Edition.* 2007;46;8699-8702.

Krebs K. The spiritual aspect of caring—an integral part of health and healing. *Nurs Adm Q.* 2001 Spring;25(3):55-60.

Kreig M. *Black Market Medicine.* New York: Bantam, 1968.

Kris-Etherton PM, Pearson TA, Wan Y, Hargrove RL, Moriarty K, Fishell V, Etherton TD. High-monounsaturated Fatty Acid Diets Lower Both Plasma Cholesterol and Triacylglycerol Concentrations. *Am J Clin Nutr.* 1999;70:1009-15

Krsnich-Shriwise S. Fibromyalgia syndrome: an overview. *Phys Ther.* 1997;77:68-75.

Kubler-Ross E. *On Life After Death.* Berkeley, CA: Celestial Arts, 1991.

Kubo I, Fujita K, Kubo A, Nihei K, Ogura T. Antibacterial activity of coriander volatile compounds against Salmonella choleraesuis. *J Agric Food Chem.* 2004 Jun 2;52(11):3329-32.

Kullo IJ, Ballantyne CM. Conditional risk factors for atherosclerosis. *Mayo Clin Proc.* 2005 Feb;80(2):219-30.

Kumar PU, Adhikari P, Pereira P, Bhat P. Safety and efficacy of Hartone in stable angina pectoris-an open comparative trial. *J Assoc Physicians India.* 1999 Jul;47(7):685-9.

Kuo FF, Kuo JJ. *Recent Advances in Acupuncture Research, Institute for Adnanced Research in Asian Science and Medicine.* Garden City, New York. 1979.

Kuuler R, Ballal S, Laike T Mikellides B, Tonello G. The impact of light and colour on psychological mood: a cross-cultral study of indoor work environments. *Ergonomics.* 2006 Nov 15;49(14):1496.

Kwang Y, Cha , Daniel P, Wirth J, Lobo R. Does Prayer Influence the Success of *in Vitro.* Fertilization–Embryo Transfer? Report of a Masked, Randomized Trial. *J Reproductive Med.* 2001;46(9).

Laaksonen M, Karkkainen M, Outila T, Vanninen T, Ray C, Lamberg-Allardt C. Vitamin D receptor gene BsmI-polymorphism in Finnish premenopausal and postmenopausal women: its association with bone mineral density, markers of bone turnover, and intestinal calcium absorption, with adjustment for lifestyle factors. *J Bone Miner Metab.* 2002;20(6):383-90.

Lad V. *Ayurveda: The Science of Self-Healing.* Twin Lakes, WI: Lotus Press.

Lafrenière, G. The material Universe is made purely out of Aether. *Matter is made of Waves.* 2002. http://www.glafreniere.com/matter.htm. Acc. 2007 June.

Lakin-Thomas PL. Transcriptional feedback oscillators: maybe, maybe not. *J Biol Rhythms.* 2006 Apr;21(2):83-92.

Lam F, Jr, Tsuei JJ, Zhao Z. Studies on the bioenergetic measurement of acupuncture points for determination of correct dosage of allopathic or homeopathic medicine in the treatment of diabetes mellitus. *Am J Acupunct.* 1990;18:127-33.

Lambing K. Biophoton Measurement as a Supplement to the Conventional Consideration of Food Quality. In: Popp F, Li K, Gu Q (eds.). *Recent Advances in Biophoton Research.* Singapore: World Scientific Publ. 1992:393-413.

Landmark K, Reikvam A. Do vitamins C and E protect against the development of carotid stenosis and cardiovascular disease? *Tidsskr Nor Laegeforen.* 2005 Jan 20;125(2):159-62.

Langhinrichsen-Rohling J, Palarea RE, Cohen J, Rohling ML. Breaking up is hard to do: unwanted pursuit behaviors following the dissolution of a romantic relationship. *Violence Vict.* 2000 Spring;15(1):73-90.

Lappe FM. *Diet for a Small Planet.* New York: Ballantine, 1971.

Latour E. Functional electrostimulation and its using in neurorehabilitation. *Ortop Traumatol Rehabil.* 2006 Dec 29;8(6):593-601.

Laura AG, Armas, B, Heaney H, Heaney R. Vitamin D_2 Is Much Less Effective than Vitamin D_3 in Humans. *J Clin Endocr & Metab.* 2004;89(11):5387-5391.

LaValle JB. *The Cox-2 Connection.* Rochester, VT: Healing Arts, 2001.

INDEX

Lazarou J, Pomeranz BH, Corey PN. Incidence of adverse drug reactions in hospitalized patients: a meta-analysis of prospective studies. *JAMA*. 1998 Apr.

Lean G. US study links more than 200 diseases to pollution. *London Independent*. 2004 Nov 14.

Leape L. Lucian Leape on patient safety in U.S. hospitals. Interview by Peter I Buerhaus. *J Nurs Scholarsh*. 2004;36(4):366-70.

Leary, PC. Rock as a critical-point system and the inherent implausibility of reliable earthquake prediction. *Geophysical Journal International*. 1997;131(3):451-466. doi:10.1111/j.1365-246X.1997.

Leder D. Spooky actions at a distance: physics, psi, and distant healing. *J Altern Complement Med*. 2005 Oct;11(5):923-30.

Lefort J, Sedivy P, Desquand S, Randon J, Coeffier E, Maridonneau-Parini I, Floch A, Benveniste J, Vargaftig BB. Pharmacological profile of 48740 R.P., a PAF-acether antagonist. *Eur J Pharmacol*. 1988 Jun 10;150(3):257-68.

Lehmann B. The vitamin D3 pathway in human skin and its role for regulation of biological processes. *Photochem Photobiol*. 2005 Nov-Dec;81(6):1246-51.

Leitzmann C. Vegetarian diets: what are the advantages? *Forum Nutr*. 2005;(57):147-56.

Lennihan B. Homeopathy: natural mind-body healing. *J Psychosoc Nurs Ment Health Serv*. 2004 Jul;42(7):30-40.

Lewis A. Rescue remedy. *Nurs Times*. 1999 May 26-Jun 1;95(21):27.

Lewis WH, Elvin-Lewis MPF. *Medical Botany: Plants Affecting Man's Health*. New York: Wiley, 1977.

Lewontin R. *The Genetic Basis of Evolutionary Change*. New York: Columbia Univ Press, 1974.

Leyel CF. *Culpeper's English Physician & Complete Herbal*. Hollywood, CA: Wilshire, 1971.

Li KH. Bioluminescence and stimulated coherent radiation. *Laser und Elektrooptik 3*. 1981:32-35.

Li N, Wang DL, Wang CW, Wu B. Discussion on randomized controlled trials about clinical researches of acupuncture and moxibustion medicine. *Zhongguo Zhen Jiu*. 2007 Jul;27(7):529-32.

Liao H, Xi P, Chen Q, Yi L, Zhao Y. Clinical study on acupuncture, moxibustion, acupuncture plus moxibustion at Weiwanxiashu (EX-B3) for treatment of diabetes. *Zhongguo Zhen Jiu*. 2007 Jul;27(7):482-4.

Lieber AL. Human aggression and the lunar synodic cycle. *J Clin Psychiatry*. 1978 May;39(5):385-92.

Lin PW, Chan WC, Ng BF, Lam LC. Efficacy of aromatherapy (Lavandula angustifolia) as an intervention for agitated behaviours in Chinese older persons with dementia: a cross-over randomized trial. *Int J Geriatr Psychiatry*. 2007 May;22(5):405-10.

Lininger S, Gaby A, Austin S, Brown D, Wright J, Duncan A. *The Natural Pharmacy*. New York: Three Rivers, 1999.

Lipkind M. Can the vitalistic Entelechia principle be a working instrument ? (The theory of the biological field of Alexander G.Gurvich). In: Popp F, Li K, Gu Q (eds.). *Recent Advances in Biophoton Research*. Singapore: World Sci Publ, 1992:469-494.

Lipkind M. Registration of spontaneous photon emission from virus-infected cell cultures: development of experimental system. *Indian J Exp Biol*. 2003 May;41(5):457-72.

Lipski E. *Digestive Wellness*. Los Angeles, CA: Keats, 2000.

Litime M, Aïssa J, Benveniste J. Antigen signaling at high dilution. *FASEB Jnl*. 1993;7: A602.

Litscher G. Bioengineering assessment of acupuncture, part 5: cerebral near-infrared spectroscopy. *Crit Rev Biomed Eng*. 2006;34(6):439-57.

Liukkonen-Lilja H, Piepponen S. Leaching of aluminium from aluminium dishes and packages. *Food Addit Contam.* 1992 May-Jun;9(3):213-23.

Livanova L, Levshina I, Nozdracheva L, Elbakidze MG, Airapetiants MG. The protective action of negative air ions in acute stress in rats with different typological behavioral characteristics. *Zh Vyssh Nerv Deiat Im I P Pavlova.* 1998 May-Jun;48(3):554-7.

Lloyd D and Murray D. Redox rhythmicity: clocks at the core of temporal coherence. *BioEssays.* 2007;29(5): 465-473.

Lloyd JU. *American Materia Medica, Therapeutics and Pharmacognosy.* Portland, OR: Eclectic Medical Publications, 1989-1983.

Lopez-Garcia E, Schulze MB, Meigs JB, Manson JE, Rifai N, Stampfer MJ, Willett WC, Hu FB. Consumption of trans fatty acids is related to plasma biomarkers of inflammation and endothelial dysfunction. *J Nutr.* 2005 Mar;135(3):562-6.

Lorenz I, Schneider EM, Stolz P, Brack A, Strube J. Sensitive flow cytometric method to test basophil activation influenced by homeopathic histamine dilutions. *Forsch Komplementarmed Klass Naturheilkd.* 2003 Dec;10(6):316-24.

Lovejoy S, Pecknold S, Schertzer D. Stratified multifractal magnetization and surface geomagnetic fields-I. Spectral analysis and modeling. *Geophysical Journal International.* 2001 145(1):112-126.

Lovelock, J. *Gaia: A New Look at Life on Earth.* Oxford: Oxford Press, 1979.

Lovely RH. Recent studies in the behavioral toxicology of ELF electric and magnetic fields. *Prog Clin Biol Res.* 1988;257:327-47.

Lu J, Cui Y, Shi R. *A Practical English-Chinese Library of Traditional Chinese Medicine: Chinese Acupuncture and Moxibustion.* Shanghai: Publishing House of the Shanghai College of Traditional Chinese Medicine, 1988.

Lucas A, Morley R, Cole T, Lister G, Leeson-Payne C. Breast milk and subsequent intelligence quotient in children born premature. Lancet. 1992;339:261-264.

Lucas WB (ed). *Regression Therapy: A Handbook for Professionals. Past-Life Therapy.* Crest Park, CA: Deep Forest Press, 1993.

Lydic R, Schoene WC, Czeisler CA, Moore-Ede MC. Suprachiasmatic region of the human hypothalamus: homolog to the primate circadian pacemaker? *Sleep.* 1980;2(3):355-61.

Lynch M, Walsh B. *Genetics and Analysis of Quantitative Traits.* Sunderland, MA: Sinauer, 1998

Lythgoe JN. Visual pigments and environmental light. *Vision Res.* 1984;24(11):1539-50.

Lytle CD, Sagripanti JL. Predicted inactivation of viruses of relevance to biodefense by solar radiation. *J Virol.* 2005 Nov;79(22):14244-52.

Maas J, Jayson, J. K.. & Kleiber, D. A. Effects of spectral differences in illumination on fatigue. *J Appl Psychol.* 1974;59:524-526.

Mabey R, ed. *The New Age Herbalist.* New York: Simon & Schuster, 1941.

Maccabee PJ, Amassian VE, Cracco RQ, Cracco JB, Eberle L, Rudell A. Stimulation of the human nervous system using the magnetic coil. *J Clin Neurophysiol.* 1991 Jan;8(1):38-55.

Macdessi JS, Randell TL, Donaghue KC, Ambler GR, van Asperen PP, Mellis CM. Adrenal crises in children treated with high-dose inhaled corticosteroids for asthma. *Med J Aust.* 2003 Mar 3;178(5):214-6.

MacDougall D. The Soul: Hypothesis Concerning Soul Substance Together with Experimental Evidence of The Existence of Such Substance. *J Am Soc Psych Res.* 1907 May.

INDEX

Machado RF, Laskowski D, Deffenderfer O, Burch T, Zheng S, Mazzone PJ, Mekhail T, Jennings C, Stoller JK, Pyle J, Duncan J, Dweik RA, Erzurum SC. Detection of lung cancer by sensor array analyses of exhaled breath. *Am J Respir Crit Care Med.* 2005 Jun 1;171(11):1286-91.

MacKay D. *Science, Chance, and Providence.* Oxford: Oxford Univ Press, 1978.

MacKay D. *The Open Mind and Other Essays.* Downer's Grove, IL: Inter-Varsity Press, 1988.

Maes HH, Silberg JL, Neale MC, Eaves LJ. Genetic and cultural transmission of antisocial behavior: an extended twin parent model. *Twin Res Hum Genet.* 2007 Feb;10(1):136-50.

Magni P, Motta M, Martini L. Leptin: a possible link between food intake, energy expenditure, and reproductive function. *Regul Pept.* 2000 Aug 25;92(1-3):51-6.

Magnusson A, Stefansson JG. Prevalence of seasonal affective disorder in Iceland. *Arch Gen Psychiatry.* 1993 Dec;50(12):941-6.

Mahachoklertwattana P, Sudkronrayudh K, Direkwattanachai C, Choubtum L, Okascharoen C. Decreased cortisol response to insulin induced hypoglycaemia in asthmatics treated with inhaled fluticasone propionate. *Arch Dis Child.* 2004 Nov;89(11):1055-8.

Makomaski Illing EM, Kaiserman MJ. Mortality attributable to tobacco use in Canada and its regions, 1998. *Can J Public Health.* 2004;95(1):38-44.

Makrides M, Neumann M, Byard R, Simmer K, Gibson R. Fatty acid composition of brain, retina, and erythrocytes in breast- and formula-fed infants. Am J Clin Nutr. 1994;60:189-94.

Makrides M, Neumann M, Gibson R. Effect of maternal docosahexaenoic acid (DHA) supplementation on breast milk composition. *Europ Jrnl of Clin Nutr.* 1996;50:352-357.

Manson JE, *et al.* Estrogen plus progestin and the risk of coronary heart disease. *NE J Med.* 2003; 349(6):523–534.

Mansour HA, Monk TH, Nimgaonkar VL. Circadian genes and bipolar disorder. *Ann Med.* 2005;37(3):196-205.

Marasanov SB, Matveev II. Correlation between protracted premedication and complication in cancer patients operated on during intense solar activity. *Vopr Onkol.* 2007;53(1):96-9.

Marcuard SP, Albernaz L, Khazanie PG. Omeprazole therapy causes malabsorption of cyanocobalamin (Vitamin B12). *Ann Intern Med.* 1994;120:211-5.

Marie PJ. Optimizing bone metabolism in osteoporosis: insight into the pharmacologic profile of strontium ranelate. *Osteoporos Int.* 2003;14 Suppl 3:S9-12.

Marie PJ. Strontium ranelate: a physiological approach for optimizing bone formation and resorption. *Bone.* 2006 Feb;38(2 Suppl 1):S10-4.

Marks C. *Commissurotomy, Consciousness, and Unity of Mind.* Cambridge: MIT Press, 1981.

Marks L. *The Unity of the Senses: Interrelations among the Modalities.* New York: Academic Press, 1978.

Martinez M. Docosahexaenoic acid therapy in docosahexaenoic acid-deficient patients with disorders of peroxisomal biogenesis. *Versicherungsmedizin.* 1996;31 Suppl:145-152

Mason D, Moore J, Green S, Liggett S. A gain-of-function polymorphism in a G-protein coupling domain of the human β1-adrenergic receptor. *J. Biol. Chem.* 1999;274:12670-12674.

Mastorakos G, Pavlatou M. Exercise as a stress model and the interplay between the hypothalamus-pituitary-adrenal and the hypothalamus-pituitary-thyroid axes. *Horm Metab Res.* 2005 Sep;37(9):577-84.

Mattix KD, Winchester PD, Scherer LR. Incidence of abdominal wall defects is related to surface water atrazine and nitrate levels. *J Pediatr Surg.* 2007 Jun;42(6):947-9.

Matutinovic Z, Galic M. Relative magnetic hearing threshold. *Laryngol Rhinol Otol.* 1982 Jan;61(1):38-

41.

Maurer HR. Bromelain: biochemistry, pharmacology and medical use. *Cell Mol Life Sci.* 2001 Aug;58(9):1234-45.

Mayr E. *Toward a New Philosophy of Biology: Observations of an evolutionist.* Boston: Belknap Press, 1988.

Mayron L, Ott J, Nations R, Mayron E. Light, radiation and academic behaviour: Initial studies on the effects of full-spectrum lighting and radiation shielding on behaviour and academic performance of school children. *Acad Ther.* 1974;10, 33-47.

McCauley B. 2005. *Achieving Great Health.* Spartan, Lansing, MI.

McConnaughey E. *Sea Vegetables.* Happy Camp, CA: Naturegraph, 1985.

McConnel JV, Cornwell PR, Clay M. An apparatus for conditioning Planaria. *Am J Psychol.* 1960 Dec;73:618-22.

McCulloch M, Jezierski T, Broffman M, Hubbard A, Turner K, Janecki T. Diagnostic accuracy of canine scent detection in early- and late-stage lung and breast cancers. *Integr Cancer Ther.* 2006 Mar;5(1):30-9.

McDougall J, McDougall M. *The McDougal Plan.* Clinton, NJ: New Win, 1983.

McTaggart L. *The Field.* New York: Quill, 2003.

Meinecke FW. Sequelae and rehabilitation of spinal cord injuries. *Curr Opin Neurol Neurosurg.* 1991 Oct;4(5):714-9.

Melzack R, Coderre TJ, Katz J, Vaccarino AL. Central neuroplasticity and pathological pain. *Ann N Y Acad Sci.* 2001 Mar;933:157-74.

Melzack R, Wall PD. Pain mechanisms: a new theory. *Science.* 1965 Nov 19;150(699):971-9.

Melzack R. Evolution of the neuromatrix theory of pain. The prithvi raj lecture: presented at the third world congress of world institute of pain, barcelona 2004. *Pain Pract.* 2005 Jun;5(2):85-94.

Melzack R. Pain: past, present and future. *Can J Exp Psychol.* 1993 Dec;47(4):615-29.

Melzack R. Pain—an overview. *Acta Anaesthesiol Scand.* 1999 Oct;43(9):880-4.

Mendoza J. Circadian clocks: setting time by food. *J Neuroendocrinol.* 2007 Feb;19(2):127-37.

Meyer A, Kirsch H, Domergue F, Abbadi A, Sperling P, Bauer J, Cirpus P, Zank TK, Moreau H, Roscoe TJ, Zahringer U, Heinz E. Novel fatty acid elongases and their use for the reconstitution of docosahexaenoic acid biosynthesis. *J Lipid Res.* 2004 Oct;45(10):1899-909.

Milke Garcia Mdel P. Ghrelin: beyond hunger regulation. *Rev Gastroenterol Mex.* 2005 Oct-Dec;70(4):465-74.

Miller GT. *Living in the Environment.* Belmont, CA: Wadsworth, 1996.

Miller JD, Morin LP, Schwartz WJ, Moore RY. New insights into the mammalian circadian clock. *Sleep.* 1996 Oct;19(8):641-67.

Miller K. Cholesterol and In-Hospital Mortality in Elderly Patients. Am Family Phys. 2004 May.

Mills A. A replication study: Three cases of children in northern India who are said to remember a previous life," *J. Sci. Explor.* 1989;3(2):133-184.

Mills A. Moslem cases of the reincarnation type in northern India: A test of the hypothesis of imposed identification, Part I: Analysis of 26 cases. *J. Sci. Exploration.* 1990;4(2):171-188.

Mindell E, Hopkins V. *Prescription Alternatives.* New Canaan CT: Keats, 1998.

Mineev VN, Bulatova NI, Fedoseev GB. Erythrocyte insulin-reactive system and carbohydrate metabolism in bronchial asthma. *Ter Arkh.* 2002;74(3):14-7.

Mishkin M, Appenzeller T. The Anatomy of Memory. *Sci. Am.* 1987 June.

Mishkin M. Memory in monkeys severely impaired by combined but not by separate removal of amygdala and hippocampus. *Nature.* 1978;273: 297-298.

Mitchell JL. *Out-of-Body Experiences: A Handbook.* New York: Ballantine Books, 1981.

Miu AC, Benga O. Aluminum and Alzheimer's disease: a new look. *J Alzheimers Dis.* 2006 Nov;10(2-3):179-201.

Modern Biology. Austin: Harcourt Brace, 1993.

Moini H, Packer L, Saris NE. Antioxidant and Prooxidant Activities of Alpha-Lipoic Acid and Dihydrolipoic Acid. *Toxicol Appl Pharmacol.* 2002;182(1):84-90.

Monod J. *Chance and Necessity.* New York: Vintage, 1972.

Monroe R. *Far Journeys.* Garden City, NY: Doubleday & Co., 1985.

Monroe R. *Journeys Out of the Body.* Garden City, NY: Anchor Press, 1977.

Montanes P, Goldblum MC, Boller F. The naming impairment of living and nonliving items in Alzheimer's disease. *J Int Neuropsychol Soc.* 1995 Jan;1(1):39-48.

Moody R. *Coming Back: A Psychiatrist Explores Past-Life Journeys.* New York: Bantam Books, 1991.

Moody R. *Life After Life.* New York: Bantam, 1975.

Moody, R. *Reflections on Life After Life: More Important Discoveries In The Ongoing Investigation Of Survival Of Life After Bodily Death.* New York: Bantam, 1977.

Moore KH. Conservative management for urinary incontinence. *Baillieres Best Pract Res Clin Obstet Gynaecol.* 2000 Apr;14(2):251-89.

Moore R. Circadian Rhythms: A Clock for the Ages. *Science* 1999 June 25;284(5423):2102 – 2103.

Moore RY, Speh JC. Serotonin innervation of the primate suprachiasmatic nucleus. *Brain Res.* 2004 Jun 4;1010(1-2):169-73.

Moore RY. Neural control of the pineal gland. *Behav Brain Res.* 1996;73(1-2):125-30.

Moore RY. Organization and function of a central nervous system circadian oscillator: the suprachiasmatic hypothalamic nucleus. *Fed Proc.* 1983 Aug;42(11):2783-9.

Morick H. *Introduction to the Philosophy of Mind: Readings from Descartes to Strawson.* Glenview, Ill: Scott Foresman, 1970.

Morse M. *Closer to the Light.* New York: Ivy Books, 1990.

Morton C. *Velocity Alters Electric Field.* www.amasci.com/ freenrg/ morton1.html. Accessed 2007 July.

Morton G. Hypothalamic Leptin Regulation of Energy Homeostasis and Glucose Metabolism. *J Physiol.* 2007 Jun 21.

Moshe M. Method and apparatus for predicting the occurrence of an earthquake by identifying electromagnetic precursors. US Patent Issued on May 28, 1996. Number 5521508.

Motoyama H. Acupuncture Meridians. *Science & Medicine.* 1999 July/August.

Motoyama H. Before Polarization Current and the Acupuncture Meridians. *Journal of Holistic Medicine.* 1986;8(1&2).

Motoyama H. Deficient/ Excessive Patterns Found in Meridian Functioning in Cases of Liver Disease. *Subtle Energy & Energy Medicine.* 2000; 11(2).

Motoyama H. Energetic Medicine: new science of healing: An interview with A. Jackson. www.shareintl.org/archives/health-healing/hh_adjenergetic.html. Acc. 2007 Oct.

Motoyama H. Smith, W. Harada T. Pre-Polarization Resistance of the Skin as Determined by the Single Square Voltage Pulse. *Psychophysiology.* 1984;21(5).

Mozafar A. Enrichment of some B-vitamin in plants with application of organic fertilizers. *Plant and Soil.* 1994;167:305-11.

Mozafar A. Is there vitamin B12 in plants or not? A plant nutritionist's view. *Vegetarian Nutrition: An International Journal.* 1997;1/2:50-52.

Müller JP, Steinegger A, Schlatter C. Contribution of aluminum from packaging materials and cooking utensils to the daily aluminum intake. *Z Lebensm Unters Forsch.* 1993 Oct;197(4):332-41.

Muhlack S, Lemmer W, Klotz P, Muller T, Lehmann E, Klieser E. Anxiolytic effect of rescue remedy for psychiatric patients: a double-blind, placebo-controlled, randomized trial. *J Clin Psychopharmacol.* 2006 Oct;26(5):541-2.

Muller H, Lindman AS, Blomfeldt A, Seljeflot I, Pedersen JI. A diet rich in coconut oil reduces diurnal postprandial variations in circulating tissue plasminogen activator antigen and fasting lipoprotein (a) compared with a diet rich in unsaturated fat in women. *J Nutr.* 2003 Nov;133(11):3422-7.

Mumby DG, Wood ER, Pinel J. Object-recognition memory is only mildly impaired in rats with lesions of the hippocampus and amygdala. *Psychobio.* 1992;20: 18-27.

Municino A, Nicolino A, Milanese M, Gronda E, Andreuzzi B, Oliva F, Chiarella F, Cardio-HKT Study Group. Hydrotherapy in advanced heart failure: the cardio-HKT pilot study. *Monaldi Arch Chest Dis.* 2006 Dec;66(4):247-54.

Murchie G. *The Seven Mysteries of Life.* Boston: Houghton Mifflin Company, 1978.

Murphy R. *Organon Philosophy Workbook.* Blacksburg, VA: HANA, 1994.

Murray M and Pizzorno J. *Encyclopedia of Natural Medicine.* 2nd Edition. Roseville, CA: Prima Publishing, 1998.

Musaev AV, Nasrullaeva SN, Zeinalov RG. Effects of solar activity on some demographic indices and morbidity in Azerbaijan with reference to A. L. Chizhevsky's theory. *Vopr Kurortol Fizioter Lech Fiz Kult.* 2007 May-Jun;(3):38-42.

Muzzarelli L, Force M, Sebold M. Aromatherapy and reducing preprocedural anxiety: A controlled prospective study. *Gastroenterol Nurs.* 2006 Nov-Dec;29(6):466-71.

Myss C. *Anatomy of the Spirit.* New York: Harmony, 1996.

Nadkarni AK, Nadkarni KM. *Indian Materia Medica.* (Vols 1 and 2). Bombay, India: Popular Pradashan, 1908, 1976.

Nakamura K, Urayama K, Hoshino Y. Lumbar cerebrospinal fluid pulse wave rising from pulsations of both the spinal cord and the brain in humans. *Spinal Cord.* 1997 Nov;35(11):735-9.

Nakamura MT, Nara TY. Structure, function, and dietary regulation of delta6, delta5, and delta9 desaturases. *Ann Rev Nutr.* 2004;24:345-76.

Nakatani K, Yau KW. Calcium and light adaptation in retinal rods and cones. *Nature.* 1988 Jul 7;334(6177):69-71.

Napoli N, Thompson J, Civitelli R, Armamento-Villareal R. Effects of dietary calcium compared with calcium supplements on estrogen metabolism and bone mineral density. *Am J Clin Nutr.* 2007;85(5): 1428-1433.

Naruszewicz M, Daniewski M, Nowicka G, Kozlowska-Wojciechowska M. Trans-unsaturated fatty acids and acrylamide in food as potential atherosclerosis progression factors. Based on own studies.

INDEX

Acta Microbiol Pol. 2003;52 Suppl:75-81.

Natarajan E, Grissom C. The Origin of Magnetic Field Dependent Recombination in Alkylcobalamin Radical Pairs. *Photochem Photobiol.* 1996;64: 286-295.

Navarro Silvera SA, Rohan TE. Trace elements and cancer risk: a review of the epidemiologic evidence. *Cancer Causes Control.* 2007 Feb;18(1):7-27.

Neeck G, Riedel W. Hormonal perturbations in fibromyalgia syndrome. *Ann N Y Acad Sci.* 1999;876:325-38.

Nestel PJ. Adulthood - prevention: Cardiovascular disease. *Med J Aust.* 2002 Jun 3;176(11 Suppl):S118-9.

Nestor PJ, Graham KS, Bozeat S, Simons JS, Hodges JR. Memory consolidation and the hippocampus: further evidence from studies of autobiographical memory in semantic dementia and frontal variant frontotemporal dementia. *Neuropsychologia.* 2002;40(6):633-54.

Netheron M. *Past Lives Therapy.* New York: Morrow, 1978.Wambach H. *Reliving Past Lives.* New York: Bantam, 1978.Fiore E. *You Have Been Here Before.* New York: Ballantine, 1978.

Newmark T, Schulick P. *Beyond Aspirin.* Prescott, AZ: Holm, 2000.

Newton M. *Destiny of Souls: New Case Studies of Life between Lives.* St. Paul: Llewellyn Publications, 2000.

Newton M. *Journey of Souls: Case Studies of Life between Lives.* St. Paul: Llewellyn Publications, 1994.

Newton PE. The Effect of Sound on Plant Grwoth. *JAES.* 1971 Mar;19(3): 202-205.

Niculescu MD, Wu R, Guo Z, da Costa KA, Zeisel SH. Diethanolamine alters proliferation and choline metabolism in mouse neural precursor cells. *Toxicol Sci.* 2007 Apr;96(2):321-6.

Nievergelt CM, Kripke DF, Remick RA, Sadovnick AD, McElroy SL, Keck PE Jr, Kelsoe JR. Examination of the clock gene Cryptochrome 1 in bipolar disorder: mutational analysis and absence of evidence for linkage or association. *Psychiatr Genet.* 2005 Mar;15(1):45-52.

Niggli H. Temperature dependence of ultraweak photon emission in fibroblastic differentiation after irradiation with artificial sunlight. *Indian J Exp Biol.* 2003 May;41:419-423.

Nishigori C, Hattori Y, Toyokuni S. Role of reactive oxygen species in skin carcinogenesis. *Antioxid Redox Signal.* 2004 Jun;6(3):561-70.

Noone EJ, Roche HM, Nugent AP, Gibney MJ. The effect of dietary supplementation using isomeric blends of conjugated linoleic acid on lipid metabolism in healthy human subjects. *Br J Nutr.* 2002 Sep;88(3):243-51.

North J. *The Fontana History of Astronomy and Cosmology.* London: Fontana Press, 1994.

O'Dwyer JJ. *College Physics.* Pacific Grove, CA: Brooks/Cole, 1990.

O'Brien SJ, Shannon JE, Gail MH. A molecular approach to the identification and individualization of human and animal cells in culture: isozyme and allozyme genetic signatures. *In Vitro.* 1980 Feb;16(2):119-35.

O'Connell OF, Ryan L, O'Brien N. Xanthophyll carotenoids are more bioaccessible from fruits than dark green vegetables. *Nutr Res.* 2007;27(5):258-264.

O'Connor J., Bensky D. (ed). *Shanghai College of Traditional Chinese Medicine: Acupuncture: A Comprehensive Text.* Seattle: Eastland Press, 1981.

Oehme FW (ed.). *Toxicity of heavy metals in the environment. Part 1.* New York: M.Dekker, 1979.

Oh CK, Lücker PW, Wetzelsberger N, Kuhlmann F. The determination of magnesium, calcium, sodium and potassium in assorted foods with special attention to the loss of electrolytes after various forms of food preparations. *Mag.-Bull.* 1986;8:297-302.

Okamura H. Clock genes in cell clocks: roles, actions, and mysteries. *J Biol Rhythms.* 2004 Oct;19(5):388-99.

Okayama Y, Begishvili TB, Church MK. Comparison of mechanisms of IL-3 induced histamine release and IL-3 priming effect on human basophils. *Clin Exp Allergy.* 1993 Nov;23(11):901-10.

Ole D. Rughede, On the Theory and Physics of the Aether. *Progress in Physics.* 2006; (1).

O'Leary KD, Rosenbaum A, Hughes PC. Fluorescent lighting: a purported source of hyperactive behavior. *J Abnorm Child Psychol.* 1978 Sep;6(3):285-9.

Olney JW, Farber NB, Spitznagel E, Robins LN. Increasing brain tumor rates: is there a link to aspartame? *J Neuropathol Exp Neurol.* 1996;55:1115-23.

Olney JW. Excitotoxins in foods. *Neurotoxicology.* 1994;15:535-44.

Onder G, Landi F, Volpato S, Fellin R, Carbonin P, Gambassi G, Bernabei R. Serum cholesterol levels and in-hospital mortality in the elderly. *Am J Med.* 2003 Sept;115:265-71

One Hundred Million Americans See Medical Mistakes Directly Touching Them as Patients, Friends, Relatives. *National Patient Safety Foundation. Press Release.* 1997 Oct 9. http://npsf.org/pr/pressrel/finalsur.htm. Acc. 2007 Mar.

Oosterga M, ten Vaarwerk IA, DeJongste MJ, Staal MJ. Spinal cord stimulation in refractory angina pectoris—clinical results and mechanisms. *Z Kardiol.* 1997;86 Suppl 1:107-13.

Ostrander S, Schroeder L, Ostrander N. *Super-Learning.* New York: Delta, 1979.

Otani S. Memory trace in prefrontal cortex: theory for the cognitive switch. *Biol Rev Camb Philos Soc.* 2002 Nov;77(4):563-77.

Otsu A, Chinami M, Morgenthale S, Kaneko Y, Fujita D, Shirakawa T. Correlations for number of sunspots, unemployment rate, and suicide mortality in Japan. *Percept Mot Skills.* 2006 Apr;102(2):603-8.

Ott J. Color and Light: Their Effects on Plants, Animals, and People (Series of seven articles in seven issues). *Internl J Biosoc Res.* 1985-1991.

Ott J. *Health and Light: The Effects of Natural and Artificial Light on Man and Other Living Things.* Self published, 1973,

Otto SJ, van Houwelingen AC, Hornstra G. The effect of supplementation with docosahexaenoic and arachidonic acid derived from single cell oils on plasma and erythrocyte fatty acids of pregnant women in the second trimester. *Prost Leuk Essent Fatty Acids.* 2000 Nov;63(5):323-8.

Ou CC, Tsao SM, Lin MC, Yin MC. Protective action on human LDL against oxidation and glycation by four organosulfur compounds derived from garlic. *Lipids.* 2003 Mar;38(3):219-24.

Packard CC. *Pocket Guide to Ayurvedic Healing.* Freedom, CA: Crossing Press, 1996.

Park AE, Fernandez JJ, Schmedders K, Cohen MS. The Fibonacci sequence: relationship to the human hand. *J Hand Surg.* 2003 Jan;28(1):157-60.

Partonen T, Haukka J, Nevanlinna H, Lonnqvist J. Analysis of the seasonal pattern in suicide. *J Affect Disord.* 2004 Aug;81(2):133-9.

Pasricha S. Cases of the reincarnation type in northern India with birthmarks and birth defects. *J. Sci. Exploration.* 1998;12(2) 259-293.

Pasricha S. *Claims of reincarnation: An Empirical Study of Cases in India.* New Delhi: Harman, 1990.

Patwardhan B, Gautam M. Botanical immunodrugs: scope and opportunities. *Drug Discov Today.* 2005 Apr 1;10(7):495-502.

Physicians' Desk Reference. Montvale, NJ: Thomson, 2003.

Pehowich DJ, Gomes AV, Barnes JA. Fatty acid composition and possible health effects of coconut constituents. West Indian Med J. 2000 Jun;49(2):128-33.

Pendell D. *Plant Powers, Poisons, and Herbcraft.* San Francisco: Mercury House, 1995.

Penn RD, Hagins WA. Kinetics of the photocurrent of retinal rods. *Biophys J.* 1972 Aug;12(8):1073-94.

Penn RD, Hagins WA. Signal transmission along retinal rods and the origin of the electroretinographic a-wave. *Nature.* 1969 Jul 12;223(5202):201-4.

Penson RT, Kyriakou H, Zuckerman D, Chabner BA, Lynch TJ Jr. Teams: communication in multidisciplinary care. *Oncologist.* 2006 May;11(5):520-6.

Perez-Galvez A, Martin HD, Sies H, Stahl W. Incorporation of carotenoids from paprika oleoresin into human chylomicrons. *Br J Nutr.* 2003 Jun;89(6):787-93.

Perl DP, Moalem S. Aluminum and Alzheimer's disease, a personal perspective after 25 years. *J Alzheimers Dis.* 2006;9(3 Suppl):291-300.

Peroxisomes from pepper fruits (Capsicum annuum L.): purification, characterisation and antioxidant activity. *J Plant Physiol.* 2003 Dec;160(12):1507-16.

Perreau-Lenz S, Kalsbeek A, Van Der Vliet J, Pevet P, Buijs RM. In vivo evidence for a controlled offset of melatonin synthesis at dawn by the suprachiasmatic nucleus in the rat. *Neuroscience.* 2005;130(3):797-803.

Perry J. *A Dialogue on Personal Identity and Immortality.* Indianapolis, IN: Hackett, 1978.

Perry J. *Personal Identity.* Berkeley: University of California Press, 1975.

Persson R, Orbaek P, Kecklund G, Akerstedt T. Impact of an 84-hour workweek on biomarkers for stress, metabolic processes and diurnal rhythm. *Scand J Work Environ Health.* 2006 Oct;32(5):349-58.

Persinger M.A., Krippner S. Dream ESP experiments and geomagnetic activity. *Journal of the American Society of Psychical Research.* 1989;83:101-106.

Persinger M.A. Psi phenomena and temporal lobe activity: The geomagnetic factor. In L.A. Henkel & R.E. Berger (Eds.), *Research in parapsychology.* (121-156). Metuchen, NJ: Scarecrow Press, 1989.

Pert C. *Molecules of Emotion.* New York: Scribner, 1997.

Petiot JF, Sainte-Laudy J, Benveniste J. Interpretation of results on a human basophil degranulation test. *Ann Biol Clin (Paris).* 1981;39(6):355-9.

Phillips M, Cataneo RN, Cummin AR, Gagliardi AJ, Gleeson K, Greenberg J, Maxfield RA, Rom WN. Detection of lung cancer with volatile markers in the breath. *Chest.* 2003 Jun;123(6):2115-23.

Piggins HD. Human clock genes. *Ann Med.* 2002;34(5):394-400.

Piluso LG, Moffatt-Smith C. Disinfection using ultraviolet radiation as an antimicrobial agent: a review and synthesis of mechanisms and concerns. *PDA J Pharm Sci Technol.* 2006 Jan-Feb;60(1):1-16.

Piolino P, Desgranges B, Belliard S, Matuszewski V, Lalevee C, De la Sayette V, Eustache F. Autobiographical memory and autonoetic consciousness: triple dissociation in neurodegenerative diseases. *Brain.* 2003 Oct;126(Pt 10):2203-19.

Piper PW. Yeast superoxide dismutase mutants reveal a pro-oxidant action of weak organic acid food preservatives. *Free Radic Biol Med.* 1999 Dec;27(11-12):1219-27.

Pitt-Rivers R, Trotter WR. *The Thyroid Gland.* London: Butterworth Publisher, 1954.

Plaut T, Jones T. *Asthma Guide for People of All Ages.* Amherst MA: Pedipress, 1999.

Plotkin H. *Darwin Machines and the Nature of Knowledge: Concerning adaptations, instinct and the evolution of intelligence.* New York: Penguin, 1994.

Plotnikoff G, Quigley J. Prevalence of Severe Hypovitaminosis D in Patients With Persistent, Nonspecific Musculoskeletal Pain. *Mayo Clin Proc.* 2003;78:1463-1470.

Poitevin B, Davenas E, Benveniste J. In vitro immunological degranulation of human basophils is modulated by lung histamine and Apis mellifica. *Br J Clin Pharmacol.* 1988 Apr;25(4):439-44.

Polkinghorne J. *Science and Providence.* Boston: Shambhala Publications, 1989.

Pongratz W, Endler PC, Poitevin B, Kartnig T. Effect of extremely diluted plant hormone on cell culture, *Proc. 1995 AAAS Ann. Meeting,* Atlanta, 1995.

Pool R. Is there an EMF-Cancer connection? *Science.* 1990;249: 1096-1098.

Popp F Chang J. Mechanism of interaction between electromagnetic fields and living organisms. *Science in China.* 2000 Series C;43(5):507-518.

Popp F, Chang J, Herzog A, Yan Z, Yan Y. Evidence of non-classical (squeezed) light in biological systems. *Physics Lett.* 2002;293:98-102.

Popp F, Yan Y. Delayed luminescence of biological systems in terms of coherent states. *Phys.Lett.* 2000;293:91-97.

Popp F. Properties of biophotons and their theoretical implications. *Indian J Exper Biology.* 2003 May;41:391-402.

Popp F. Molecular Aspects of Carcinogenesis. In Deutsch E, Moser K, Rainer H, Stacher A (eds.). *Molecular Base of Malignancy.* Stuttgart: G.Thieme, 1976:47-55.

Popper KR, Eccles, JC. *The Self and Its Brain.* London: Routledge, 1983.

Postlethwait EM. Scavenger receptors clear the air. *J Clin Invest.* 2007 Mar;117(3):601-4.

Poulos LM, Toelle BG, Marks GB. The burden of asthma in children: an Australian perspective. *Paediatr Respir Rev.* 2005 Mar;6(1):20-7.

Prescott J. Alienation of Affection. *Psych Today.* 1979 Dec.

Prescott J. The Origins of Human Love and Violence. *Pre- and Perinatal Psych J. 1*996;10(3):143-188.

Pribram K. *Brain and perception: holonomy and structure in figural processing.* Hillsdale, N. J.: Lawrence Erlbaum Assoc., 1991.

Pronina TS. Circadian and infradian rhythms of testosterone and aldosterone excretion in children. *Probl Endokrinol.* 1992 Sep-Oct;38(5):38-42.

Protheroe WM, Captiotti ER, Newsom GH. *Exploring the Universe.* Columbus, OH: Merrill, 1989,

Provalova NV, Suslov NI, Skurikhin EG, Dygaï AM. Local mechanisms of the regulatory action of Scutellaria baicalensis and ginseng extracts on the erythropoiesis after paradoxical sleep deprivation. *Eksp Klin Farmakol.* 2006 Sep-Oct;69(5):31-5.

Puthoff H, Targ R, May E. Experimental Psi Research: Implication for Physics. AAAS Proceedings of the 1979 Symposium on the Role of Consciousness in the Physical World. 1981.

Puthoff H, Targ R. A Perceptual Channel for Information Transfer Over Kilometer distances: Historical Perspective and Recent Research. Proc. *IEEE.* 1976;64(3):329-254.

Radin D. *The Conscious Universe.* San Francisco: HarperEdge, 1997.

Rahman K. Garlic and aging: new insights into an old remedy. *Ageing Res Rev.* 2003 Jan;2(1):39-56.

Raiten DJ, Talbot JM, Fisher KD, eds. Life Sciences Research Office Report. Executive summary from the report. Analysis of adverse reactions to monosodium glutamate (MSG). *J Nutr.* 1995;125 (suppl).:2892-906.

INDEX

Rodale R. *Our Next Frontier.* Emmaus, PA: Rodale, 1981.

Rodermel SR, Smith-Sonneborn J. Age-correlated changes in expression of micronuclear damage and repair in Paramecium tetraurelia. *Genetics.* 1977 Oct;87(2):259-74.

Rodgers JT, Puigserver P. Fasting-dependent glucose and lipid metabolic response through hepatic sirtuin 1. *Proc Natl Acad Sci USA.* 2007 Jul 31;104(31):12861-6.

Rosenfeldt V, Benfeldt E, Nielsen SD, Michaelsen KF, Jeppesen DL, Valerius NH, Paerregaard A. Effect of probiotic Lactobacillus strains in children with atopic dermatitis. *J Allergy Clin Immunol.* 2003 Feb;111(2):389-95.

Rosenlund M, Picciotto S, Forastiere F, Stafoggia M, Perucci CA. Traffic-related air pollution in relation to incidence and prognosis of coronary heart disease. *Epidemiology.* 2008 Jan;19(1):121-8.

Rosenthal N, Blehar M (Eds.). *Seasonal affective disorders and phototherapy.* New York: Guildford Press, 1989.

Rossouw JE, Prentice RL, Manson JE, Wu L, Barad D, Barnabei VM, Ko M, LaCroix AZ, Margolis KL, Stefanick ML. Postmenopausal hormone therapy and risk of cardiovascular disease by age and years since menopause. *JAMA.* 2007 Apr 4;297(13):1465-77.

Routasalo P, Isola A. The right to touch and be touched. *Nurs Ethics.* 1996 Jun;3(2):165-76.

Rowland AS, Baird DD, Long S, Wegienka G, Harlow SD, Alavanja M, Sandler DP. Influence of medical conditions and lifestyle factors on the menstrual cycle. *Epidemiology.* 2002 Nov;13(6):668-74.

Roy M, Kirschbaum C, Steptoe A. Intraindividual variation in recent stress exposure as a moderator of cortisol and testosterone levels. Ann Behav Med. 2003 Dec;26(3):194-200.

Roybal K, Theobold D, Graham A, DiNieri JA, Russo SJ, Krishnan V, Chakravarty S, Peevey J, Oehrlein N, Birnbaum S, Vitaterna MH, Orsulak P, Takahashi JS, Nestler EJ, Carlezon WA Jr, McClung CA. Mania-like behavior induced by disruption of CLOCK. *Proc Natl Acad Sci USA.* 2007 Apr 10;104(15):6406-11.

Rubenowitz E, Molin I, Axelsson G, Rylander R. (2000) Magnesium in drinking water in relation to morbidity and mortality from acute myocardial infarction. *Epidemiology.* 2000;11:416-421.

Rubin E and Farber J. *Pathology 3rd Edition.* Lippincott-Raven, Philadelphia, PA, 1999.

Russ MJ, Clark WC, Cross LW, Kemperman I, Kakuma T, Harrison K. Pain and self-injury in borderline patients: sensory decision theory, coping strategies, and locus of control. *Psychiatry Res.* 1996 Jun 26;63(1):57-65.

Russek LG, Schwartz GE. Narrative descriptions of parental love and caring predict health status in midlife: a 35-year follow-up of the Harvard Mastery of Stress Study. *Altern Ther Health Med.* 1996 Nov;2(6):55-62.

Russell IJ. Advances in fibromyalgia: possible role for central neurochemicals. *Am J Med Sci.* 1998;315:377-84.

Russell RM, Golner BB, Krasinski SD, Sadowski JA, Suter PM, Braun CL. Effect of antacid and H2 receptor antagonists on the intestinal absorption of folic acid. *J Lab Clin Med.* 1988;112:458-63.

Russo PA, Halliday GM. Inhibition of nitric oxide and reactive oxygen species production improves the ability of a sunscreen to protect from sunburn, immunosuppression and photocarcinogenesis. *Br J Dermatol.* 2006 Aug;155(2):408-15.

Saarijarvi S, Lauerma H, Helenius H, Saarilehto S. Seasonal affective disorders among rural Finns and Lapps. *Acta Psychiatr Scand.* 1999 Feb;99(2):95-101.

Sabom M. *Light and Death: One Doctor's Fascinating Account of Near Death Experiences.* Grand Rapids, MI: Zondervan Publishing, 1998.

INDEX

Sabom M. *Recollections of Death: A Medical Investigation.* New York: Harper and Row, 1982.

Sacks O. *The Man Who Mistook his Wife for a Hat and Other Clinical Tales.* New York: Simon & Schuster, 1998.

Sahlin C, Pettersson FE, Nilsson LN, Lannfelt L, Johansson AS. Docosahexaenoic acid stimulates non-amyloidogenic APP processing resulting in reduced Abeta levels in cellular models of Alzheimer's disease. *Eur J Neurosci.* 2007 Aug;26(4):882-9.

Sainte-Laudy J, Belon P. Analysis of immunosuppressive activity of serial dilutions of histamine on human basophil activation by flow cytometry. *Inflam Rsrch.* 1996 Suppl. 1: S33-S34.

Sakugawa H, Cape JN. Harmful effects of atmospheric nitrous acid on the physiological status of

Salem N, Wegher B, Mena P, Uauy R. Arachidonic and docosahexaenoic acids are biosynthesized from their 18-carbon precursors in human infants. *Proc Natl Acad Sci.* 1996;93:49-54.

Salom IL, Silvis SE, Doscherholmen A. Effect of cimetidine on the absorption of vitamin B12. *Scand J Gastroenterol.* 1982;17:129-31.

Sanders R. Slow brain waves play key role in coordinating complex activity. *UC Berkeley News.* 2006 Sep 14.

Sarah Janssen S, Solomon G, Schettler T. Chemical Contaminants and Human Disease:A Summary of Evidence. *The Collaborative on Health and the Environment.* 2006. http://www.healthandenvironment.org. Acc. 2007 Jul.

Saran, S., Gopalan, S. and Krishna, T. P. Use of fermented foods to combat stunting and failure to thrive. *Nutrition.* 2002;8:393-396.

Sarveiya V, Risk S, Benson HA. Liquid chromatographic assay for common sunscreen agents: application to in vivo assessment of skin penetration and systemic absorption in human volunteers. *J Chromatogr B Analyt Technol Biomed Life Sci.* 2004 Apr 25;803(2):225-31.

Sato TK, Yamada RG, Ukai H, Baggs JE, Miraglia LJ, Kobayashi TJ, Welsh DK, Kay SA, Ueda HR, Hogenesch JB. Feedback repression is required for mammalian circadian clock function. *Nat Genet.* 2006 Mar;38(3):312-9.

Satyanarayana S, Sushruta K, Sarma GS, Srinivas N, Subba Raju GV. Antioxidant activity of the aqueous extracts of spicy food additives-evaluation and comparison with ascorbic acid in in-vitro systems. *J Herb Pharmacother.* 2004;4(2):1-10.

Sauvant M, Pepin D. Drinking water and cardiovascular disease. *Food Chem Toxicol.* 2002;40:1311-1325.

Schenk BE, Festen HP, Kuipers EJ, Klinkenberg-Knol EC, Meuwissen SG. Effect of short-and long-term treatment with omeprazole on the absorption and serum levels of cobalamin. *Aliment Pharmacol Ther.* 1996;10:541-5.

Schirber M. Earth as a Giant Pinball Machine. *LiveScience.* 2004; 19 Nov 19. http://www.livescience.com/ environment/041119_earth_layers.html. Acc. 2006 Nov.

Schlebusch KP, Maric-Oehler W, Popp FA. Biophotonics in the infrared spectral range reveal acupuncture meridian structure of the body. *J Altern Complement Med.* 2005 Feb;11(1):171-3.

Schlumpf M, Cotton B, Conscience M, Haller V, Steinmann B, Lichtensteiger W. In vitro and in vivo estrogenicity of UV screens. *Environ Health Perspect.* 2001 Mar;109(3):239-44.

Schmidt H, Quantum processes predicted? *New Sci.* 1969 Oct 16.

Schmitt B, Frölich L. Creative therapy options for patients with dementia—a systematic review. *Fortschr Neurol Psychiatr.* 2007 Dec;75(12):699-707.

Schonberger B. Bladder dysfunction and surgery in the small pelvis. Therapeutic possibilities. *Urologe A.* 2003 Dec;42(12):1569-75.

Schulz T, Zarse K, Voigt A, Urban N, Birringer M, Ristow M. Glucose Restriction Extends Caenorhabditis elegans Life Span by Inducing Mitochondrial Respiration and Increasing Oxidative Stress. *Cell Metabolism.* 2007 Oct 3;6:280-293.

Schumacher P. *Biophysical Therapy Of Allergies.* Stuttgart: Thieme, 2005.

Schwartz GG, Skinner HG. Vitamin D status and cancer: new insights. *Curr Opin Clin Nutr Metab Care.* 2007 Jan;10(1):6-11.

Schwartz S, De Mattei R, Brame E, Spottiswoode S. Infrared spectra alteration in water proximate to the palms of therapeutic practitioners. In: Wiener D, Nelson R (Eds.): *Research in parapsychology 1986.* Metuchen, NJ: Scarecrow Press, 1987:24-29.

Schwellenbach LJ, Olson KL. McConnell KJ, Stolepart RS, Nash JD, Merenich JA. The triglyceride-lowering effects of a modest dose of docosahexaenoic acid alone versus in combination with low dose eicosapentaenoic acid in patients with coronary artery disease and elevated triglycerides. *J Am Coll Nutr.* 2006;25(6):480-485.

Scoville WB, Milner B. Loss of recent memory after bilateral hippocampal lesions. *J Neurol Neurosurg Psychiatry.* 1957;20:11-21.

Semenza C. Retrieval pathways for common and proper names. *Cortex.* 2006 Aug;42(6):884-91.

Senekowitsch F, Endler PC, Pongratz W, Smith CW. Hormone effects by CD record /replay. *FASEB J.* 1995:A12025.

Senior F. Fallout. *New York Mag.* 2003 Fall.

Seo K, Jung S, Park M, Song Y, Choung S. Effects of leucocyanidines on activities of metabolizing enzymes and antioxidant enzymes. *Biol Pharm Bull.* 2001 May;24(5):592-3.

Serra-Valls A. Electromagnetic Industrion and the Conservation of Momentum in the Spiral Paradox. *Cornell University Library.* http://arxiv.org/ftp/physics/papers/0012/0012009.pdf. Acc. 2007 Jul.

Serway R. *Physicis For Scientists & Engineers.* Philadelphia: Harcourt Brace, 1992.

Shaffer D. *Developmental Psychology: Theory, Research and Applications.* Monterey, CA: Brooks/Cole, 1985.

Shafik A. Role of warm-water bath in anorectal conditions. The "thermosphincteric reflex". *J Clin Gastroenterol.* 1993 Jun;16(4):304-8.

Shankar R. *My Music, My Life.* New York: Simon & Schuster, 1968.

Sharp KC. *After the Light.* New York: William Morrow & Co., 1995.

Shearman LP, Zylka MJ, Weaver DR, Kolakowski LF Jr, Reppert SM. Two period homologs: circadian expression and photic regulation in the suprachiasmatic nuclei. *Neuron.* 1997 Dec;19(6):1261-9.

Shen YF, Goddard G. The short-term effects of acupuncture on myofascial pain patients after clenching. *Pain Pract.* 2007 Sep;7(3):256-64.

Shevelev IA, Kostelianetz NB, Kamenkovich VM, Sharaev GA. EEG alpha-wave in the visual cortex: check of the hypothesis of the scanning process. *Int J Psychophysiol.* 1991 Aug;11(2):195-201.

Shupak NM, Prato FS, Thomas AW. Human exposure to a specific pulsed magnetic field: effects on thermal sensory and pain thresholds. *Neurosci Lett.* 2004 Jun 10;363(2):157-62.

Shutov AA, Panasiuk IIa. Efficacy of rehabilitation of patients with chronic primary low back pain at the spa Klyuchi using balneopelotherapy and transcranial electrostimulation. *Vopr Kurortol Fizioter Lech Fiz Kult.* 2007 Mar-Apr;(2):16-8.

Sicher F, Targ E, Moore D, Smith H. A Randomized Double-Blind Study of the Effect of Distant Healing in a Population With Advanced AIDS. Western Journal of Medicine. 1998;169 Dec::356-363.

INDEX

Siegfried J. Electrostimulation and neurosurgical measures in cancer pain. *Recent Results Cancer Res.* 1988;108:28-32.

Simpson G. *The Major Features of Evolution.* New York: Columbia Univ Press, 1953.

Sin DD, Man J, Sharpe H, Gan WQ, Man SF. Pharmacological management to reduce exacerbations in adults with asthma: a systematic review and meta-analysis. *JAMA.* 2004 Jul 21;292(3):367-76.

Skoczylas A, Wiecek A. Ghrelin, a new hormone involved not only in the regulation of appetite. *Wiad Lek.* 2006;59(9-10):697-701.

Skwerer RG, Jacobsen FM, Duncan CC, Kelly KA, Sack DA, Tamarkin L, Gaist PA, Kasper S, Rosenthal NE. Neurobiology of Seasonal Affective Disorder and Phototherapy. *J Biolog Rhyth.* 1988;3(2):135-154.

Sloan F and Gelband (ed). Cancer Control Opportunities in Low- and Middle-Income Countries. Committee on Cancer Control in Low- and Middle-Income Countries. 2007.

Smith CW. Coherence in living biological systems. *Neural Network World.* 1994:4(3):379-388.

Smith MJ. "Effect of Magnetic Fields on Enzyme Reactivity" in Barnothy M.(ed.), *Biological Effects of Magnetic Fields.* New York: Plenum Press, 1969.

Smith MJ. *The Influence on Enzyme Growth By the 'Laying on of Hands: Dimensions of Healing.* Los Altos, California: Academy of Parapsychology and Medicine, 1973.

Smith T. *Homeopathic Medicine: A Doctor's Guide.* Rochester, VT: Healing Arts, 1989.

Smith-Sonneborn J. Age-correlated effects of caffeine on non-irradiated and UV-irradiated Paramecium Aurelia. *J Gerontol.* 1974 May;29(3):256-60.

Smith-Sonneborn J. DNA repair and longevity assurance in Paramecium tetraurelia. *Science.* 1979 Mar 16;203(4385):1115-7.

Snyder K. Researchers Produce Firsts with Bursts of Light: Team generates most energetic terahertz pulses yet, observes useful optical phenomena. *Press Release: Brookhaven National Laboratory.* 2007 July 24.

Soler M, Chandra S, Ruiz D, Davidson E, Hendrickson D, Christou G. A third isolated oxidation state for the Mn12 family of singl molecule magnets. *ChemComm;* 2000; Nov 22.

Soni MG, Carabin IG, Burdock GA. Safety assessment of esters of p-hydroxybenzoic acid (parabens). *Food Chem Toxicol.* 2005 Jul;43(7):985-1015.

Soul Has Weight, Physician Thinks. *The New York Times.* 1907 March 11:5.

Southgate, D. Nature and variability of human food consumption. *Philosophical Transactions of the Royal Society of London.* 1991;B(334): 281-288.

Spanagel R, Rosenwasser AM, Schumann G, Sarkar DK. Alcohol consumption and the body's biological clock. *Alcohol Clin Exp Res.* 2005 Aug;29(8):1550-7.

Speed Of Light May Not Be Constant, Physicist Suggests. *Science Daily.* 1999 Oct 6. www.sciencedaily.com/releases/1999/10/991005114024.htm. Acc. 2007 Jun.

Spence A. *Basic Human Anatomy.* Menlo Park, CA: Benjamin/Commings, 1986.

Spetner L. *Not By Chance! -Shattering The Modern Theory of Evolution.* New York: The Judaica Press, 1997.

Spillane M. Good Vibrations, A Sound 'Diet' for Plants. *The Growing Edge.* 1991 Spring.

Spiller G. *The Super Pyramid.* New York: HRS Press, 1993.

Squire LR, Zola-Morgan S. The medial temporal lobe memory system. *Science.* 1991;253(5026):1380-1386.

St Hilaire MA, Klerman EB, Khalsa SB, Wright KP Jr, Czeisler CA, Kronauer RE. Addition of a non-photic component to a light-based mathematical model of the human circadian pacemaker. *J Theor Biol.* 2007 Aug 21;247(4):583-99.

Stachowska E, Dolegowska B, Chlubek D, Wesolowska T, Ciechanowski K, Gutowski P, Szumilowicz H, Turowski R. Dietary trans fatty acids and composition of human atheromatous plaques. *Eur J Nutr.* 2004 Oct;43(5):313-8.

Stahler C. 1994. How many vegetarians are there?" *Veget Jnl.* 1994: July/August.

Stamets P. *Mycelium Running.* Berkeley, CA: Ten Speed Press, 2005.

Stampfer MJ, Willett WC, Colditz GA, Rosner B, Speizer FE, Hennekens CH. A prospective study of postmenopausal estrogen therapy and coronary heart disease. *N Engl J Med.* 1985 Oct 24;313(17):1044-9.

Stanford, C. B. The hunting ecology of wild chimpanzees: Implications for the evolutionary ecology of Pliocene hominids. *American Anthropologist.* 1996;98: 96-113.

Steck B. Effects of optical radiation on man. *Light Resch Techn.* 1982;14:130-141.

Steiner R. *Agriculture.* Kimberton, PA: Bio-Dynamic Farming, 1924-1993.

Stevenson I, Samararatne G. Three new cases of the reincarnation type in Sri Lanka with written records made before verification. *J. Sci. Exploration.* 1988;2(2): 217-238.

Stevenson I. American children who claim to remember previous lives. *J. Nervous and Mental Disease.* 1983;171:742-748.

Stevenson I. *Cases of the Reincarnation Type.* Charlottesville, VA: Univ Virginia Press. Vol. 1: *Ten Cases in India,* 1975. Vol. 2: *Ten Cases in Sri Lanka,* 1977. Vol. 3: *Twelve Cases in Lebanon and Turkey,* 1980. Vol. 4: *Twelve Cases in Thailand and Burma,* 1983.

Stevenson I. *Children Who Remember Previous Lives: A Question of Reincarnation.* Charlottesville, VA: Univ Virginia Press, 1987.

Stevenson I. *European Cases of the Reincarnation Type.* Jefferson, NC: McFarland and Co., 2003.

Stevenson I. *Reincarnation and Biology: A Contribution to the Etiology of Birthmarks and Birth Defects.* (2 volumes). Westport, CN: Praeger Publishers, 1997.

Stevenson I. *Twenty Cases Suggestive of Reincarnation.* New York: American Society for Psychical Research, 1967.

Stevenson I. *Where Reincarnation and Biology Intersect.* Westport, CN: Praeger, 1997.

Stojanovic MP, Abdi S. Spinal cord stimulation. *Pain Physician.* 2002 Apr;5(2):156-66.

Stoupel E, Babyev E, Mustafa F, Abramson E, Israelevich P, Sulkes J. Acute myocardial infarction occurrence: Environmental links - Baku 2003-2005 data. *Med Sci Monit.* 2007 Aug;13(8):BR175-179.

Stoupel E, Kalediene R, Petrauskiene J, Gaizauskiene A, Israelevich P, Abramson E, Sulkes J. Monthly number of newborns and environmental physical activity. *Medicina Kaunas.* 2006;42(3):238-41.

Stoupel E, Monselise Y, Lahav J. Changes in autoimmune markers of the anti-cardiolipin syndrome on days of extreme geomamagnetic activity. *J Basic Clin Physiol Pharmacol.* 2006;17(4):269-78.

Stoupel EG, Frimer H, Appelman Z, Ben-Neriah Z, Dar H, Fejgin MD, Gershoni-Baruch R, Manor E, Barkai G, Shalev S, Gelman-Kohan Z, Reish O, Lev D, Davidov B, Goldman B, Shohat M. Chromosome aberration and environmental physical activity: Down syndrome and solar and cosmic ray activity, Israel, 1990-2000. *Int J Biometeorol.* 2005 Sep;50(1):1-5.

Strange BA, Dolan RJ. Anterior medial temporal lobe in human cognition: memory for fear and the unexpected. *Cognit Neuropsychiatry.* 2006 May;11(3):198-218.

INDEX

Streitberger K, Ezzo J, Schneider A. Acupuncture for nausea and vomiting: an update of clinical and experimental studies. *Auton Neurosci.* 2006 Oct 30;129(1-2):107-17.

Sulman FG, Levy D, Lunkan L, Pfeifer Y, Tal E. New methods in the treatment of weather sensitivity. *Fortschr Med.* 1977 Mar 17;95(11):746-52.

Sulman FG. Migraine and headache due to weather and allied causes and its specific treatment. *Ups J Med Sci Suppl.* 1980;31:41-4.

Suppes P, Han B, Epelboim J, Lu ZL. Invariance of brain-wave representations of simple visual images and their names. *Proc Natl Acad Sci Psych-BS.* 1999;96(25):14658-14663.

Suzuki Y, Kondo K, Ichise H, Tsukamoto Y, Urano T, Umemura K. Dietary supplementation with fermented soybeans suppresses intimal thickening. *Nutrition.* 2003 Mar;19(3):261-4.

Szyf M, McGowan P, Meaney MJ. The social environment and the epigenome. *Environ Mol Mutagen.* 2008 Jan;49(1):46-60.

Tan DX, Manchester LC, Reiter RJ, Qi WB, Karbownik M, Calvo JR. Significance of melatonin in antioxidative defense system: reactions and products. *Biol Signals Recept.* 2000 May-Aug;9(3-4):137-59.

Tanagho EA. Principles and indications of electrostimulation of the urinary bladder. *Urologe A.* 1990 Jul;29(4):185-90.

Tang G, Serfaty-Lacronsniere C, Camilo ME, Russell RM. Gastric acidity influences the blood response to a beta-carotene dose in humans. *Am J Clin Nutr.* 1996;64:622-6.

Taoka S, Padmakumar R, Grissom C, Banerjee R. Magnetic Field Effects on Coenzyme B-12 Dependent Enzymes: Validation of Ethanolamine Ammonia Lyase Results and Extension to Human Methylmalonyl CoA Mutase. *Bioelectromagnetics.* 1997;18: 506-513.

Tapiero H, Ba GN, Couvreur P, Tew KD. Polyunsaturated fatty acids (PUFA) and eicosanoids in human health and pathologies. *Biomed Pharmacother.* 2002 Jul;56(5):215-22.

Tapsell LC, Hemphill I, Cobiac L, Patch CS, Sullivan DR, Fenech M, Roodenrys S, Keogh JB, Clifton PM, Williams PG, Fazio VA, Inge KE. Health benefits of herbs and spices: the past, the present, the future. *Med J Aust.* 2006 Aug 21;185(4 Suppl):S4-24.

Taraban M, Leshina T, Anderson M, Grissom C. Magnetic Field Dependence and the Role of electron spin in Heme Enzymes: Horseradish Peroxidase. *J. Am. Chem. Soc.* 1997;119: 5768-5769.

Targ R, Katra J, Brown D, Wiegand W. Viewing the future: A pilot study with an error-detecting protocol. *J Sci Expl.* 9:3:367-380, 1995.

Targ R, Puthoff H. Information transfer under conditions of sensory shielding. *Nature.* 1975;251:602-607.

Tassone F, Broglio F, Gianotti L, Arvat E, Ghigo E, Maccario M. Ghrelin and other gastrointestinal peptides involved in the control of food intake. *Mini Rev Med Chem.* 2007 Jan;7(1):47-53.

Tauchert M. Efficacy and safety of crataegus extract WS 1442 in comparison with placebo in patients with chronic stable New York Heart Association class-III heart failure. *Am Heart J.* 2002 May;143(5):910-5.

Taussig SJ, Batkin S. Bromelain, the enzyme complex of pineapple (Ananas comosus) and its clinical application. An update. *J Ethnopharmacol.* 1988 Feb-Mar;22(2):191-203.

Taylor A. *Soul Traveler: A Guide to Out-of-Body Experiences and the Wonders Beyond.* New York: Penguin, 2000.

Teitelbaum J. *From Fatigue to Fantastic.* New York: Avery, 2001.

Termanini B, Gibril F, Sutliff VE, Yu F, Venzon DJ, Jensen RT. Effect of long-term gastric acid suppressive therapy on serum vitamin B12 levels in patients with Zollinger-Ellison syndrome. *Am J*

Med. 1998 May;104(5):422-30.

Tevini M, ed. *UV-B Radiation and Ozone Depletion: Effects on humans, animals, plants, microorganisms and materials.* Boca Raton: Lewis Pub, 1993.

Thakur CP, Sharma D. Full moon and crime. *Br Med J.* 1984 December 22; 289(6460): 1789-1791.

Thaut MH. The future of music in therapy and medicine. *Ann N Y Acad Sci.* 2005 Dec;1060:303-8.

The Mystery of Smell. Howard Hughes Medical Instit. http://www.hhmi.org/senses/d110.html. Acc. 2007 Jul.

The Timechart Company. *Timetables of Medicine.* New York: Black Dog & Leventhal, 2000.

Thie J. *Touch for Health.* Marina del Rey, CA: Devorss Publications, 1973-1994.

Thomas MK, Lloyd-Jones DM, Thadhani RI, Shaw AC, Deraska DJ, Kitch BT, Vamvakas EC, Dick IM, Prince RL, Finkelstein JS. Hypovitaminosis D in medical inpatients. *N Engl J Med.* 1998 Mar 19;338(12):777-83

Thomas Y, Litime H, Benveniste J. Modulation of human neutrophil activation by "electronic" phorbol myristate acetate (PMA). *FASEB Jnl.* 1996;10: A1479.

Thomas Y, Schiff M, Belkadi L, Jurgens P, Kahhak L, Benveniste J. Activation of human neutrophils by electronically transmitted phorbol-myristate acetate. *Med Hypoth.* 2000;54: 33-39.

Thomas Y, Schiff M, Litime M, Belkadi L, Benveniste J. Direct transmission to cells of a molecular signal (phorbol myristate acetate, PMA) via an electronic device. *FASEB Jnl.* 1995;9: A227.

Thomas-Anterion C, Jacquin K, Laurent B. Differential mechanisms of impairment of remote memory in Alzheimer's and frontotemporal dementia. *Dement Geriatr Cogn Disord.* 2000 Mar-Apr;11(2):100-6.

Thompson D. *On Growth and Form.* Cambridge: Cambridge University Press, 1992.

Thorogood M, Mann J, Appleby P, McPherson K. Risk of death from cancer and ischaemic heart disease in meat and non-meat eaters. *BMJ.* 1994 June 25;308:1667-1670.

Threlkeld DS, ed. Central Nervous System Drugs, Analeptics, Caffeine. *Facts and Comparisons Drug Information.* St. Louis, MO: Facts and Comparisons. 1998 Feb: 230-d.

Threlkeld DS, ed. Gastrointestinal Drugs, Proton Pump Inhibitors. *Facts and Comparisons Drug Information.* St. Louis, MO: Facts and Comparisons. 1998 Apr: 305r.

Tian FS, Zhang HR, Li WD, Qiao P, Duan HB, Jia CX. Study on acupuncture treatment of diabetic neurogenic bladder. *Zhongguo Zhen Jiu.* 2007 Jul;27(7):485-7.

Tierra L. *The Herbs of Life.* Freedom, CA: Crossing Press, 1992.

Tierra M. *The Way of Herbs.* New York: Pocket Books, 1990.

Timofeev I, Steriade M. Low-frequency rhythms in the thalamus of intact-cortex and decorticated cats. *J Neurophysiol.* 1996 Dec;76(6):4152-68.

Ting W, Schultz K, Cac NN, Peterson M, Walling HW. Tanning bed exposure increases the risk of malignant melanoma. Int J Dermatol. 2007 Dec;46(12):1253-7.

Tisserand R. *The Art of Aromatherapy.* New York: Inner Traditions, 1979.

Tiwari M. *Ayurveda: A Life of Balance.* Rochester, VT: Healing Arts, 1995.

Todd GR, Acerini CL, Ross-Russell R, Zahra S, Warner JT, McCance D. Survey of adrenal crisis associated with inhaled corticosteroids in the United Kingdom. *Arch Dis Child.* 2002 Dec;87(6):457-61.

Tompkins, P, Bird C. *The Secret Life of Plants.* New York: Harper & Row, 1973.

Toomer G. "Ptolemy". *The Dictionary of Scientific Biography*. New York: Gale Cengage, 1970.

Triglia A, La Malfa G, Musumeci F, Leonardi C, Scordino A. Delayed luminsecence as an indicator of tomato fruit quality. *J Food Sci*. 1998;63:512-515.

Trivedi B. Magnetic Map" Found to Guide Animal Migration. *Natl Geogr Today*. 2001 Oct 12.

Tsinkalovsky O, Smaaland R, Rosenlund B, Sothern RB, Hirt A, Steine S, Badiee A, Abrahamsen JF, Eiken HG, Laerum OD. Circadian variations in clock gene expression of human bone marrow CD34+ cells. *J Biol Rhythms*. 2007 Apr;22(2):140-50.

Tsong T. Deciphering the language of cells. *Trends in Biochem Sci*. 1989;14: 89-92.

Tsuei JJ, Lam Jr. F, Zhao Z. Studies in Bioenergetic Correlations-Bioenergetic Regulatory Measurement Instruments and Devices. *Am J Acupunct*. 1988;16:345-9.

Tsuei JJ, Lehman CW, Lam F, Jr, Zhu D. A food allergy study utilizing the EAV acupuncture technique. *Am J Acupunct*. 1984;12:105-16.

Tubek S. Role of trace elements in primary arterial hypertension: is mineral water style or prophylaxis? *Biol Trace Elem Res*. 2006 Winter;114(1-3):1-5.

Tucker J. *Life Before Life: A Scientific Investigation of Children's Memories of Previous Lives*. New York: St. Martin's Press, 2005.

Tweed K. Study: Conceiving in Summer Lowers Baby's Future Test Scores. *Fox News*. 2007 May 9, 2007. (Study done by: Winchester P. 2007. Pediatric Academic Societies annual meeting.)

Udermann H, Fischer G. Studies on the influence of positive or negative small ions on the catechol amine content in the brain of the mouse following shorttime or prolonged exposure. *Zentralbl Bakteriol Mikrobiol Hyg*. 1982 Apr;176(1):72-8.

Ulett G. Electroacupuncture: mechanisms and clinical application. *Biological Psychiatry*. 1998;44(2):129-138.

Ullman D. Controlled clinical trials evaluating the homeopathic treatment of people with human immunodeficiency virus or acquired immune deficiency syndrome *J Altern Complement Med*. 2003 Feb;9(1):133-41.

Ullman D. *Discovering Homeopathy*. Berkeley, CA: North Atlantic, 1991.

Unger RH. Leptin physiology: a second look. *Regul Pept*. 2000 Aug 25;92(1-3):87-95.

Vallance A. Can biological activity be maintained at ultra-high dilution? An overview of homeopathy, evidence, and Bayesian philosophy. *J Altern Complement Med*. 1998 Spring;4(1):49-76.

Van Cauter E, Leproult R, Plat L. Age-related changes in slow wave sleep and REM sleep and relationship with growth hormone and cortisol levels in healthy men. *JAMA*. 2000 Aug 16;284(7):861-8.

van den Berg H, Dagnelie P, van Staveren W. Vitamin B12 and seaweed. *Lancet*. 1988;1:242-3.

van den Eeden SK, Koepsell TD, Longstreth WT, van Belle G, Daling JR, McKnight B. Aspartame ingestion and headache: a randomized crossover trial. *Neurology*. 1994;44:1787-93.

Van Wijk R, Wiegant FAC. *Cultured mammalian cells in homeopathy research: the similia principle in self-recovery*. Utrecht: University Utrecht Publ, 1994.

Vandenbroucke JP. Should you eat meat, or are you confounded by methodological debate? *BMJ*. 1994 Jun 25;308(6945):1671.

Vaquero JM, Gallego MC. Sunspot numbers can detect pandemic influenza A: the use of different sunspot numbers. *Med Hypotheses*. 2007;68(5):1189-90.

Vargha-Khadem F, Polkey CE. A review of cognitive outcome after hemidecortication in humans. *Adv*

Exp Med Biol. 1992;325:137-51.

Vauthier JM, Lluch A, Lecomte E, Artur Y, Herbeth B. Family resemblance in energy and macronutrient intakes: the Stanislas Family Study. *Int J Epidemiol.* 1996 Oct;25(5):1030-7.

Vescelius E. *Music and Health.* New York: Goodyear Book Shop, 1918.

Vickers A. Botanical medicines for the treatment of cancer: rationale, overview of current data, and methodological considerations for phase I and II trials. *Cancer Invest.* 2002;20(7-8):1069-79.

Vickers AJ, Kuo J, Cassileth BR. Unconventional anticancer agents: a systematic review of clinical trials. *J Clin Oncol.* 2006 Jan 1;24(1):136-40.

Vidgren HM, Agren JJ, Schwab U, Rissanen T, Hanninen O, Uusitupa MI. Incorporation of n-3 fatty acids into plasma lipid fractions, and erythrocyte membranes and platelets during dietary supplementation with fish, fish oil, and docosahexaenoic acid-rich oil among healthy young men. *Lipids.* 1997 Jul;32(7):697-705.

Vierling-Claassen D, Siekmeier P, Stufflebeam S, Kopell N. Modeling GABA alterations in schizophrenia: a link between impaired inhibition and altered gamma and beta range auditory entrainment. *J Neurophysiol.* 2008 May;99(5):2656-71.

Vigny P, Duquesne M. *On the fluorescence properties of nucleotides and polynucleotides at room temperature.* In. Birks J (ed.). Excited states of biological molecules. London-NY: J Wiley, 1976:167-177.

Volkmann H, Dannberg G, Kuhnert H, Heinke M. Therapeutic value of trans-esophageal electrostimulation in tachycardic arrhythmias. *Z Kardiol.* 1991 Jun;80(6):382-8.

Voll R. The phenomenon of medicine testing in elecroacupuncture according to Voll. *Am J Acupunct.* 1980;8:97-104.

Voll R. Twenty years of electroacupuncture diagnosis in Germany: a progressive report. *Am J Acupunct.* 1975;3:7-17.

von Schantz M, Archer SN. *Clocks, genes and sleep. J R Soc Med.* 2003 Oct;96(10):486-9.

Vyasadeva S. *Srimad Bhagavatam.* Approx rec 4000 BCE.

Wachiuli M, Koyama M, Utsuyama M, Bittman BB, Kitagawa M, Hirokawa K. Recreational music-making modulates natural killer cell activity, cytokines, and mood states in corporate employees. *Med Sci Monit.* 2007 Feb;13(2):CR57-70.

Wade N. From Ants to Ethics: A Biologist Dreams of Unity of Knowledge. Scientist at Work, Edward O. Wilson. *New York Times.* 1998 May 12.

Walker AF, Marakis G, Morris AP, Robinson PA. Promising hypotensive effect of hawthorn extract: a randomized double-blind pilot study of mild, essential hypertension. *Phytother Res.* 2002 Feb;16(1):48-54.

Walker M. *The Power of Color.* Gujarat, India: Jain Publ., 2002.

Wang R, Jiang C, Lei Z, Yin K. The role of different therapeutic courses in treating 47 cases of rheumatoid arthritis with acupuncture. *J Tradit Chin Med.* 2007 Jun;27(2):103-5.

Wang XY, Shi X, He L. Effect of electroacupuncture on gastrointestinal dynamics in acute pancreatitis patients and its mechanism. *Zhen Ci Yan Jiu.* 2007;32(3):199-202.

Waser M, *et al.* PARSIFAL Study team. Inverse association of farm milk consumption with asthma and allergy in rural and suburban populations across Europe. *Clin Exp Allergy.* 2007 May;37(5):661-70.

Watnick S. Pregnancy and contraceptive counseling of women with chronic kidney disease and kidney transplants. *Adv Chronic Kidney Dis.* 2007 Apr;14(2):126-31.

Watson L. *Beyond Supernature.* New York: Bantam, 1987.

Watson L. *Supernature*. New York: Bantam, 1973.

Wauters M, Considine RV, Van Gaal LF. Human leptin: from an adipocyte hormone to an endocrine mediator. *Eur J Endocrinol.* 2000 Sep;143(3):293-311.

Wayne R. *Chemistry of the Atmospheres*. Oxford Press, 1991.

WB Saunders; 1982, Fishman HC. Notalgia paresthetica. *J Am Acad Dermatol.* 1986;15:1304-1305

Weatherley-Jones E, Thompson E, Thomas K. The placebo-controlled trial as a test of complementary and alternative medicine: observations from research experience of individualised homeopathic treatment. *Homeopathy.* 2004 Oct;93(4):186-9.

Weaver J, Astumian R. The response of living cells to very weak electric fields: the thermal noise limit. *Science.* 1990;247: 459-462.

Wee K, Rogers T, Altan BS, Hackney SA, Hamm C. Engineering and medical applications of diatoms. *J Nanosci Nanotechnol.* 2005 Jan;5(1):88-91.

Weikl A, Assmus KD, Neukum-Schmidt A, Schmitz J, Zapfe G, Noh HS, Siegrist J. Crataegus Special Extract WS 1442. Assessment of objective effectiveness in patients with heart failure (NYHA II). *Fortschr Med.* 1996 Aug 30;114(24):291-6.

Weinberger P, Measures M. The effect of two audible sound frequencies on the germination and growth of a spring and winter wheat. *Can. J. Bot.* 1968;46(9):1151-1158.

Weiner MA. *Secrets of Fijian Medicine*. Berkeley, CA: Univ. of Calif., 1969.

Weinert D, Waterhouse J. The circadian rhythm of core temperature: effects of physical activity and aging. *Physiol Behav.* 2007 Feb 28;90(2-3):246-56.

Weiss B. *Many Lives, Many Masters*. New York: Simon & Schuster, 1988.

Weiss RF. *Herbal Medicine*. Gothenburg, Sweden: Beaconsfield, 1988.

Weller A, Weller L. Menstrual synchrony between mothers and daughters and between roommates. *Physiol Behav.* 1993 May;53(5):943-9.

Weller L, Weller A, Roizman S. Human menstrual synchrony in families and among close friends: examining the importance of mutual exposure. *J Comp Psychol.* 1999 Sep;113(3):261-8.

Welsh D, Yoo SH, Liu A, Takahashi J, Kay S. Bioluminescence Imaging of Individual Fibroblasts Reveals Persistent, Independently Phased Circadian Rhythms of Clock Gene Expression. *Current Biology.* 2004;14:2289-2295.

Werbach M. *Nutritional Influences on Illness*. Tarzana, CA: Third Line Press, 1996.

West P. *Surf Your Biowaves*. London: Quantum, 1999.

West R. Risk of death in meat and non-meat eaters. *BMJ.* 1994 Oct 8;309(6959):955.

Westman M, Eden D. Effects of a respite from work on burnout: vacation relief and fade-out. *J Appl Psychol.* 1997 Aug;82(4):516-27.

Wetterberg L. Light and biological rhythms. *J Intern Med.* 1994 Jan;235(1):5-19.

Wheeler FJ. *The Bach Remedies Repertory*. New Canaan, CN: Keats, 1997.

White AR, Rampes H, Ernst E. Acupuncture for smoking cessation. *Cochrane Database Syst Rev.* 2002;(2):CD000009.

White J, Krippner S (eds). *Future Science: Life Energies & the Physics of Paranormal Phenomena*. Garden City: Anchor, 1977.

White S. *The Unity of the Self*. Cambridge: MIT Press, 1991.

Whiten, A. and E. M. Widdowson (eds.). *Foraging Strategies and Natural Diet of Monkeys, Apes and Humans.* Oxford: Clarendon Press, 1991.

Whitfield KE, King G, Moller S, Edwards CL, Nelson T, Vandenbergh D. Concordance rates for smoking among African-American twins. *J Natl Med Assoc.* 2007 Mar;99(3):213-7.

Whittaker E. *History of the Theories of Aether and Electricity.* New York: Nelson LTD, 1953.

Whitton J. *Life Between Life.* New York: Warner, 1986.

WHO. *Guidelines for Drinking-water Quality.* 2nd ed, vol. 2. Geneva: World Health Organization, 1996.

WHO. How trace elements in water contribute to health. *WHO Chronicle.* 1978;32: 382-385.

Wilkinson SM, Love SB, Westcombe AM, Gambles MA, Burgess CC, Cargill A, Young T, Maher EJ, Ramirez AJ. Effectiveness of aromatherapy massage in the management of anxiety and depression in patients with cancer: a multicenter randomized controlled trial. *J Clin Oncol.* 2007 Feb 10;25(5):532-9.

Williams A. Electron microscopic changes associated with water absorption in the jejunum. *Gut.* 1963;4:1-7.

Williams G. *Natural Selection: Domains, levels, and challenges.* Oxford: Oxford Univ Press, 1992.

Wilson L. *Nutritional Balancing and Hair Mineral Analysis.* Prescott, AZ: LD Wilson, 1998.

Winchester AM. *Biology and its Relation to Mankind.* New York: Van Nostrand Reinhold, 1969.

Winfree AT. *The Timing of Biological Clocks.* New York: Scientific American, 1987.

Winstead DK, Schwartz BD, Bertrand WE. Biorhythms: fact or superstition? *Am J Psychiatry.* 1981 Sep;138(9):1188-92.

Wittenberg JS. *The Rebellious Body.* New York: Insight, 1996.

Wixted JT. A Theory About Why We Forget What We Once Knew. *CurrDir Psychol Sci.* 2005;14(1):6-9.

Wolf, M. Beyond the Point Particle - *A Wave Structure for the Electron. Galilean Electrodynamics.* 1995 Oct;6(5): 83-91.

Wolverton BC. *How to Grow Fresh Air: 50 House Plants that Purify Your Home or Office.* New York: Penguin, 1997.

Wood M. *The Book of Herbal Wisdom.* Berkeley, CA: North Atlantic, 1997.

Woolger R. *Other Lives, Other Selves.* New York: Bantam, 1988.

World Cancer Research Fund, American Institute for Cancer Research. *Food, Nutrition and the Prevention of Cancer: A Global Perspective.* 1997: 509.

Worwood VA. *The Complete Book of Essential Oils & Aromatherapy.* San Rafael, CA: New World, 1991.

Wright ML. Melatonin, diel rhythms, and metamorphosis in anuran amphibians. *Gen Comp Endocrinol.* 2002 May;126(3):251-4.

Wyart C, Webster WW, Chen JH, Wilson SR, McClary A, Khan RM, Sobel N. Smelling a single component of male sweat alters levels of cortisol in women. *J Neurosci.* 2007 Feb 7;27(6):1261-5.

Yadav H, Jain S, Sinha PR. Antidiabetic effect of probiotic dahl containing Lactobacillus acidophilus and Lactobacillus casei in high fructose fed rats. *Nutrition.* 2007 Jan;23(1):62-8.

Yadav VS, Mishra KP, Singh DP, Mehrotra S, Singh VK. Immunomodulatory effects of curcumin. *Immunopharmacol Immunotoxicol.* 2005;27(3):485-97.

Yamaoka Y. Solid cell nest (SCN) of the human thyroid gland. *Acta Pathol Jpn.* 1973 Aug;23(3):493-506.

INDEX

Yan YF, Wei YY, Chen YH, Chen MM. Effect of acupuncture on rehabilitation training of child's autism. *Zhongguo Zhen Jiu.* 2007 Jul;27(7):503-5.

Yang HQ, Xie SS, Hu XL, Chen L, Li H. Appearance of human meridian-like structure and acupoints and its time correlation by infrared thermal imaging. *Am J Chin Med.* 2007;35(2):231-40.

Yeager S. *The Doctor's Book of Food Remedies.* Emmaus, PA: Rodale Press, 1998.

Yeung JW. A hypothesis: Sunspot cycles may detect pandemic influenza A in 1700-2000 A.D. *Med Hypotheses.* 2006;67(5):1016-22.

Yokoi S, Ikeya M, Yagi T, Nagai K. Mouse circadian rhythm before the Kobe earthquake in 1995. *Bioelectromagnetics.* 2003 May;24(4):289-91.

Yoshioka M, Doucet E, Drapeau V, Dionne I, Tremblay A. Combined effects of red pepper and caffeine consumption on 24 h energy balance in subjects given free access to foods. *Br J Nutr.* 2001 Feb;85(2):203-11.

Yu XM, Zhu GM, Chen YL, Fang M, Chen YN. Systematic assessment of acupuncture for treatment of herpes zoster in domestic clinical studies. *Zhongguo Zhen Jiu.* 2007 Jul;27(7):536-40.

Yuan SY, Lun X, Liu DS, Qin Z, Chen WT. Acupoint-injection of BCG polysaccharide nuclear acid for treatment of condyloma acuminatum and its immunoregulatory action on the patient. *Zhongguo Zhen Jiu.* 2007 Jun;27(6):407-11.

Zaets VN, Karpov PA, Smertenko PS, Blium IaB. Molecular mechanisms of the repair of UV-induced DNA damages in plants. *Tsitol Genet.* 2006 Sep-Oct;40(5):40-68. Review.

Zamora JL. Chemical and microbiologic characteristics and toxicity of povidone-iodine solutions. *Am J Surg.* 1986 Mar;151(3):400-6.

Zarate G, Gonzalez S, Chaia AP. *Assessing survival of dairy propionibacteria in gastrointestinal conditions and adherence to intestinal epithelia.* Centro de Referencia para Lactobacilos-CONICET. Tucuman, Argentina: Humana Press. 2004.

Zhang C, Popp, F., Bischof, M.(eds.). *Electromagnetic standing waves as background of acupuncture system. Current Development in Biophysics - the Stage from an Ugly Duckling to a Beautiful Swan.* Hangzhou: Hangzhou University Press, 1996.

Zimecki M. The lunar cycle: effects on human and animal behavior and physiology. *Postepy Hig Med Dosw.* 2006;60:1-7.

Zizza, C. The nutrient content of the Italian food supply 1961-1992. *European Journal of Clinical Nutrition.* 1997;51: 259-265.

Zou Z, Li F, Buck L. Odor maps in the olfactory cortex. *Proc Natl Acad of Sci.* 2005;102(May 24):7724-7729.